BIOSECURITY INTERVENTIONS

Biosecurity Interventions

GLOBAL HEALTH & SECURITY IN QUESTION

Edited by Andrew Lakoff and Stephen J. Collier

COLUMBIA UNIVERSITY PRESS — NEW YORK

A COLUMBIA / SSRC BOOK

COLUMBIA UNIVERSITY PRESS
Publishers Since 1893
New York   Chichester, West Sussex

Library of Congress Cataloging-in-Publication Data

Biosecurity interventions : global health and security in
practice / edited by Andrew Lakoff and Stephen J. Collier.
    p.   cm.
    Includes bibliographical references and index.
    ISBN 978-0-231-14606-7 (cloth : alk. paper)—
    ISBN 978-0-231-51177-3 (e-book)
    1. World health. 2. Biological warfare—Prevention.
    3. Communicable diseases—Prevention.
    4. Bioterrorism—Prevention. 5. National security.
    I. Lakoff, Andrew, 1970– II. Collier, Stephen J.
    [DNLM: 1. World Health. 2. Bioterrorism—prevention
    & control. 3. Communicable Diseases, Emerging—
    prevention & control. 4. Disease Outbreaks—
    prevention & control. 5. Food Contamination—
    prevention & control. 6. Health Policy.
    WA 530.1 B616 2008]

RA441.B56 2008
363.325'3—dc22
                                        2008020099

Columbia University Press books are printed on
permanent and durable acid-free paper. This book
is printed on paper with recycled content.
Printed in the United States of America

C 10 9 8 7 6 5 4 3 2 1

References to Internet Web sites (URLs) were accurate
at the time of writing. Neither the editors nor Columbia
University Press is responsible for URLs that may have
expired or changed since the manuscript was prepared.

Design by Julie Fry

CONTENTS

CHAPTER ONE

The Problem of Securing Health

Stephen J. Collier and Andrew Lakoff

Biosecurity Interventions

In 2007 the World Health Organization (WHO) issued its annual World Health Report, entitled "A Safer Future: Global Public Health Security in the 21st Century."[1] The report began by noting the success of public health measures during the twentieth century in dealing with great microbial scourges such as cholera and smallpox. But in recent decades, it continued, there has been an alarming shift in the "delicate balance between humans and microbes."[2] A series of factors—demographic changes, economic development, global travel and commerce, and conflict—have "heightened the risk of disease outbreaks," ranging from emerging infectious diseases such as HIV/AIDS and drug-resistant tuberculosis to food-borne pathogens and bioterrorist attacks.[3]

The WHO report proposed a framework for responding to this new landscape of threats, which it called "public health security." The framework is striking in its attempt to bring together previously distinct technical problems and political domains. Some of the biological threats discussed in the report—particularly the use of bioweapons—have traditionally been taken up under the rubric of "national security," and approached by organizations concerned with national defense. Others, such as infectious disease, have generally been managed as problems of public health, whose history, though certainly not unrelated to conflict and military affairs, has been institutionally separate.[4] The WHO proposal also sought to reconfigure the spatial and temporal frame of existing approaches to ensuring health. The report emphasized a space of "global health" that is distinct from the predominantly national organization of both biodefense and public health. "In the globalized world of the 21st century," it argued, simply stopping disease at national borders is not adequate. Nor is it sufficient to respond to diseases after they have become established in a population. Rather, it is necessary to prepare for unknown outbreaks in advance, something that can be achieved only "if there is immediate alert and response to disease outbreaks and other incidents that could spark epidemics or spread globally and if there are national systems in place for detection and response should such events occur across international borders."[5]

The WHO report is one among a range of recent proposals for securing health against new or newly recognized biological threats. Other prominent examples include recent "Pandemic and All-Hazards Preparedness" legislation in the U.S., reports on "global biological threats" from think tanks such as the RAND Corporation, new research facilities such as the National Biodefense Analysis and Countermeasures Center (NBACC), and ambitious global initiatives such as the Global Fund to Fight AIDS, Tuberculosis, and Malaria, and the President's Emergency Plan for AIDS Relief (PEPFAR). These initiatives build on a growing perception among diverse actors—life scientists and public health officials, policymakers and security analysts—that new biological threats challenge existing ways of understanding and managing collective health and security. From the vantage point of such actors, the global scale of these threats crosses and confounds the boundaries of existing regulatory jurisdictions. Moreover, their pathogenicity and mutability pushes the limits of current technical capacities to detect and treat disease. And the diverse sources of these perceived threats—biomedical laboratories, the industrial food system, global trade and travel—suggest a troubling growth of "modernization risks" that are produced by institutions meant to promote health, security, and prosperity. In response, proposals for new interventions seek to bring various actors and institutions into a common strategic framework.

The aim of this volume is to map this emerging field of "biosecurity interventions." As we use the term here, "biosecurity" does not refer exclusively—or even primarily—to practices and policies associated with "national security," that is, to military defense against enemy attack. Rather, we refer to the various technical and political interventions—efforts to "secure health"—that have been formulated in response to new or newly perceived pathogenic threats. In examining these interventions, the chapters that follow do not focus on the character of health threats per se, or on the social factors that exacerbate disease risk, but rather on the *forms of expertise* and the *knowledge practices* through which disease threats are understood and managed. As such, the chapters bring into view not only the complex ecologies of pathogenicity in which threats to health have emerged, but also the ecologies of experts and organizations that are being assembled in new initiatives to link health and security—public health officials, policy experts, humanitarian activists, life scientists, multilateral agencies such as WHO, national health agencies such as the Centers for Disease Control (CDC), national security experts, physicians, veterinarians, and government officials—and the practices in which they are engaged.[6] Through close examination of concrete settings in which biosecurity interventions are being articulated, these chapters show that ways of understanding and intervening in contemporary threats to health are still in formation: "biosecurity" does not name stable or clearly defined understandings and strategies, but rather a number of overlapping and rapidly changing problem areas.

Domains of Biosecurity

The current concern with new microbial threats has developed in at least four overlapping but distinct domains: emerging infectious disease; bioterrorism; the cutting-edge life sciences; and food safety. The first of these domains, "emerging infectious disease," initially drew the attention of public health experts in the late 1980s, in response to the AIDS crisis and the appearance of drug-resistant strains of tuberculosis and malaria.[7] Alarm about these emerging or reemerging diseases emanated from various quarters, including scientific reports by prominent organizations such as the National Academy of Science's Institute of Medicine, the reporting of science journalists such as Laurie Garrett, and the scenarios of novelists such as Richard Preston.[8] For many observers, the emerging disease threat—particularly when combined with weakening public health systems—marked a troubling reversal in the history of public health. At just the moment when it seemed that infectious disease was about to be conquered, and that the critical health problems of the industrialized world now involved chronic disease and diseases of lifestyle, experts warned, we were witnessing a "return of the microbe." This judgment seemed to be confirmed in ensuing years by the appearance of new diseases such as West Nile virus and SARS, by the intensification of the AIDS crisis, and by the current specter of an influenza pandemic.[9] After considerable delay, we have recently seen the implementation of large-scale responses to these new infectious disease threats that bring together governmental, multilateral, and philanthropic organizations.

A second area in which microbial threats have received renewed attention as a technical and political problem is in response to the prospect of bioterrorism. U.S. national security officials began to focus on this threat in the wake of the Cold War, hypothesizing an association between rogue states, global terrorist organizations and the proliferation of weapons of mass destruction.[10] Revelations during the 1990s about Soviet and Iraqi bioweapons programs, along with the Aum Shinrikyo subway attack in 1995 and the anthrax letters of 2001, lent a sense of credibility and urgency to calls for biodefense measures focused on bioterrorism. Early advocates of such efforts, including infectious disease experts such as D. A. Henderson and national security officials such as Richard Clarke, argued that adequate preparation for a biological attack would require a massive infusion of resources into both biomedical research and public health response capacity.[11] More broadly, they claimed, it would be necessary to incorporate the agencies and institutions of the life sciences and public health into the national security establishment. The eventual success of their campaign is reflected in the exponential increase in total U.S. government spending on civilian biodefense research between 2001 and 2005, from $294.8 million to $7.6 billion.[12]

Third, developments in the cutting-edge life sciences have generated new concerns about the proliferation of technical capacities to create lethal organisms, particularly in light of recent developments in fields like synthetic biology that promise dramatic advances in techniques of genetic manipulation.[13] Security experts and some life scientists worry that existing biosafety protocols focused on material controls in laboratories will not be sufficient as techniques of genetic manipulation become more powerful and routine, and as expertise in molecular biology becomes increasingly widespread. A number of new biosafety regulations have been imposed on research dealing with potentially dangerous pathogens. Meanwhile, intensive discussions about how to regulate the production of knowledge are underway among policy planners, life scientists and security officials;

and lawmakers have put in place new oversight mechanisms such as the National Science Advisory Board for Biosecurity (NSABB).

Fourth, and with more pronounced effects in Europe than in the United States, a series of food safety crises has sparked anxieties about agricultural biosecurity and the contamination of the food supply. In Europe, outbreaks of mad cow disease and foot-and-mouth disease in the 1990s drew attention to the side effects of industrial meat production. In the wake of these outbreaks, controversies raged both about the failures of the regulatory system in detecting new pathogens and about the mass culling measures that were mobilized in response. Also in Europe, environmental activists put the problem of regulating genetically modified food at the top of the political agenda. In the U.S., meanwhile, public outcry over food safety has been provoked by outbreaks of *E. coli* and by the presence of sick animals in the food supply, which led in early 2008 to the largest beef recall in the history of the meat industry.

In each of these four domains, a series of events has turned the attention of policymakers, health experts, civic groups, and the media to new biological threats. At one level, these may usefully be seen as "focusing events" in Thomas Birkland's sense: they have raised public awareness of threats to health, and catalyzed action on the part of governments and other actors.[14] But this characterization elides the fact that the meaning of such "focusing" events is not self-evident; indeed, these events are characterized by substantial ambiguity. In all of them, we find that health experts, policy advocates, and politicians have competing visions about how to characterize the problem of biosecurity and about what constitutes the most appropriate response. Thus, the question is not just *whether* certain events (or potential events) have been characterized as "biosecurity" threats that require attention; we also need to ask what *kind* of biosecurity problem they are seen to pose, what techniques are used to assess them, and how certain kinds of responses to them are justified.

In this light, it is worth examining more closely how these new or newly perceived threats to health have been *problematized*.[15] Problematization is a term that suggests a particular way of analyzing an event or situation: not as a given but as a question. As Michel Foucault writes, "a problematization does not mean the representation of a pre-existent object nor the creation through discourse of an object that did not exist. It is the ensemble of discursive and non-discursive practices that make something enter into the play of true and false and constitute it as an object of thought (whether in the form of moral reflection, scientific knowledge, political analysis, etc.)."[16] The reason that problematizations are problematic, he argues, is that "something prior must have happened to introduce uncertainty, a loss of familiarity; that loss, that uncertainty is the result of difficulties in our previous way of understanding, acting, relating."[17]

This mode of inquiry into problematizations is not that of a first-order actor who seeks, as Rabinow puts it, to proceed directly toward intervention and repair of the situation's discordance.[18] Rather, it is that of a second-order observer whose task is to achieve a "modal change from seeing a situation not only as a given but equally as a question, to understand how, in a given situation, there are multiple constraints at work...but multiple responses as well."[19] This analytical approach, when turned to the field of biosecurity, makes neither broad prescriptions for the improvement of health and security, nor blanket denunciations of new biosecurity interventions. Rather, it examines how policymakers, scientists, and security planners have constituted potential future events as biosecurity threats, and have responded by criticizing, redeploying, or reworking existing apparatuses.

The chapters in this volume provide a guide to the various ways in which the field of biosecurity is being problematized today. On the one hand, they examine the different *political and normative frameworks* through which the problem of biosecurity is approached: national defense, public health, and humanitarianism, for example. On the other hand, they examine the *styles of reasoning* through which uncertain threats to health are transformed into risks that can be known and acted upon: public health practices based on cost-benefit analysis, preparedness strategies that emphasize the mitigation of vulnerabilities, and precautionary approaches that seek to avoid potentially catastrophic threats.[20] And the chapters show how, in fields such as public health and biomedical research, existing apparatuses are being reconfigured to shape new assemblages of organizations, techniques, and forms of expertise.

Toward National Preparedness

We first turn to one field in which an existing set of practices, understandings, and institutions has been refigured as experts perceive and respond to new microbial threats: public health. To simplify a very complex story: the field of public health developed in the eighteenth and nineteenth centuries as a new way to understand and manage disease. In contrast to prior understandings of disease as an unexpected and unpredictable misfortune that beset human communities from without, public health traced disease to the immanent properties of the social field—sanitation practices, water supplies, forms of habitation and circulation—using statistical analysis of the incidence and severity of disease events across a population over time. Public health also provided an approach to evaluating a given response to disease events in a population. For example, as Foucault showed in his classic analysis of "the security of the population," beginning in the early nineteenth century statistical techniques were used to evaluate inoculation strategies by weighing the probability of disease outbreaks against the probability of adverse effects from inoculation.[21] Such "cost-benefit" analyses became the norm for assessing public health interventions.

Public health institutions consolidated after World War II, but simultaneously, in parallel domains such as biodefense, experts began to point to possible limits to the public health approach. Thus, Lyle Fearnley has shown that in the U.S. after World War II, as officials perceived endemic disease to be increasingly well managed, some biodefense experts, concerned about bioweapons attack, began to conceptualize outbreaks of infectious disease as anomalous events—that is, novel occurrences about which historical data do not exist, and about which little is known.[22] And yet, as Andrew Lakoff (chapter 2) points out, well into the post–World War II period techniques had not been established for assessing or managing such uncertain disease "events." Thus, in responding to a possible swine flu epidemic in 1976, U.S. public health authorities did not have a paradigm for managing a future event whose likelihood and consequence was unknown, and therefore had a difficult time agreeing on appropriate response measures—for example, whether to undertake mass vaccination of the population.

In recent decades, newly perceived threats to health—including bioterrorist threats such as a smallpox attack and emerging infectious diseases such as avian flu—have placed greater pressure on public health departments and national security officials to develop an approach to disease events not easily managed through the traditional paradigm of public health. As Lakoff shows, one significant response

13

to these new threats has been the articulation of *preparedness* practices among local public health jurisdictions in the U.S. In contrast to classic public health, preparedness does not draw on statistical records of past events. Rather, it employs imaginative techniques of enactment such as scenarios, exercises, and analytical models to simulate uncertain future threats.[23] The aim of such techniques is not to manage known disease but to address vulnerabilities in health infrastructure by, for example, strengthening hospital surge capacity, stockpiling drugs, exercising response protocols, and vaccinating first responders. Approaches based on preparedness may not be guided by rigorous cost-benefit analysis. Rather, they are aimed at developing the capability to respond to various types of potentially catastrophic biological events.

The demand for "public health preparedness" escalated as public health institutions faced mounting concerns about, first, a possible bioterrorist attack and then, beginning in 2005, a devastating influenza pandemic. The U.S. Congress's 2006 "Pandemic and All-Hazards Preparedness Act" delegated a number of new health preparedness functions to local and national public health authorities. According to the Center for Biosecurity, the legislation marked "a major milestone in improving public health and hospital preparedness for bioterrorist attacks, pandemics, and other catastrophes and for improving the development of new medical countermeasures, such as medicines and vaccines, against biosecurity threats."[24] Preparedness has thus become a crucial interface between public health and national security.

But increased attention and funding to health preparedness by no means implies consensus around a single approach. The existing institutions of public health are not easily reconciled with the new demands and norms of health preparedness and there is considerable disagreement about the appropriate way to achieve preparedness. One question is whether preparedness measures should focus on specific interventions against known agents such as anthrax and smallpox, or instead on generic measures that would be effective against currently unknown pathogens.[25] Another debate surrounds the "dual use" potential of biodefense measures.[26] Advocates of increased health preparedness argue that even in the absence of a bioterrorist attack, resources spent on strengthening the public health infrastructure will be useful for managing other unexpected events, such as the outbreak of a "naturally" occurring infectious disease. However, the ideal of dual use faces many difficulties, in part because public health professionals often do not agree with security experts about which problems deserve attention, and how interventions should be implemented.[27] Such disagreements point to broader tensions provoked by the current intersection of public health and national security.[28] Public health officials and national security experts promoting preparedness strategies have very different ways of evaluating threats and responses. As a result, programs that depend on coordination between these groups may often founder.

Take, for example, the 2002–2003 Smallpox Vaccination Program examined here by Dale Rose (chapter 4). The Smallpox Vaccination Program, whose goal was to vaccinate up to ten million "first responders," was initiated, in part, in response to imaginative enactments of the type Lakoff describes (chapter 2). A June 2001 scenario-based exercise called "Dark Winter" convinced officials that the U.S. was highly vulnerable to smallpox attack. This focus on smallpox intensified in the run-up to the second Iraq war, as White House security officials became concerned that Iraq might retaliate against a U.S. invasion with a smallpox attack in the U.S. The vaccination campaign, Rose notes, was meant to "take smallpox off the table" as a threat to national security. But here a problem arose around conflicting styles of reasoning—as well as conflicting political positions. Public health experts are trained to weigh the risks of disease against risks posed by vaccines. From this perspective, the expert committee charged with making vaccination recommendations to the CDC had trouble gauging the costs and benefits of smallpox vaccination. The likelihood of a smallpox attack was unknown, while the side effects of the vaccine could be fatal. As a consequence, the committee could not develop a credible recommendation. What is more, the program faced resistance from public health workers—particularly hospital medical and nursing personnel—who were skeptical about the likelihood of a smallpox attack and who, in many cases, were reluctant to be enrolled in national security efforts. In the absence of convincing cost-benefit data about the program, they were unwilling to take the risks associated with vaccination. As a result of such conflicts, the vaccination program faltered.[29]

A similar problem of normative conflict combined with political distrust, described by Lyle Fearnley (chapter 3), has hindered federal efforts to build a nationwide health monitoring system based on so-called "syndromic" surveillance. Initially developed by local public health departments in response to an

E. coli outbreak that went undetected by physicians, syndromic surveillance uses sources other than physicians' diagnostic reports—such as over-the-counter drug sales—to alert health authorities of possible disease outbreaks. In the late 1990s, national security experts began to explore the possibility of using this kind of system to detect a biological attack, given that physicians might not immediately recognize the symptoms caused by an unexpected or unknown pathogen. It soon became apparent, however, that national security planners at the federal level and local public health officials had very different priorities in designing the system's algorithm—its mechanism for distinguishing normal from anomalous fluctuations in syndrome incidence. Rather than data quality and predictive value—emphasized by public health officials, who were accustomed to dealing with known, regularly occurring diseases—national security planners wanted a highly sensitive algorithm that would ensure the rapid detection of a wider range of potential disease outbreaks. While most signals from anomalous events would be insignificant, they believed each must be considered potentially catastrophic. Local public health officials argued that they did not have the epidemiological capacity to investigate a high number of signals and that resources needed to address existing health problems would be wasted chasing after false positives. As one early developer of syndromics put it, in a trenchant critique of the contradictions inherent to the program, "We have 80 percent of the nation covered but we really have nothing covered"—since, in the absence of adequate local epidemiological capacity, even a highly sophisticated syndromic surveillance program is useless.

Global Health and Emergency Response

"Global health" is a second field in which health threats have been problematized in new ways. Contemporary articulations of global health typically share two elements. First, they focus on "globalization" processes as a key source of pathogenicity, claiming that the intensifying global circulation of humans, animals, and agricultural products—as well as knowledge and technologies—encourages the spread of novel and dangerous new diseases. Second, there is the problem of regulation and responsibility: given the global scale of biological threats and their multiple sources, it is often unclear who has regulatory jurisdiction or responsibility for managing a given disease event. A good example of such an articulation of global health comes from an influential 2002 RAND Corporation report, *The Global Threat of New and Reemerging Infectious Disease*. The report defines emerging disease as one among a number of new threats to security that "do not stem from the actions of clearly defined individual states but from diffuse issues that transcend sovereign borders and bear directly on the effects of increasing globalization that challenge extant frameworks for thinking about national and international security."[30]

Proposed responses to this new "global threat" have come from various kinds of organizations, with diverse agendas. International health agencies such as WHO are developing new preparedness-based approaches to potential outbreaks of infectious disease; humanitarian organizations such as *Médecins Sans Frontières* focus on the immediate problem of reducing human suffering in the context of emergencies; and philanthropic ventures such as the Gates Foundation seek to manage global health threats by developing and disseminating low-cost interventions. Despite differences in their approaches, these efforts to respond to urgent global disease threats share what we might call an emergency modality of intervention. The emergency modality does not involve long-term intervention into the social and economic determinants of disease. Rather, it emphasizes practices such as rapid medical response, standardized protocols for managing global health crises, surveillance and reporting systems, or simple technological fixes like mosquito nets or drugs. Such emergency management techniques are characterized by their mobility: at least in principle, they can be deployed anywhere, regardless of the distinctive characteristics of a given setting.

There are various reasons why organizations in the field of global health are drawn to an emergency modality. One is that emergencies galvanize public attention and resources in a way that long-term problems do not. Another is that— at least from the vantage of first-order actors—measures focused on mitigating potential emergencies are easier to implement than longer-term structural interventions. As Nicholas King writes, short-term, technically focused emergency measures have "the advantage of immensely reducing the scale of intervention, from global political economy to laboratory investigation and information management."[31] And as Michael Barnett notes, such measures seem to avoid the complex entanglements implied by longer term interventions in development and public health that "are political because they aspire to restructure underlying social relations."[32]

For these reasons, even experts who understand that social issues such as poverty and deteriorating health infrastructure are critical determinants of disease risk may propose narrower technical measures given the difficulty of implementing more ambitious schemes. In 1996, for example, Nobel Prize winner Joshua Lederberg noted the connections between global inequality and threats to U.S. health security: "World health is indivisible, [and] we cannot satisfy our most parochial needs without attending to the health conditions of all the globe."[33] But the concrete interventions Lederberg advocated, such as networks of reference laboratories and global disease surveillance systems, were modest and, as he put it, "selfishly motivated"—that is, focused on protecting the U.S. from outbreaks rather than on addressing major problems of political and economic transformation. Medical anthropologist Daniel Halperin has pointed to the tendency of global health organizations to self-consciously avoid investment in public health infrastructures despite the awareness that such investments would reduce mortality. While billions of dollars have been earmarked to fight what are seen as disease emergencies, he notes, basic public health issues are often not of interest to major donors. "Shortages of food and basic health services like vaccinations, prenatal care and family planning contribute to large family size and high child and maternal mortality. Major donors like the President's Emergency Plan for AIDS Relief, known as PEPFAR, and the Global Fund to Fight AIDS, Tuberculosis and Malaria have not directly addressed such basic health issues. As the Global Fund's director acknowledged, 'We are not a global fund that funds local health.'"[34]

The emergency management approach thus seeks to develop techniques for managing health emergencies that can work independently of political context and of socioeconomic conditions. As several chapters in the volume show, this approach has become an increasingly central way of thinking about and intervening in global health threats. For example, Erin Koch (chapter 5) describes the implementation of a TB-control program called DOTS (for "Directly-Observed Treatment, Short-Course") in post-Soviet Georgia. Part of the attraction of DOTS for nonstate funders is that it can seemingly be implemented without treating longer-term issues of social and economic development. Thus Koch quotes a doctor from a U.S.–based

NGO, who says: "[With DOTS] your TB program works under whatever conditions: in refugee camps, in prison, wherever.... If you do your program you can forget about the big social economic approach." Peter Redfield (chapter 6) describes the impressive logistical capabilities of *Médecins Sans Frontières*, which enable the humanitarian NGO to rapidly respond to health emergencies around the globe. Redfield focuses on the container-sized "humanitarian kit," a ready-made device, transported in shipping containers, for immediate intervention irrespective of place that has proven its efficacy in acute health emergencies. And Nick Bingham and Steve Hinchliffe (chapter 7) describe a WHO-prescribed program of massive poultry culling in Cairo to mitigate the risk of avian flu contagion. The program, based on an emergency-oriented protocol designed to be implemented automatically in the event of disease detection, is an example of the effort to develop a "standard, worldwide approach to dealing with 'out of place' biological entities."

However, there are serious limitations to forms of intervention that focus only on emergency response—whether such response is based on a humanitarian imperative of sympathy for suffering strangers or on a security-based logic seeking to avert the spread of emergencies. As Craig Calhoun has recently noted in an essay on the rise of emergency as a mode of justification for urgent global intervention, and on the limitations to such intervention, "There is a tension between responses rooted in simply providing care and responses linked to broader notions of human progress."[35] This tension relates to a difference in aims but also in forms of intervention: emergency response is acute, short-term, focused on alleviating what is conceived as a temporally circumscribed event; whereas "social" interventions—such as those associated with development policy—focus on transforming political-economic structures over the long term. Thus, in global health initiatives we find a contrast between possible modalities of intervention that parallels the one already described in U.S.–based biosecurity efforts: between acute emergency measures on the one hand and long-term approaches to health and welfare on the other.

One common problem in emergency-oriented response is that highly mobile protocols or devices are often implemented without attention to what is necessary in order for these protocols to function in concrete settings. Thus, Koch shows that the DOTS protocol for treatment of drug-resistant TB in "resource poor" settings like post-Soviet Georgia faces major hurdles. The economic situation has led to a massive deterioration of the public health infrastructure, making adherence to DOTS' strict diagnostic and treatment regimen nearly impossible. Compounding the problem in Georgia, the professional norms of Soviet-trained doctors are incommensurable with the practices required by DOTS: most doctors in Georgia have been trained in very different methods for managing TB and are therefore unwilling or unable to comply with the protocol's directives. The implication, Koch notes, is not necessarily that DOTS is the "wrong" answer, but that it cannot be successfully implemented without attention to a broader range of questions concerning social development and health infrastructure.

Redfield, meanwhile, shows that the very strength of the humanitarian kit and of the emergency modality more generally—its independence from social and political context—becomes a weakness as soon as *Médecins Sans Frontières* seeks to manage longer-term problems. Redfield points to the challenges posed by a new MSF initiative to provide sustained treatment to patients with HIV/AIDS in Uganda: to what extent can the kit—and the ostensibly apolitical humanitarian project it is associated with—be assimilated to chronic disease? Given its traditional focus on acute intervention, MSF struggles to provide the long-term care necessary to adequately treat HIV/AIDS. The organization is not equipped to deal with social and economic problems that are outside the scope of biomedical intervention. As Redfield writes: "Finding jobs and forging new relationships were matters of keen interest for members of patient support groups I encountered. Although sympathetic, MSF was poorly equipped to respond to matters of poverty, unemployment and family expectations. The translation of treatment from rich to poor countries could not alter the structural imbalance between contexts in economic terms. That particular crisis exceeded the boundaries of a shipping container."

The fact that emergency-oriented measures do not take into account the social realities of the contexts in which they are applied often undermines the effectiveness of such measures. Thus Bingham and Hinchliffe point out that WHO–prescribed culling measures in Cairo do not attend to the distinctive political and economic characteristics of the setting. Subsistence farmers' dependence on their poultry stocks for their livelihood, along with their lack of trust in the government, meant that they were unlikely to comply with the mass culling directive: "Householders skeptical of the government's promises or level of compe nsation...successfully hid their birds, unwilling to let such valuable possessions be needlessly culled." More broadly, Bingham and Hinchliffe argue, the "contemporary project of worldwide integration and harmonization of biosecurity measures," exemplified by such mass culling programs, "is fraught with risks however appealing it might sound": it may fail to decrease the likelihood of a flu pandemic, while exacerbating problems of hunger and poverty. They suggest that the uncertainties endemic to contemporary biosecurity threats such as avian flu point to the need to develop new ways of living with and managing the possibility of outbreaks that are more nuanced than current attempts to achieve absolute security at the expense of local well being.

Health Security and Modernization Risks

The regulation of what Ulrich Beck calls "modernization risks" comprises a third field in which biosecurity has been newly problematized. As Beck has argued, increasing dependence on complex systems and technical innovations for health and welfare has "systematically produced" new risks.[36] In the domain of health, modernization risks have been linked to processes such as expanding trade, industrial food production, or advances in the life sciences. Of course, these problems are not entirely new. But, following Beck, the recent intensification of such processes has created new uncertainties about the forms of expertise appropriate to understand and mitigate these risks.

To illustrate, we can take the area of food safety. Again, to simplify a complex story: the modernization of food production over the last century through industrial agriculture and food processing has, in the richest countries, provided access to an abundant and predictable supply of food. But this increase in "food security" through industrialization and rationalization has consistently generated new risks, and, in response, new efforts to manage these risks. Thus, the first wave of food industrialization in the late nineteenth century led to abuses and scandals that were addressed in the United States by progressive era reforms, including the founding of the Food and Drug Administration and an expansion of the responsibilities of the U.S. Department of Agriculture.

For a variety of reasons, however, the food safety risks that have emerged in recent decades challenge such existing apparatuses of regulation. First, the globalization of industrial food production has posed new difficulties, such as the problem of maintaining quality control over global food and drug production chains, as indicated by recent scandals over the regulation of ingredients for pet food, toothpaste, or blood thinner that are imported from China.[37] Second, emerging pathogens such as BSE and virulent new strains of *E. coli* have cast doubt on the adequacy of existing protocols and organizations for regulating food safety.[38] Third, intervention into agricultural production at the molecular level (e.g. genetically modified [GM] soy and corn) has led to disputes about proper forms of regulation, particularly in areas where risks are unknown.

As Beck notes, modernization risks are often associated with disputes over the authority of expert knowledge.[39] In the field of biosecurity, such disputes are characterized by technical disagreements over how to evaluate threats: cost-benefit analyses versus "precautionary" approaches that emphasize worst-case scenarios, for example, or different models for assessing the risk of certain experiments in the life sciences. In the area of food safety, one well known case concerns the regulation of GM foods. In the 1990s the European Union sought to ban the import of GM foods, influenced by a movement toward "precautionary" regulation which argued that new technologies could be restricted even in the absence of conclusive evidence about the risks they posed. The U.S., which beginning in the 1980s instituted the use of cost-benefit analysis for addressing environmental and health risks, challenged the European Union's policy in the World Trade Organization, insisting that without quantitative risk assessment, the ban constituted an illegal restraint on trade.[40]

Similar questions about risk assessment have played out in national regulatory systems. For example, Frédéric Keck (chapter 8) shows how the outbreak of spongiform encephalopathy (known as mad cow disease, or BSE) in France cast doubt on existing approaches to regulating food safety. In the French regulatory system, he notes, food safety had previously been the responsibility of veterinarians, who sought to manage diseases that occurred regularly in animal populations. But the scandals around BSE triggered a reproblematization of food safety. Human mortality had to be avoided at all costs, pushing the government to favor a precautionary approach that emphasized uncertain but potentially catastrophic threats—replacing, at least in part, the cost-benefit approach of traditional public health. In response to the BSE crisis, the existing authority of veterinarians was supplanted by a new French Food Safety Agency in which physicians played a leading role. In his research into these events, Keck finds that "the controversy between veterinarians and physicians on animal diseases profoundly structures the field of food safety, and gives a specific meaning to the term 'biosecurity' as it emerges in this field."

While these conflicts appear in technical disputes about methods of risk assessment, they often have much broader social and economic consequences: the "politics of expertise" relates to questions about the distribution of social goods—and, as Beck points out, of social "bads."[41] In their chapter, Hinchliffe and Bingham show that the WHO consensus that avian flu can be traced to the interaction of wild bird migration and domestic poultry has meant that measures to counteract avian flu—particularly culling techniques—have disproportionately harmed the poor and benefited large-scale poultry farms that international officials assume to be biosecure. An alternative theory—that the spread of avian flu can be traced to the international circulation of poultry through legal or illegal trade, and to industrial poultry production and processing—has been largely ignored in international protocols to contain the disease, but would imply a very different set of measures.[42]

Conflicting frameworks for assessing and managing modernization risks are also found in debates around regulation of the life sciences, particularly in light of concerns that new techniques of genetic manipulation could become instruments of bioterrorism. Debates about the regulation of the life sciences are not new—they can be traced at least to the 1970s, when civic and environmental groups in the U.S. raised questions about the "social and ethical implications" of scientific research at a number of levels. The "social responsibility" of scientists was scrutinized, particularly in light of physicists' contributions to military research. Meanwhile, biomedical scandals such as the Tuskegee Syphilis Experiment shaped an emergent field of bioethics, and the environmental movement drew attention to the risks of an accidental release of new pathogens created in laboratory environments. As Susan Wright has shown, life scientists managed to fend off these critiques, in part by shifting attention from the possibility of a pathogen release outside of the lab to questions of laboratory safety.[43] From this perspective, leading biologists argued, the most relevant measures were material controls in laboratories, and self-regulation by scientists, who claimed that they were best able to judge the potential danger of experiments, thus excluding others from the assessment of risks.

More recently, however, this regime of material controls and self-regulation has been called into question. This is due in part to advances in techniques of genetic manipulation that have made it ever easier to engineer dangerous new pathogens. But it is also due to the increasing attention paid to bioterrorism, which has shifted the discussion about regulating science in significant ways. In the 1970s civic groups focused on whether well meant scientific experiments could have unintended consequences. Today, by contrast, the focus is on the intentional malevolent use of scientific knowledge, a concern that has been voiced by some scientists, but which has predominantly come from the national security establishment, including think tanks such as the Center for Strategic and International Studies (CSIS).[44] From the national security perspective, advanced research in the life sciences may in the future make it possible to detect, characterize, and mitigate the effects of a bioterrorist attack. But such research may also introduce new threats. The question, for security officials, is no longer one of material controls and self-regulation, but of regulating the production and circulation of dangerous knowledge.

In this context, disputes have taken shape over how to assess the threat posed by research in the life sciences. These disputes often pit security planners, oriented to precautionary measures in the face of worst-case scenarios, against scientists, who cling to autonomy and free inquiry against what they perceive to be, as Carlo Caduff notes (chapter 10), "provisional rules, vague obligations, and impossible demands [that] are systematically imposed on biomedical research in the name of national security." Underlying these explicit debates are often divergent assumptions about how scientific knowledge works, and what might make it "dangerous." Security planners tend to see scientific knowledge as easily abstracted from its context of production: once it is developed, they fear, it can be used anywhere to reproduce pathogenic organisms. As chapters by Caduff and Kathleen Vogel demonstrate, however, experiments considered "dangerous" may in fact depend on highly specific contexts that are difficult to reproduce.

Thus, Vogel (chapter 9) argues that most participants in discussions about the regulation of potentially dangerous scientific knowledge assume that both the knowledge produced in advanced labs and the materials that they employ could easily be used elsewhere. She cites a report from CSIS that claims that if the results of research in the life sciences "are published openly, they become available to all—including those who may seek to use those results maliciously."[45] She also points to a 2004 National Academy of Sciences report, *Biotechnology Research in an Age of Terrorism,* which argued that "it is unrealistic to think that biological technologies...can somehow be isolated within the borders of a few countries."[46] But on the basis of three case studies—the Soviet anthrax program, the 2003 poliovirus synthesis, and the 2003 synthesis of phiX bacteriophage—Vogel shows that, in fact, the replication of such feats of biological engineering is extremely challenging, depending on tacit knowledge and complex research apparatuses. She proposes an alternative approach to assessing "dangerous knowledge" not in terms of isolated materials and knowledge but in terms of the sociotechnical assemblies required to make experiments actually work.

Caduff makes a similar point in his study of the laboratory synthesis of the 1918 flu virus at the Centers for Disease Control, which was conducted under stringent biosafety controls. Media coverage focused on the possibility that the publication of results from these experiments could arm potential bioterrorists. Echoing Vogel, Caduff notes that such concerns rested on a questionable model of pathogenicity. Viral pathogenicity is a property not of a virus in isolation, but of an interaction between the virus and the "host"—that is, human beings. Since humans are not, with respect to the 1918 virus, a naïve population (influenza viruses of the H1N1 subtype are still circulating today), it is unlikely that a release of the virus would have the same effects as it did 90 years ago.

Nonetheless, Caduff shows, just as "biosafety" transformed the practice of science in the 1970s, biosecurity practices are transforming it today. Scientists involved in the synthesis of the 1918 flu virus faced a demand to demonstrate that their experiments did not raise biosecurity issues. Thus, "anticipating biosecurity"— focusing not on the threats themselves but rather on *concerns* about the threats—has become a central part of scientific work in fields like virology. In the case of the 1918 flu virus synthesis, experiments to demonstrate that current vaccines and antiviral drugs are effective against the 1918 virus were conducted simultaneously with the synthesis itself. As Caduff notes, "By enrolling a few recombinant viruses, some tissue culture, and a couple of inbred mice a truth was performed to open up rather than close down the future of a research project." In other words, scientists sought to anticipate biosecurity concerns through an experimental demonstration that the knowledge they were producing was not as dangerous as the media might suggest.

Toward Critical, Reflexive Knowledge

Although there is a great sense of urgency to address contemporary biosecurity problems—and while impressive resources have been mobilized to do so—there is no consensus about how to conceptualize these threats, nor about what the most appropriate measures are to deal with them. This situation is recognized by some of the more reflective observers in the fields in question here. Thus, as Richard Danzig has argued in the case of bioterrorism, despite the striking increase in funding for biodefense in the U.S., there is still no "common conceptual framework" that might bring various efforts together and make it possible to assess their adequacy.[47] Similarly, Laurie Garrett has noted, in a recent commentary on ambitious new initiatives to fight infectious disease on a global scale, that health leaders are just beginning to ask: "Who should lead the fight against disease? Who should pay for it? And what are the best strategies and tactics to adopt?"[48]

There is no shortage of attempts to answer these questions. As we have seen, the field of biosecurity is filled with actors laying claim to authoritative knowledge about the most serious threats to health, and about the most appropriate responses to these threats. Political elites and policy experts make urgent calls to enact new biosecurity measures, whether for reasons of national security, of global health, or in the name of a moral imperative to alleviate suffering. Meanwhile, experts of various stripes, engaged in developing and implementing interventions, debate how to evaluate and improve existing measures. In studying the work of these first-order actors, the second-order observation conducted by the authors in this volume addresses the problem of health and security in a different register. The authors do not advance claims about the urgency (or nonurgency) of biological threats; nor do they offer direct solutions to biosecurity problems. Rather, they take the conflicting claims of first-order actors—and the disputatious claimants—as objects of analysis.

A key insight of such second-order observation is that there are different kinds of biosecurity—that is, there are diverse ways that biosecurity can be problematized—and these different kinds of biosecurity entail not only different technical understandings of threats, but different underlying values.[49] From this vantage many of the disputes that emerge in the field are not simply matters of technical disagreement, of finding the right protocol, the right drug, or the right approach to risk assessment. Rather, these disputes revolve around questions that cannot be settled—or, indeed, even posed—by technical experts alone. One of the contributions of this volume, in this light, is to make these values—and tensions over conflicting values—more explicit as objects of reflection.[50]

Thus, Keck notes that culling programs imply a judgment about the value of human versus animal life: animals, it is assumed, can be sacrificed on a massive scale to avert deadly human disease, even if the risk of widespread outbreaks in humans is unknown. In a similar vein, Hinchliffe and Bingham show that WHO protocols implicitly assume that the economic costs of culling domestic poultry in Cairo—a cost that falls disproportionately on the poor—is a "reasonable" price to pay for measures that may avert a global pandemic. But are such programs in fact reasonable, particularly when experts disagree about how effective culling will be in mitigating the risk of an influenza pandemic? "Reasonable" will mean different things depending, in part, on the standard of rationality used in making assessments. But it will also depend on political and ethical judgments about how the costs and harms of biosecurity interventions can be justly distributed when the benefits are uncertain or highly diffused. Thus, the dispute over the smallpox vaccination program is in part a dispute about technical risk assessment. But it is also a dispute about the politics of risk that cannot be resolved in purely technical terms. How should known risks taken by first responders be weighed against the unknown benefits of the program for the national population in the event of a smallpox attack? How, as in the case of syndromic surveillance programs, should the resources of government be directed, and where does its responsibility lie? Is the primary imperative to respond through public health measures to known and regularly occurring disease? Or to take measures that may avert uncertain but catastrophic outbreaks? Such problems are most acute, perhaps, when the field of regulation is global. How to decide which measures to undertake in situations with tremendous needs, and limited resources—such as the TB crisis amid the crumbling health infrastructure of post-Soviet Georgia?

These kinds of questions are crucial to address today, when responses to the problem of health and security are still taking shape. Doing so requires critical and reflexive knowledge that examines how technical efforts to increase biosecurity relate to the political and ethical challenges of what might be called "living with risk." Security—the freedom from fear or risk—always suggests an absolute demand; security has, as Foucault wrote, no principle of limitation. There is no such thing as being "too secure."[51] Living with risk, by contrast, acknowledges a more complex calculus. It requires new forms of political and ethical reasoning that take into account questions that are often only implicit in discussions of biosecurity interventions. We hope the contributions in this volume provide an initial guide to developing such forms of reasoning.

NOTES

Acknowledgment: We are grateful for the suggestions made by Carlo Caduff, Lyle Fearnley, Paul Rabinow, Dale Rose, and Anthony Stavrianakis on earlier drafts of this chapter.

1   World Health Organization, *The World Health Report 2007: A Safer Future. Global Public Health Security in the 21st Century* (Geneva: World Health Organization, 2007).

2   Ibid., 1.

3   Ibid.

4   For discussions of the historical relationships between public health and national security see Lyle Fearnley, "Pathogens and the Strategy of Preparedness," ARC Working Paper, Anthropology of the Contemporary Research Collaboratory, Berkeley, California, 2005; and Nicholas B. King, "Security, Disease, Commerce: Ideologies of Postcolonial Global Health," *Social Studies of Science* 32, no. 5–6 (2002): 763–789.

5   *The World Health Report 2007*, 11.

6   See Aihwa Ong and Stephen J. Collier, *Global Assemblages: Technology, Politics, and Ethics as Anthropological Problems* (Malden, MA: Blackwell Publishing, 2005); and Paul Rabinow, "Diffusion of the Human Thing: Virtual Virulence, Preparedness, Dignity" (Berkeley, California, unpublished manuscript, 2006).

7   King, "Security, Disease, Commerce."

8   Institute of Medicine, *Emerging Infections: Microbial Threats to Health in the United States* (Washington, DC: National Academy Press, 1992); Laurie Garrett, *The Coming Plague: Newly Emerging Diseases in a World out of Balance* (New York: Farrar, Straus and Giroux, 1994); Richard Preston, *The Cobra Event* (New York: Ballantine, 1998).

9   There has been a lively anthropological critique which argues that the "emerging infectious disease" discourse ignores the role social and political factors such as poverty and inequality play in fostering disease. See, for example, Paul Farmer, *Infections and Inequalities: The Modern Plagues* (Berkeley; London: University of California Press, 2001); Vinh-Kim Nguyen, "Emerging Infectious Disease," *Encyclopedia of Medical Anthropology: Health and Illness in the World's Cultures,* edited by Carol R. Ember and Melvin Ember (New York, Kluwer Academic, 2004).

10   Judith Miller, Stephen Engelberg and William J. Broad, *Germs: Biological Weapons and America's Secret War* (New York: Simon & Schuster, 2001); Ken Alibek and Stephen Handelman, *Biohazard: The Chilling True Story of the Largest Covert Biological Weapons Program in the World, Told from Inside by the Man Who Ran It* (New York: Random House, 1999); Jeanne Guillemin, *Biological Weapons from the Invention of State-Sponsored Programs to Contemporary Bioterrorism* (New York: Columbia University Press, 2005).

11   For a detailed review of the developing concern with bioterrorism in the 1990s, see Susan Wright, "Terrorists and Biological Weapons," *Politics and the Life Sciences* 25, no. 1 (2006): 57–115. As Wright argues, the very use of the term "weapons of mass destruction" to link nuclear weapons to biological weapons was a strategic act on the part of biodefense advocates.

12   It then declined slightly, to $5.37 billion, in 2006. See Clarence Lam, Crystal Franco, and Ari Schuler, "Billions for Biodefense: Federal Agency Biodefense Funding, FY2006–FY2007," in *Biosecurity and Bioterrorism: Biodefense Strategy, Practice, and Science* 4 (2006): 2.

13   Michele S. Garfinkel, Drew Endy, Gerald L. Epstein and Robert M. Friedman, "Synthetic

Genomics: Options for Governance," *Industrial Biotechnology* 3, no. 4 (2007): 333–365.

14 Thomas A. Birkland, "Focusing Events, Mobilization, and Agenda Setting," *Journal of Public Policy* 18 (1998): 54.

15 Stephen J. Collier, Andrew Lakoff and Paul Rabinow, "Biosecurity: Towards an Anthropology of the Contemporary," *Anthropology Today* 20, no. 5 (2004): 3–7.

16 Michel Foucault, *Dits et Ecrits, 1954–1988* (Paris: Gallimard, 1994), 670.

17 Ibid., 598.

18 Paul Rabinow, *Anthropos Today: Reflections on Modern Equipment* (Princeton, NJ: Princeton University Press, 2003), 18.

19 Ibid., 18–19. For an analysis of second-order observation see Niklas Luhmann, *Risk: A Sociological Theory* (New York: Aldine de Gruyter, 1993).

20 For a discussion of diverse styles of reasoning in scientific practice, see Ian Hacking, *Historical Ontology* (Cambridge, MA and London: Harvard University Press, 2002).

21 Michel Foucault, *Security, Territory, Population: Lectures at the Collège de France, 1977–78* (New York: Palgrave Macmillan, 2007). Important histories of public health include William Coleman, *Death Is a Social Disease: Public Health and Political Economy in Early Industrial France* (Madison: University of Wisconsin Press, 1982); and George Rosen, *A History of Public Health* (Baltimore: Johns Hopkins University Press, 1993).

22 Lyle Fearnley, "Pathogens," 2005.

23 For discussions of preparedness and enactment see Andrew Lakoff, "Preparing for the Next Emergency," *Public Culture* 19, no. 2 (2007); Stephen J. Collier, "Enacting Catastrophe: Preparedness, Insurance, Budgetary Rationalization," *Economy and Society* 37, no. 2 (2008): 224–250; Stephen J. Collier and Andrew Lakoff,

"Distributed Preparedness: The Spatial Logic of Domestic Security in the United States," *Environment and Planning D: Society and Space* 26, no. 1 (2008).

24 Michael Mair, Beth Maldin and Brad Smith, "Passage of S. 3678: The Pandemic and All-Hazards Preparedness Act," UPMC, Center for Biosecurity, December 20, 2006.

25 See Fearnley, "From Chaos to Controlled Disorder," and Roger Brent, "In the Shadow of the Valley of Death," Working Paper, Cambridge, MA: Massachusetts Institute of Technology, 2006, accessed at http://dspace.mit.edu/bitstream/1721.1/34914/1/Valley2006.pdf.

26 In these discussions "dual use" refers, somewhat confusingly, to two distinct questions: first, the possible malign use of bioscience; second, the use of certain programs for multiple policy objectives, such as public health and national defense. Here we refer to the latter.

27 See, for example, H. W. Cohen, R. M. Gould and V. W. Sidel, "Bioterrorism Initiatives: Public Health in Reverse?" *American Journal of Public Health* 89, no. 2 (1999): 1629–1631.

28 The relationship between public health and national security is not, of course, new (see King, "Security, Disease, Commerce"). But the specific programs and contexts around which this intersection is organized are significantly changed and intensified today.

29 This explanation diverges from usual understandings of the Smallpox Vaccination Program's failure, which tend to emphasize problems in execution or the misguided perceptions of risk among health workers.

30 Jennifer Brower and Peter Chalk, *The Global Threat of New and Reemerging Infectious Diseases: Reconciling U.S. National Security and Public Health Policy* (Santa Monica: RAND Science and Technology, 2003), 3.

31 Nicholas B. King, "The Scale Politics of Emerg-

ing Diseases," *Osiris* 19 (2004): 69.

32 Michael Barnett, "Humanitarianism Transformed," *Perspectives on Politics* 3, 2005, 723–740. Similarly, Craig Calhoun notes that "the field of international humanitarian action grew not merely in the development of new organizations and better techniques to address emergencies but in some considerable and warranted skepticism about master plans to end all conflict, poverty, and injustice." Craig Calhoun, "The Imperative to Reduce Suffering: Charity, Progress, and Emergencies in the Field of Humanitarian Action," in *Humanitarianism in Question: Power, Politics, Ethics,* eds. Michael Barnett and Thomas G. Weiss (Ithaca: Cornell University Press, 2008), 22.

33 Joshua Lederberg, "Infection Emergent," *Journal of the American Medical Association* 275, no. 3 (1996): 243–245; cited in King, "The Scale Politics of Emerging Diseases," 65.

34 Daniel Halperin, "Putting a Plague in Perspective," *New York Times,* January 1, 2008. Emphasis added.

35 Calhoun, "The Imperative to Reduce Suffering."

36 Ulrich Beck, *Risk Society: Towards a New Modernity* (London: Sage Publications, 1992), 19.

37 In early 2008 the U.S. media reported on medical complications from the blood thinner herapin that were due to problems in the Chinese supply of pig intestines, a raw material for the drug. David Barboza and Walt Bogdanovich, "Twists in Chain of Supply for Blood Drug," *New York Times,* February 28, 2008.

38 For example, as Elizabeth Dunn notes, an outbreak of a deadly new strain of *E. coli* in the U.S. was "the product of a particular agroindustrial configuration which is highly concentrated and which produces an astronomical amount of food." Elizabeth Dunn, *"Escherichia coli,* Corporate Discipline and the Failure of the Sewer State," *Space and Polity* 11, no. 1

(2007): 35–53.

39 As Beck has written, risk society is characterized by "competing rationality claims, struggling for acceptance" (ibid., 30).

40 For an analysis of the GM food debates see Sheila Jasanoff, *Designs on Nature: Science and Democracy in Europe and the United States* (Princeton, N.J.: Princeton University Press, 2005). Other recent analyses have called into question the strict divide between European "precaution" and U.S. "risk assessment," and noted a significant shift in the European discussion away from precaution with the emergence of the "better regulation" agenda. See Jonathan B. Weiner, "Precaution in a Multirisk World," in *Human and Ecological Risk Assessment: Theory and Practice,* ed. Dennis Paustenbach (New York: John Wiley and Sons, 2002): 1509–1531; Ragnar E. Lofstedt, "The Swing of the Regulatory Pendulum in Europe: From Precautionary Principle to (Regulatory) Impact Analysis," AEI–Brookings Joint Center Working Paper 04-07, 2004.

41 Beck, *Risk Society.*

42 For a critical analysis of the migratory bird hypothesis of avian influenza transmission, see M. Gauthier-Clerc, C. Lebarbenchon, and F. Thomas, "Recent Expansion of Highly Pathogenic Avian Influenza H5N1: A Critical Review," *Ibis* 149 (2007): 202–214.

43 Susan Wright, "Molecular Biology or Molecular Politics? The Production of Scientific Consensus on the Hazards of Recombinant DNA Technology," *Social Studies of Science* 16, no. 4 (1986): 593–620. See also Sheldon Krimsky, "From Asilomar to Industrial Biotechnology: Risks, Reductionism and Regulation," *Science as Culture* 14 (2005): 309–323.

44 See, for example, Garfinkel et al. For a critique of Garfinkel et al. see Paul Rabinow, Gaymon Bennett, and Anthony Stavrianakis,

"Response to 'Synthetic Genomics: Options for Governance,'" ARC Concept Note No. 10. Anthropology of the Contemporary Research Collaboratory. Berkeley, California, 2006.

45 Center for Strategic and International Studies, *Security Controls on Scientific Information* (June 2005), accessed on July 25, 2007 at http://thefdp.org/CSIS_0506_cscans.pdf.

46 National Research Council, Committee on Research Standards and Practices to Prevent the Destructive Application of Biotechnology. *Biotechnology Research in an Age of Terrorism* (Washington, DC: National Academies Press 2004).

47 Richard Danzig, *Catastrophic Bioterrorism: What Is to Be Done?* (Washington, DC, Center for Technology and National Security Policy, National Defense University, 2003).

48 Laurie Garrett, "The Challenge of Global Health," *Foreign Affairs* Jan/Feb 2007.

49 The chapters share a concern with developing critical knowledge about contemporary biosecurity interventions. But they suggest that there is no single critical lens that would enable us to arrive at an overarching diagnosis of "biosecurity" today. In this sense, they diverge from critical studies that denounce what is claimed to be the increasing "securitization" or "militarization" of health. For basic texts on "securitization" see Ronnie Lipschutz, ed., *On Security* (New York: Columbia University Press, 1995).

50 Collier and Lakoff, "Distributed Preparedness: Space, Security and Citizenship in the United States." The proposition that critical analysis of technical expertise can yield insight into value-orientations is a classic Weberian position. See Max Weber, *Methodology of the Social Sciences* (New York: Free Press, 1949).

51 Michel Foucault, "The Risks of Security," in Paul Rabinow, ed., *Power: Essential Works of Foucault, 1954–1984*, vol. 3 (New York: The New Press, 2000), 365–382.

CHAPTER TWO

From Population to Vital System

NATIONAL SECURITY AND THE CHANGING OBJECT OF PUBLIC HEALTH

Andrew Lakoff

In early 1976, health officials warned the Ford administration that a new strain of influenza had appeared in the United States and threatened to become a deadly pandemic. A soldier had died in Fort Dix, and others at the base were infected with the virus. Experts and officials gathered and quickly recommended a plan of action to the president: an urgent, intensive program to immunize the entire U.S. population before the next flu season, at an estimated cost of $135 million. Such a program had never been tried before—indeed, it had only recently become technically feasible. But given the perceived scale of the swine flu threat and the new possibility of intervention, public health experts were nearly unanimous about the rational course of action: mass vaccination. "If we believe in preventive medicine," as one infectious disease expert said, "we have no choice."[1]

Three decades later, in the fall of 2005, the attention of the U.S. government was again focused on the threat of pandemic influenza. This time the threat did not come suddenly; public health officials had been warning of its danger with increasing urgency since the appearance of a deadly strain of the virus in Hong Kong in 1997. But it seemed that now a major initiative was possible: in part because of an increasing perception of the seriousness of the threat, as the virus spread globally through poultry stocks and migratory birds; in part as a result of fallout from the administration's widely perceived failure to respond to Hurricane Katrina. President Bush described the combination of urgency and uncertainty posed by avian flu: "Scientists and doctors cannot tell us where or when the next pandemic will strike, or how severe it will be, but most agree: at some point, we are likely to face another pandemic."[2] Or, as a concerned senator put it: "Experts no longer ask if such a pandemic could occur, rather they question when it will occur."[3]

In November, the administration unveiled a $7.1 billion pandemic preparedness strategy described by the secretary of health as "the most robust proposal ever made for public health at one time."[4] The plan included funds for disease surveillance, stockpiling antiviral medicine, and new methods of vaccine production. The details of the administration's plan were sharply criticized in the public health world as overly focused on pharmaceutical interventions, and as underemphasizing the needs of state and local health agencies. But among various commentators, there was remarkable accord on several points. First, that pandemic planning was a matter of urgent concern; second, that the nation was currently far from adequately prepared for it; and third, that whether or not a pandemic occurred, the process of preparing for it would strengthen readiness for other potential threats. As the senator put it, "even if we are spared from a flu pandemic, the work that we do today will serve us all well in the event of any national emergency."[5]

Indeed, the flu threat had become a vehicle for a more general form of planning—one oriented toward a variety of potential threats. The assistant secretary of health said: "Preparedness for a pandemic makes us a nation better prepared for any and all hazards, manmade or natural." But, he warned, such a condition would not come quickly or easily: "Preparedness is a journey, not a destination. It's a journey that must be nationwide; involve federal, state, and local leaders in partnership; and include every sector of society."[6] As the secretary put it, "We're overdue and we're not as well prepared as we need to be. We're better prepared than we were yesterday. We'll be better prepared tomorrow than we are today. It's a continuum of preparedness."[7] The states' organization of health officers agreed: "Are we fully prepared? Absolutely not. We are more prepared than we were several years ago but not prepared enough."[8]

Over the course of three decades, a new way of thinking about and acting on disease threat had emerged: it was no longer a question only of prevention, but also—and perhaps even more—one of preparedness. How did this shift happen? How, in other words, did a norm of preparedness come to structure thought about threats to public health, and how did a certain set of responses to these threats become possible? The story is a complex one, involving the migration of techniques initially developed in the military and civil defense to other areas of governmental intervention.

My analysis is centered not on widespread public discussion of biological threats, but rather on particular sites of expertise where a novel way of understanding and intervening in threats was developed and deployed. In what follows, I focus on one particular technique, the scenario-based exercise. I argue that this technique served two important functions: first, to generate an affect of urgency in the absence of the event itself; and second, to generate knowledge about vulnerabilities in response capability that could then guide intervention. The scenario-based exercise, I suggest, is exemplary of the rationality underlying the contemporary articulation of national security and public health in the United States.

Scenario-based planning can be usefully contrasted with quantitative methods for managing uncertainty: risk assessment and insurance are examples of techniques that calculate the *probability* of future events in order to guide rational action in the present. They rely on historical patterns of incidence to make such calculations. For this form of planning, the future is the product of calculated decisions made in the present, based on a limited number of possibilities: the past contains the elements of what is to come. However, the problem of *catastrophe*—the event whose likelihood cannot be known, and whose consequences cannot be managed—seems to defy such calculations.[9] This leads to the question I want to focus on in what follows: How, among national security and public health experts in the U.S., is the future prospect of catastrophe brought into the present as an object of knowledge and intervention?

National Security and Public Health

In his 2006 congressional testimony on avian flu preparedness, former White House Homeland Security Advisor Richard Falkenrath said: "When viewed in comparison to all other conceivable threats to U.S. national security, the catastrophic disease threat is and for the foreseeable future will remain the greatest danger we face."[10] Given Falkenrath's background as an expert in counterterrorism and nuclear proliferation, this was a striking statement—a clear affirmation that national security strategists must turn their attention to a subject that, until recently, had been mostly under the purview of public health.

As Nicholas King and others have shown, this was by no means the first time U.S. national security concerns had been linked to public health.[11] To understand the specific implications of Falkenrath's claim—and its distinction from prior such conjunctures—it is important to analytically disaggregate the concept of "national security." In other words, to ask: What *type* of security is meant? What are its political objectives and what are its technical methods? In this context, as we will see, experts who were concerned with the catastrophic disease threat did not for the most part articulate a logic of interdiction.[12] Nor could their approach best be described in terms of a rationality of prevention. Rather, they were engaged in formulating a distinctive way of approaching biological threats—one of ongoing, vigilant readiness for potential disaster.

To show this, it will be useful to introduce a set of analytic distinctions among forms of collective security.[13] *Sovereign state security* dates from the monarchical states of the seventeenth century, and refers to practices oriented to the defense of territorial sovereignty against foreign enemies using military means. *Population security,* which emerged in the nineteenth century, involves the protection of the national population against regularly occurring internal threats, such as illness, industrial accident, or infirmity. Its exemplary knowledge forms include epidemiology and demography, and its interventions range from social insurance and public health to urban infrastructure development.

However, a number of current security initiatives—such as pandemic preparedness or "critical infrastructure protection"—do not fit neatly into either one of these familiar security frameworks. In recent years, a third form, which we can term *vital systems security,* has become increasingly central to the politics of security. This form of security is oriented to a distinctive type of threat: the event whose probability cannot be calculated, but whose consequences are potentially catastrophic. Its object of protection is not the national territory or the population but rather the critical systems that underpin social and economic life. Vital systems security does not develop knowledge about an enemy or about regularly occurring events, but rather uses techniques of imaginative enactment to generate knowledge about system vulnerabilities. Its interventions are not focused on protecting against

Figure 2.1: Forms Of Collective Security

	SOVEREIGN STATE SECURITY	POPULATION SECURITY	VITAL SYSTEMS SECURITY
MOMENT OF ARTICULATION	17th century monarchies	19th century urban hygiene	Mid-20th century civil defense
NORMATIVE RATIONALITY	Interdiction	Prevention	Preparedness
TYPES OF THREATS	Adversaries	Regularly occurring events	Unpredictable, potentially catastrophic events
EXEMPLARY FORM OF KNOWLEDGE	Strategy	Epidemiology, demography	Imaginative enactment
OPERATION	Deter or defend against enemy	Distribute risk	Gauge vulnerability, develop capability

foreign enemies or modulating the living conditions of the population; instead, they seek to assure the continuous functioning of critical systems in the event of emergency (see figure 2.1).[14]

Vital systems security came out of one practice of sovereign state security—civil defense—beginning in the 1960s. Its techniques were initially developed to approach the threat of nuclear attack, but were gradually extended to approach other potential catastrophes, ranging from natural disasters to technological accidents, terrorist attacks, and epidemics of infectious disease. As we will see, when infectious disease is approached as a problem of population security, interventions are structured by a logic of prevention; whereas when it is taken up from the vantage of vital systems security, the guiding logic is one of preparedness.

It should be underlined that these distinctions do not mark epochal shifts: it is not that there has been an overarching transformation from one form of security to another, but rather that these forms operate in dynamic relation to one another—so, for example, the very systems that were developed as the *means* of population security have now, in some cases, become the *targets* of vital systems security. In what follows, I will describe how this has occurred in the case of public health—how a public health preparedness system has been constituted in response to the rise of what Falkenrath called "the catastrophic disease threat."

Swine Flu: The Limits of Population Security

The central object of knowledge and intervention for public health is the population, described by Foucault as "a global mass affected by overall pressures of birth, death, production, illness." As he noted, "these are phenomena that are aleatory and unpredictable when taken in themselves or individually, but which, at the collective level, display constants that are easy, or at least possible, to establish." Statistical knowledge makes such collective regularities visible. Health interventions seek to know and manage these regularities, to decrease mortality and increase longevity, to "optimize a state of life."[15]

Thus modern public health interventions are based on the analysis of historical patterns of disease in a population. The case of nineteenth-century Britain is instructive. As George Rosen has shown, British public health reformers carefully tracked the incidence of disease according to differential social locations to make the argument that "health was affected for better or worse by the state of the physical or social environment."[16] Such knowledge was cumulative and calculative. Reformers gathered and analyzed vital statistics—rates of birth, death, and illness among various classes—in order to demonstrate the economic rationality of disease-prevention measures such as the provision of clean water or the removal of waste from streets. Thus, as Chadwick's famous 1842 inquiry into living conditions among the working classes argued, "the expenditures necessary to the adoption and maintenance of measures of prevention would ultimately amount to less than the cost of disease now constantly expanded."[17]

If this initial mode of public health intervention emphasized social conditions—sanitation, nutrition, the safety of factories—a next iteration worked more directly on the bodies of the collectivity. The rise of bacteriology in the late nineteenth century led to the systematic practice of immunization against infectious disease. But again, making rational public health interventions required knowledge about the historical pattern of disease incidence in the population. For example, as Rosen notes, in designing New York City's vaccination campaign against diphtheria among schoolchildren in the 1920s, it was "necessary to know the natural history of diphtheria within the community: How many children of different ages had already acquired immunity, how many were well carriers, and what children were highly susceptible?"[18] Such data were gathered in order to make decisions based on the balance between the expected costs and benefits of a given intervention.

Given this type of rationality, public health expertise has difficulty in approaching events that cannot be mapped through statistical means. What happens when experts are faced with the threat of a singular event—one whose probability is not known, but whose consequences could be catastrophic?

THE SWINE FLU FIASCO

Let me return to the event with which I began: the apparent outbreak of swine flu in 1976. As we will see, the guiding logic of public health structured the way that the threat was taken up—and led to an eventual "fiasco." In January 1976, the Centers for Disease Control reported that a soldier at Fort Dix had died of an unfamiliar strain of swine flu. Moreover, there were several other cases of the same flu, and so the virus seemed to be both virulent and capable of human-to-human transmission. Was a pandemic on the horizon? At the time, some experts believed that antigenic shifts leading to deadly pandemics occurred approximately once per decade. The last one had occurred in 1968. In the worst case, this strain might be comparable to the 1918 Spanish flu, which, it was estimated, had killed over fifty million people worldwide.[19]

The possibility of pandemic flu had not been part of the planning process for U.S. health officials. For this reason, it was not immediately clear what options were available. A catastrophe on the scale of 1918 was not predictable, but was possible. Leading influenza experts warned health officials to plan for an imminent health emergency. Given the tools available, there seemed to be only one possible course of action: vaccination of the entire U.S. population. Such an option would be both expensive and practically daunting. It would mean producing and distributing enough vaccine to immunize over two hundred million people by the next flu season. This was a new technical possibility: only recently could enough flu vaccine be produced in a given year to envision mass immunization. But a decision would have to be made immediately. And there was no way of knowing whether the cases at Fort Dix were signs of an imminent pandemic or a fluke.

Health officials were thus faced—for the first time—with the possibility of intervening in advance of a potential flu pandemic. This situation presented a problem for public health expertise. As we have seen, modern public health institutions had been set up in response to actual, rather than potential, disease incidence. Indeed, they relied on archival knowledge of the timing and location of outbreaks to design effective interventions. For this reason, as the swine flu affair demonstrates, experts had difficulty in approaching a foreseeable, but not statistically calculable event.

On March 10, officials at the Centers for Disease Control (CDC) met with the Advisory Committee on Immunization Practices (ACIP). Each year the committee recommended which viruses to vaccinate against, and which groups to target for vaccination. Since the general population did not have any immunity to this new strain, a vaccination plan could not be limited to high-risk groups.[20] At the meeting, the group observed: first, there was evidence of a new strain with human-to-human transmission; second, all previous new strains had been followed by pandemics; and third, for the first time there was both knowledge and time to provide for mass immunization, given developments in vaccine production techniques. Some experts also saw an opportunity to demonstrate the importance of preventive medicine, to "strike a blow for epidemiology in the interest in humanity."[21] If the plan were immediately put in motion, inoculation could begin by the summer.

One question was raised, but not pursued: Under what circumstances might it make sense to produce and then stockpile the vaccine rather than moving straight to mass vaccination? The CDC's director David Sencer argued that the virus would spread too quickly and that distribution logistics were too difficult to consider waiting for evidence of an epidemic before beginning vaccination. There was also a concern about future blame: if officials chose not to vaccinate and then there was a deadly pandemic, they would face biting criticism. It would be said that "they had the opportunity to save life," but didn't take it.[22]

Following the meeting, Sencer wrote a strongly worded memorandum to his superiors at the Department of Health summarizing the committee's advice. Given what he called a "strong possibility" of widespread swine influenza that could be highly virulent, the committee recommended a plan to immunize 213 million people in three months, at a cost of $134 million. The memo's tone was urgent: "The situation is one of 'go or no go'...there is barely enough time.... A decision must be made now."[23] The secretary of health then wrote a note to President Ford. In the note, he shifted Sencer's conditional to the future tense, from possibility into apparent certainty:

> There is evidence there will be a major epidemic this coming fall. The indication
> is that we will see a return of 1918 flu virus that is the most virulent form of flu.
> In 1918 a half a million people died. The projections are that this virus will kill
> one million Americans in 1976.[24]

Ford consulted a number of leading experts in virology and public health, including Jonas Salk, who urged mass vaccination.[25] The president publicly announced the vaccination plan on March 24, saying: "No one knows exactly how serious this threat could be. Nevertheless, we cannot afford to take a chance with the health of the nation."[26]

Outside of the administration and its circle of experts there was criticism of the program. The New Jersey state epidemiologist publicly warned of dangerous side effects. *New York Times* editorials were repeatedly skeptical, accusing the administration of engaging in politics at the expense of science. In advance of a major meeting of program participants in Atlanta, one cautious expert wrote to Sencer to recommend an alternative to mass vaccination: stockpiling vaccines, "along the lines of military defense," and developing "well-worked-out contingency plans."[27] The idea would be to create a period of potential intervention in anticipation of the event, rather than engaging in immediate intervention. Such an approach would have provided an alternative to mass vaccination. The proposal was not taken seriously: as I will argue below, this type of "preparedness" measure was not, at this stage, part of the tool kit of public health.

The goal of the program was to start immunizations in August and finish before the end of winter. Field trials of the vaccine were launched in April.[28] An unexpected blow to the program came in the summer: vaccine manufacturers announced that they would not bottle the vaccine without liability insurance.

Insurers were unwilling to offer such coverage, given uncertainties about the health risks of the vaccination program.[29] For the program to begin, the government would have to find a way to assure manufacturers that liability risk would be covered.[30] Once this problem was solved and the program finally began, there were major problems with logistics at the federal level, and wide variability in individual states' capacity to actually implement the program.

What then became clear was that the CDC had not seriously considered how to manage the risk of side effects. When several elderly vaccine recipients died shortly after receiving their shot, CDC simply announced that a certain number of such deaths were to be "expected." Despite these problems, by December forty million people had been immunized, though they were oddly distributed given the variation in individual states' execution of the plan. In the middle of the month, however, Minnesota health officials reported multiple cases of Guillain-Barré Syndrome, a severe neurological condition, among vaccinees. At this point it was clear that the expected epidemic was not coming, and the program was immediately suspended. A *New York Times* op-ed piece declared, "Swine Flu Fiasco."[31]

A later report on the program did not fault the decision to go ahead with it; experts were, after all, unanimous. But it did suggest that one source of failure was its administrators' lack of foresight. Health officials did not have contingency plans in place, and so reacted in an ad hoc manner. Thus they were not able to make available to themselves a solution that could have helped: stockpiling vaccine in advance, and then—if the epidemic did develop—applying advanced logistics to design an efficient method of distribution. Moreover, they did not envision and plan for potential problems such as manufacturers' liability, variations in state distribution capacities, and side effects. Given the rationality of public health prevention, there was "no choice" but to go forward with mass vaccination. Public health officials did not have a mechanism with which to engage in responsible, but limited, action under conditions of urgency and uncertainty.

Crisis Management and the Vulnerable System

Interestingly, around the same time a systematic method for dealing flexibly with potential crises was being developed in a very different domain of government.

Civil defense had extended its purview from a focus on nuclear catastrophe to a more general form of preparedness for emergencies. In this section I describe the articulation of crisis management as a novel approach to uncertain but potentially catastrophic threats. Although in its inception it was completely separate from public health, crisis management would eventually extend its purview to manage the threat of catastrophic disease.

Much of this development initially took place in federal government agencies devoted to planning for nuclear attack. An exemplary figure was Robert Kupperman, an applied mathematician who worked in Nixon's Office of Emergency Preparedness (OEP) in the early 1970s. Kupperman's task was to quantitatively analyze the operations of large sociotechnical systems, such as energy, transportation, and industrial production. Based in the Systems Evaluation Division of OEP, Kupperman was involved in governmental response to a number of crises in the early 1970s, including the wage-price freeze, Hurricane Agnes, a rash of terrorist attacks, and the energy crisis.

In this context Kupperman developed an interest in the common structure of crisis situations, and in the development of techniques that could be used to prepare for them. He argued that crises, however diverse, shared some common problems: the paucity of accurate information, the difficulty of communication among decision makers, and a confusing array of authorities seeking to take charge of the situation. Such situations involved uncertainty about what was unfolding, coupled with an urgent demand for immediate action to alleviate the crisis. Flexibility for decision makers depended on the extent to which the crisis manager had forecast the situation and invested in preparation for it. The apparent recent increase in numbers of crises demonstrated the contemporary importance of such foresight. "As we begin to recognize the complex problems that threaten every nation with disaster," he and two colleagues from OEP asked, "can we continue to trust the ad hoc processes of instant reaction to muddle through?"[32]

Kupperman's background was in operations research (OR), a relatively new field dating from World War II efforts to introduce quantitative analysis to military practice. OR developed tools for analyzing and optimizing complex systems. This meant first of all seeing multiple, heterogeneous elements as part of a coherent system whose behavior was, as Jay Forrester put it, "a consequence of the interaction of its parts."[33] For example, in studying the efficiency of allied bombing strategy during World War II, OR analysts gathered detailed data on specific bombing runs, looking at the interconnection and interaction of multiple variables such as altitude, speed, number and formation of bombers, weather, and light. "In general," as historian Thomas Hughes writes, "advocates of the systems approach perceived, conceived of, or created a world made up of systems."[34] The systems view gained prominence in the 1950s and 1960s in settings including the RAND Corporation and the Department of Defense under Robert McNamara.

If early operations researchers were interested in the optimization of systems, Kupperman was most concerned with their potential failure. His experience in the OEP led him toward an emphasis on the vulnerability of critical systems to sudden, unexpected events. After leaving the OEP, he continued to think about how to systematize governmental response to crisis, especially through his work at the Center for Strategic and International Studies (CSIS). He was coauthor, with R. James Woolsey, of a 1984 CSIS report on "crisis management in a society of networks" called *America's Hidden Vulnerabilities*. The report argued that the United States relied for its survival on a sophisticated and intricate set of systems, or networks, for energy distribution, communication, and transportation. It noted recent disruptions of these systems, and warned: "A serious potential exists...for much more serious disabling of networks crucial to life support, economic stability, and national defense."[35]

At CSIS, Kupperman and his colleagues sought to persuade national security officials of the problem of system vulnerability, and the need to develop techniques of contingency planning. One of their approaches was to hold scenario-based simulations of crisis situations, and invite officials to participate.[36] The emergency exercise was a tool for demonstrating to leaders the vulnerabilities of vital systems. As he and Woolsey wrote:

> If planning has involved the operating teams and managers (as it always should) these critical personnel gain an increased understanding of how the system works and, particularly valuable, how it is likely to behave under abnormal conditions. Training with crisis games and emergency exercises will augment this benefit significantly.[37]

America's Hidden Vulnerabilities listed a number of measures to ensure the continued functioning of vital systems in the event of emergency, including: improving system resilience, building in redundancy, stockpiling spare parts, performing risk analysis as a means of prioritizing resource allocation, and running scenario-based exercises. A final key element of crisis management, according to the report, was the specification in advance of responsibilities during the crisis situation itself.[38]

There is, of course, a long history of reflection on how to approach specific crisis situations—extending from early modern quarantine plans to Cold War civil defense. And the military practice of training simulations or "war games" also has a long history. What was perhaps distinctive about Kupperman's approach was the application of the method of imaginative enactment to the *generic* crisis situation in order to generate knowledge about internal system vulnerabilities. The CSIS method of crisis simulation would eventually help convince national security planners to think seriously about biological threats. It would also make visible the elements of a new object: the public health infrastructure.

Military Medicine and Tropical Disease

How were the two strands we have so far been looking at—public health on the one hand, and crisis management on the other—brought together? The first conjuncture I want to follow is an encounter between military medicine and international health. At a conference of tropical disease specialists in Honolulu in 1989, Col. Llewellyn Legters ran a table-top exercise simulating the outbreak of a deadly and highly contagious virus. Legters, then head of preventive medicine at the Uniformed Services Hospital, had been a special forces doctor in Vietnam, where he had treated the first reported case of drug-resistant malaria in 1964.[39] His exercise in Honolulu focused on the lack of international public health resources to manage a dangerous outbreak. It was designed to convince participants of the urgency of the problem of emerging infectious disease.

The premise of the exercise was that a pandemic of a novel and horrifying virus—an "airborne Ebola"—had broken out among refugees in a war-torn African republic. As the epidemic extended to humanitarian aid workers, initial public health response was tepid, and the disease spread rapidly to the United States, with devastating results. Participants in the exercise saw that there was no system in place to contain such an outbreak if it occurred. After the exercise, Legters announced that "the outbreak has confirmed, in a very dramatic way, just how ill-prepared we are to detect global epidemic disease threats in a timely fashion, and, once detected, to respond appropriately."[40]

Experts in the field were alarmed. As journalist Laurie Garrett reported:

> "I found this scenario very realistic," said Dr. William Reeves, professor emeritus from the University of California at Berkeley and one of the world's experts on disease-carrying insect control. "You could take any disease as a model—Ebola, malaria, whatever—and it would reveal the same thing. We aren't ready. Where are the people? The expertise? The equipment? Some planning needs to be done on this."[41]

Legters' exercise framed the closing chapter of Garrett's 1994 bestseller, *The Coming Plague*. "What the war games revealed," she wrote, "was an appalling state of nonreadiness. Overall, the mood in Honolulu after five hours was grim, even nervous. The failings, weaknesses, and gaps in preparedness were enormous."[42]

The exercise was exemplary of the problematic of "emerging infectious disease" as it was articulated in the late 1980s and early 1990s.[43] Also in 1989, virologist Stephen Morse and Nobel Prize winner Joshua Lederberg hosted a major conference on the topic, which led to the landmark volume, *Emerging Viruses*.[44] Participants in the conference warned of a dangerous intersection: On the one hand, there were a number of new disease threats, including emerging viruses such as AIDS and Ebola as well as newly antimicrobial resistant strains of diseases such as tuberculosis and malaria. On the other hand, public health systems had been left to decay, beginning in the late 1960s with the assumption that infectious disease had effectively been conquered. Moreover, the emergence of dangerous new infectious diseases could be expected to continue due to a number of global processes, such as increased travel, urbanization, civil wars and refugee crises, and environmental destruction.

In his contribution to *Emerging Viruses* epidemiologist D. A. Henderson argued that novel pathogen emergence was inevitable: "mutation and change are facts of nature...the world is increasingly interdependent, and...human health and survival will be challenged, ad infinitum, by new and mutant microbes, with unpredictable pathophysiological manifestations." As a result, he said, "we are uncertain as to what we should keep under surveillance, or even what we should look for." What we need, Henderson argued, is a system that can detect novelty: in the case of AIDS, such a detection system could have warned early of a new virus and put measures in place to prevent its spread. He proposed a system of global surveillance units to be run by CDC, and located in peri-urban areas in major cities in the tropics, which could provide a "window on events in surrounding areas."[45]

Legters also contributed to this volume, using the results of the exercise in Honolulu to make the case for a rejuvenation of the field of tropical medicine as the generation trained in World War II retired. He pointed to declining U.S. capability in epidemiology, diagnosis, and treatment of tropical disease. The chapter identified both the sources of the new disease threat, along the lines of Morse and Lederberg, and institutional responses that would be necessary to manage it: a global surveillance system to identify the outbreak; a laboratory system to characterize the agent; a reporting system to alert the world health community; and academic training of a new generation of tropical disease experts.

Garrett's vision of the source of the problem was broader than that of scientists such as Legters or Henderson. On the one hand, she diagnosed a collapse of the public health system. Problems included discrepancies in capabilities between different health departments, widespread deficiencies in disease-reporting systems, few staff for disease surveillance, and suffering health department laboratories. At the same time, Garrett argued that global living conditions—poverty, civil war, lack of basic healthcare—were the source of the emerging disease threat, and that these social problems would need to be addressed in order to provide security against emerging pathogens. She quoted former CDC director William Foege, who argued that new disease emergence was linked to "thirdworldization": the overall status of healthcare, immunizations, sanitation, and education.[46] But in policy discussions, this "population security" orientation to the threat of emerging disease was mostly overshadowed by a more narrow technical focus on developing a global system for detecting and managing outbreaks.

Disease as a National Security Threat

At this stage, "emerging infectious disease"—although widely taken up as a public health and biomedical issue—was not yet conceptualized as a problem of national security. This changed over the following decade, when the emerging infectious disease problematic combined with increased anxiety about bioterrorism. Scenario-based exercises were central to this process. In the late 1990s, accounts began to circulate of a massive, secret Soviet bioweapons program that had continued throughout the Cold War, and which had employed scores of scientists whose whereabouts were now unknown.[47] D. A. Henderson was one of the experts who linked the new bioterrorist threat to the problem of emerging diseases. He argued that his proposed global disease surveillance system would be useful for both types of threat—from emerging diseases and from proliferating bioweapons knowledge. In 1998, Henderson founded the Johns Hopkins Center for Civilian Biodefense Strategies, which became a leading site of knowledge production around the new biological threat.

The CDC developed a number of initiatives in response to the bioterrorist threat—one of which was a program of global disease surveillance akin to Henderson's proposal. Another was the Office of Bioterrorism Preparedness and Response, which distributed $40 million per year in bioterrorism grants to local public health departments. However, critics such as Tara O'Toole of the Hopkins biodefense center argued that these measures were not nearly enough.[48] The question for such critics was how to convince officials of the urgent need to address the problem. This threat was different from what public health experts were accustomed to dealing with: there was no historical record on which to estimate its likelihood of occurrence, or to calculate the most effective intervention measures. Nor was infectious disease a problem that national security officials were trained to think about. What kind of experience could convey a sense of urgency and generate knowledge about necessary interventions?

With O'Toole's lead, the Hopkins biodefense center entered into a collaboration with Kupperman's former think tank, the Center for Strategic and International Studies, to design a table-top exercise simulating a smallpox attack on the United States.[49] The exercise, called "Dark Winter," took place at Andrews Air Force Base in June 2001. It was aimed at influential national security experts and government officials. Participants included Sam Nunn as the president, David Gergen as national security advisor, and James Woolsey as director of the CIA. The exercise took place in three segments over two days, depicting a time span of two weeks after the initial attack. While designers used historical data on the patterns of smallpox outbreaks to design the exercise, the point of using this epidemiological information was not to accurately model probability, but rather to create a plausible scenario.[50]

The exercise began with a meeting of the National Security Council. The scenario laid out the situation for the council members. There were reports of an outbreak of smallpox in Oklahoma City, assumed to be the result of a terrorist attack. Initial questions for the council were technical: "With only twelve million doses of vaccine available, what is the best strategy to contain the outbreak? Should there be a national or a state vaccination policy? Is ring vaccination or mass immunization the best policy?" The problem was that there was not enough information about the scale of the attack to come up with a solution. By the second meeting, the situation looked grim. "Only 1.25 million doses of vaccine remain, and public unrest grows as the vaccine supply dwindles," read the scenario. "Vaccine distribution efforts vary from state to state, are often chaotic, and lead to violence in some areas." International borders were closed, leading to food shortages. Meanwhile simulated twenty-four-hour news coverage, shown to participants as video clips, sharply criticized the government's response. Graphic photographs of American smallpox victims were also displayed.

As vaccine stock dwindled further, the prospect of using the National Guard to enforce containment was broached. But who had the authority to make emergency decisions? In one sequence, an NSC member advised the president to federalize the National Guard, as states had begun to seal their borders. Governor Keating of Oklahoma objected:

> *Keating:* "That's not your function."
>
> *George Terwilliger (playing the Attorney General):* "Mr. President, this question got settled at Appomattox. You need to federalize the National Guard."
>
> *Nunn:* "We're going to have absolute chaos if we start having war between the federal government and the state government."

Meanwhile civil unrest grew. "With vaccine in short supply, increasingly anxious crowds mob vaccination clinics," the scenario continued. "Riots around a vaccination site in Philadelphia left two dead. At another vaccination site, angry citizens overwhelmed vaccinators."[51] By the third meeting, there had been thousands of deaths, and the situation was growing still worse. The exercise ended as the disaster continued to escalate: there was no vaccine remaining and none was expected for four weeks. As CSIS Director John Hamre later narrated the final stage: "In the last forty-eight hours there were fourteen thousand cases. We now have over one thousand dead, another five thousand that we expect to be dead within weeks. There are two hundred people who died from the vaccination, because there is a small percentage [of risk], and we have administered twelve million doses.... At this stage the medical system is overwhelmed completely."[52]

At the congressional hearings on the exercise, participants reported on their experience of "Dark Winter." For example, Sam Nunn reflected on the debate over using the National Guard: "It is a terrible dilemma. Because you know that your vaccine is going to give out, and you know the only other strategy is isolation, but you don't know who to isolate. That is the horror of this situation." Hamre added: "We thought that we were going to be spending our time with the mechanisms of government. We ended up spending our time saying, 'How do we save democracy in America?' Because it is that serious, and it is that big."[53]

The point of the exercise was to give national security officials a *feeling* of how an unprecedented event might unfold. Its circle of influence extended outward through a series of briefings featuring a realistic video portraying the events as they unfolded. Vice President Cheney, DHS Secretary Tom Ridge, and key congressional leaders were among those briefed. At the congressional hearing, where the video was about to be shown, Rep. Christopher Shays asked Hamre about its affective qualities:

> Mr. Shays: Now, I understand there may be some graphic display here.
> Mr. Hamre: Sir, there will be graphics as well as some video. This will be shown on these side monitors.
> Mr. Shays: I'm told that some of it is not pleasant.
> Mr. Hamre: It is not pleasant. Let me also emphasize, sir, this is a simulation. This had frightening qualities of being real, as a matter of fact too real.

And because we have television cameras here broadcasting, we want to tell everyone, this did not happen, it was a simulation. But, it had such realism, and we are going to try to show you the sense of realism that came from that today.[54]

Indeed, Shays did react strongly to the video, noting afterwards how nervous he had felt while watching it:

I felt like I've been in the middle of a movie, and maybe that's why I was anxious. I wanted to know how it turned out. And so I asked my staff how did we finally get a handle on it, you know, twelve million vaccines out, the disease spreading? And the response was we did not get a handle on it. They stopped the exercise before resolution. Kind of scary, huh?

The exercise was successful in that it convinced participants (and later briefing audiences) of the urgent need to plan for a bioattack. Keating was stunned at the lack of preparedness demonstrated by the exercise: "We think an enemy of the United States could attack us with smallpox or with anthrax…and we really don't prepare for it, we have no vaccines for it—that's astonishing." As Woolsey noted, this was a new type of enemy: "We are used to thinking about health problems as naturally occurring problems outside the framework of a malicious actor." With disease as tool of attack, "we are in a world we haven't ever really been in before."[55]

The exercise demonstrated a number of vulnerabilities. First, officials did not have real-time understanding—"situational awareness"—of the various aspects of the crisis while it unfolded. As the scenario designers wrote, "this lack of information, critical for leaders' situational awareness in 'Dark Winter,' reflects the fact that few systems exist that can provide a rapid flow of the medical and public health information needed in a public health emergency."[56] Second, without adequate stockpiles of medical countermeasures, leaders could not properly manage the crisis. Third, there was a gulf between public health and national security expertise: "It isn't just [a matter of] buying more vaccine," said Woolsey. "It's a question of how we integrate these public health and national security communities in ways that allow us to deal with various facets of the problem."[57]

Participants had concrete suggestions for improvement. Nunn argued for vaccination of first responders in advance of an attack: "Every one of those people you are trying to mobilize is going to have to be vaccinated. You can't expect them to go in there and expose themselves and their family to smallpox or any other deadly disease without vaccinations."[58] Jerome Hauer, a former New York City emergency manager, spoke of the problem of distributing vaccines in cities: "The logistical infrastructure necessary to vaccinate the people of New York City, Los Angeles, Chicago is just—would be mind-boggling." But the broader lesson was the need to enact the event in order to plan for it.[59] As Hamre said, "We didn't have the strategy at the table on how to deal with this, because we have never thought our way through it before, and systematically thinking our way through this kind of a crisis is now going to become a key imperative. It clearly is going to require many more exercises."[60]

The Scenario-Event: Hurricane Katrina

Until 2005, U.S. biological preparedness efforts were mostly focused on specific threat agents such as smallpox and anthrax. These efforts were reoriented by the failed governmental response to Hurricane Katrina. For thinkers of preparedness, Katrina served as a "live action" exercise demonstrating gaps in the system of preparedness. The disaster also suggested that while homeland security planners had been focused on the threat of terrorism, the problematic of emergency was much broader: the rubric of "all-hazards planning" that had originally structured the Federal Emergency Management Agency (FEMA) came to the fore. Washington, DC, was in a "post-Katrina, prepandemic" moment, as anthropologist Monica Schoch-Spana noted.[61] As a member of the House Committee on Homeland Security said, "the pandemic flu scenario is affording us much more time to prepare, but as of today it appears that the nation is poised to repeat a grave error by not heeding the lessons learned from Katrina."[62]

The problem of avian flu now appeared in a new light—in terms of the vulnerability of the nation's public health infrastructure. For Sen. Richard Burr, chairman of the Subcommittee on Public Health Preparedness, Katrina "exposed an unstable public health infrastructure at all levels of government during an emergency event." According to Burr, the challenge at hand was akin to the project of constructing the national highway infrastructure in the 1950s. "For the purpose of national public health and defense we need a national standardized public health system," he said. Such a system would have to do more than prepare for known threats: "The question is, are we smart enough to design a template that enables us to address the threats that we don't know about for tomorrow?"[63]

What were the necessary elements of such a system? These could be seen through an analysis of current gaps in response. Experts and officials collaborated to constitute the necessary elements of a national public health system, based on knowledge of its vulnerabilities. "There are multiple holes in our capacity to respond," said Rep. Henry Waxman. "We need to increase our vaccine production capacity, strengthen our public health infrastructure, create adequate hospital surge capacity, and draft contingency plans that will ensure the continued operation of important government functions."[64]

For many analysts, the most serious problem Katrina had exposed was that of the locus of responsibility in an emergency situation. For some, the problem was the incompetence of federal leadership; for others, it was that local authorities were not up to the task of coordinating response. Former Homeland Security Advisor Richard Falkenrath argued that state and local health authorities would be incapable of coordinating an adequate response to a catastrophic disease event. The Department of Health and Human Services (HHS), he testified, "is simply not going to be able to meet the American people's expectation of the federal government in a truly catastrophic disease contingency such as a high lethal pandemic or major bioterrorist attack." He was especially concerned about civil unrest resulting from "shortages in vital, life-saving countermeasures to the disease in question"—the premise of "Dark Winter." "I mean something very, very specific, which is to prepare to distribute life-saving medications to extremely large populations, very, very quickly, when they are afraid, because there is a communicable disease out there that they do not know how to deal with."

Falkenrath cited evidence from scenario-based exercises to validate his claim that the HHS did not have the operational capabilities to distribute medical supplies in a crisis: "This extraordinary national deficiency was first revealed during the first TOPOFF exercise in May 2000 at which I was an observer," and "in a wide variety of smaller-scale tabletop exercises and simulations." He continued: "The implication is inescapable: the plans, if put to the severe test of a catastrophic disease scenario in the near future, will fail." There was a clear policy implication: the National Response Plan should be amended to assign Emergency Support Function #8 to the military in a catastrophic disease incident, at the order of the president: "Only the Department of Defense has the planning, logistics, and personnel resources needed to conduct nationwide medical relief operations in a full-scale catastrophic disease scenario."[65]

O'Toole drew a different lesson from Katrina: "What we have to do, and what the main point of planning is, as we have learned in all of the emergency preparedness done so far, is that we have to start talking with each other."[66] She disagreed with Falkenrath. "I think it would be a big mistake to…plan to put DoD in charge whenever we have a big bad thing happening." While it is necessary to "rethink federalism," she argued, the federal role is one of creating infrastructure to enable local response: "What the feds have to do is create the capacity to plug in and that's [what] they ought to be focusing on. But I don't think we want the DoD to suddenly become everybody's responder in cases of dire need."[67]

One thing that everyone agreed on was that health agencies should carry out more exercises. A representative of the American College of Emergency Physicians said: "We need to train the hospital and healthcare workers to more long-term pandemic scenarios. And then we need to take these lessons learned, the best practices and lessons learned, and disseminate."[68] The commissioner of health of Duchess County New York testified: "I think over the last five years we've built the framework of a system that we can carry forward…but we need to strengthen that and continue to have strategic exercises community wide, not just public health departments, but every single community drill to include as many partners as possible so that we can learn from each other."[69] And a Virginia state emergency health preparedness official said: "We have been working very closely with [the Department of Homeland Security] in terms of developing metrics as well as with the CDC and HHS, but we need to assure that we have the exercises and events to test our plans and that's really the test of preparedness. What we've done in Virginia is we've used every event as an opportunity to test our plans and we've had many."[70]

By the end of the year, Congress had moved to address the problem of preparedness in a more sustained, integrated way, with the passage of the Pandemic and All-Hazards Preparedness Act of 2006. Even critics of the prior year's plan hailed the bill's passage as a "milestone" piece of public health legislation.[71] The act included a range of measures, from the reorganization of federal health administration, to funding for local and state health agencies, the training of epidemiological investigators, and a novel biomedical research initiative. A key issue the act sought to address was how to create an integrated "system" of public health preparedness, one that extended from disease detection to vaccine production to the relations among the various government agencies that would be charged with response. Such a system would be focused not specifically on pandemic flu, but on a generic form of threat: the unpredictable, but potentially catastrophic, disease event.

There was broad agreement that addressing this threat was not simply a matter of public health, but one of national security. Although the link between national security and public health was not in itself new, what was distinctive about these measures was the attempt to integrate the institutions, forms of knowledge, and techniques of intervention developed in the period of modern public health into a more general system of preparedness, in the context of a broader security problematic that focused on the vulnerability of "critical infrastructures" to potentially catastrophic events.

In closing, let me return to the comparison, outlined above, between the 1976 swine flu campaign and the "pandemic preparedness" measures enacted three decades later.[72] Along with the contrast in their scale, the two technopolitical responses differed profoundly in their approach to disease threat (see figure 2.2). First, in the way of conceptualizing the threat to be managed: the 2005–2006 measures were focused not only on the specific threat of a new and virulent strain of influenza, but on the generic "catastrophic disease threat." Second, the site of intervention differed: whereas the 1976 campaign was aimed at the national population using classical methods of public health, the later plans were aimed at multiple elements of the "public health infrastructure," both within the United States and globally, including disease surveillance capacity, the ability to produce and distribute countermeasures, and the administrative organization of response. And third, the

Figure 2.2: Swine Flu vs. Pandemic Preparedness

	SWINE FLU (1976)	PANDEMIC PREPAREDNESS (2006)
TYPE OF THREAT	Specific	Generic
NORMATIVE RATIONALITY	Prevention	Preparedness
TARGET	National population	Public health infrastructure
FORM OF KNOWLEDGE	Risk calculation	Imaginative enactment
TECHNIQUE OF INTERVENTION	Mass vaccination	Capacity building

prominent form of knowledge used to authorize expert claims about needed interventions had changed: rather than the statistical calculation of risk based on the historical incidence of disease, the emphasis of experts was on knowledge gathered through the imaginative enactment of singular events.

We can see in contrasting these cases that a vital systems approach emerges at the limit point of population security—but that it is constrained in the type of problems it can approach. It is not that the two forms of security are necessarily in conflict or mutually exclusive: rather, vital systems security operates in reflexive relation to population security, working to define its elements as a "critical infrastructure" whose vulnerabilities must be mitigated. However, if political attention focuses only on vital systems security at the expense of population security, only certain types of problems become visible as possible targets of intervention. Whereas Laurie Garrett had pointed to global living conditions—poverty, access to healthcare, decent housing—as a key source of the threat of emerging infectious disease, the eventual preparedness measures enacted in response to avian flu focused only on technical response to the potential outbreak. From the vantage of vital systems security, whose task is to prepare for potential emergencies, the ongoing living conditions of members of the population are not a salient political problem.

NOTES

1   Richard E. Neustadt and Harvey V. Fineberg, *The Epidemic That Never Was: Policy Making and the Swine Flu Scare* (New York: Vintage Books, 1983), 26.

2   White House, "President Outlines Pandemic Influenza Preparedness and Response," Press Release, November 1, 2005.

3   Senator Herb Kohl, U.S. Senate Special Committee on Aging, *Hearing on Preparation for Pandemic Flu*, 109th Cong., 2nd sess., Serial No. 109-24, May 25, 2006.

4   Michael O. Leavitt, Pandemic Planning: Convening of the States, "Remarks to the Convening of the States on Pandemic Influenza Preparedness," December 5, 2005.

5   Kohl, *Hearing on Preparation for Pandemic Flu*.

6   John Agwunobi, Testimony to House of Representatives, Committee on Government Reform, *Hearing on Working through an Outbreak: Pandemic Flu Planning and Continuity of Operations*, 109th Cong., 2nd sess., Serial No. 109-155, May 11, 2006.

7   Michael O. Leavitt, Testimony to U.S. Senate Special Committee on Aging, *Hearing on Preparation for Pandemic Flu*, 109th Cong., 2nd sess., Serial No. 109-24, May 25, 2006.

8   Mary Selecky, Testimony to U.S. House of Representatives Committee on Homeland Security, *Hearing on Avian Influenza*, February 8, 2006.

9   See Niklas Luhmann, "Describing the Future," in *Observations on Modernity* (Stanford: Stanford University Press, 1998).

10 Richard A. Falkenrath, Testimony to U.S. Senate Committee on Health, Education, Labor and Pensions, *Hearing on Enhancing Public Health and Medical Preparedness: Reauthorization of the Public Health Security and Bioterrorism Preparedness and Response Act*, March 16, 2006.

11 For example, one might look at the role of army malaria prevention during World War II in the institutional history of the Centers for Disease Control. Nicholas B. King, "Security, Disease, Commerce: Postcolonial Ideologies of Global Health," *Social Studies of Science* 32 (2002): 763–89.

12 Of course there were other, more visible actors in the U.S. government who did treat biological threats this way, for example in the lead-up to the war in Iraq. For a discussion, see Melinda Cooper, "Preempting Emergence: The Biological Turn in the War on Terror," *Theory, Culture and Society* 23, no. 4 (2006): 113–35.

13 The initial contrast is based on the distinction that Foucault draws between sovereignty and governmentality in his 1978 lectures at the Collège de France. Michel Foucault, *Sécurité, territoire, population. Cours au Collège de France, 1977–78*, ed. Michel Senellart (Paris: Seuil/Gallimard, 2004).

14 Its objects are similar to the kinds of threats Ulrich Beck describes as central to "world risk society." However, from the vantage of vital systems security, such threats do not lead to a politics of precaution; the task, rather, is to envision and plan for the occurrence of the potentially catastrophic event. Ulrich Beck, *World Risk Society* (Cambridge: Polity, 1999).

15 Michel Foucault, *"Society Must Be Defended": Lectures at the Collège de France, 1975–76*, ed. Mauro Bertani and Alessandro Fontana (New York: Picador, 2003), 243.

16 George Rosen, *A History of Public Health* (Baltimore: Johns Hopkins University Press, 1993), 185. For the French case, see François Delaporte, *Disease and Civilization: The Cholera in Paris, 1832* (Cambridge, MA: The MIT Press, 1986), and Paul Rabinow, *French*

Modern: Norms and Forms of the Social Environ-ment (Cambridge, MA: The MIT Press, 1989).

17 Edwin Chadwick, *Report...On an Inquiry into the Sanitary Conditions of the Labouring Population of Great Britain* (London, 1842), cited in Rosen, *History of Public Health*, 187. Ian Hacking looks to this period to find the moment when a "laws of sickness" were discovered, in part through the use of benefit societies' actuarial tables; see *The Taming of Chance* (Cambridge [England]; New York: Cambridge University Press, 1990).

18 Rosen, *History of Public Health*, 312.

19 This account is based on Neustadt and Fine-berg, *The Epidemic That Never Was.*

20 As CDC Director David Sencer later said: "Most people were at risk.... An epidemic spreading into a pandemic had to be considered as a pos-sibility"; from the vantage of preventive medi-cine, "something had to be done." Ibid., 25.

21 Ibid., 26.

22 Ibid., 28.

23 Ibid., 30. The memo would prove politically impossible to ignore, given the later possibility of a leak.

24 Ibid., 35.

25 Ibid. Salk saw the program as an "opportunity to fill part of the 'immunity gap'"—that is, the gap between environmental antigens and populations without antibodies.

26 Ibid., 46.

27 Ibid., 60.

28 By June, the epidemic had not yet appeared. At an ACIP meeting in Bethesda that month, virologist Alfred Sabin suggested stockpiling the vaccine.

29 Neustadt and Fineberg write: "These questions defied actuaries. There was no experience.... They were in the business to spread risk, not take it." Ibid., 77.

30 The matter was settled by the outbreak of a fatal illness at the Legionnaires Convention in Philadelphia. Although the illness turned out not to be swine flu, alarm around the episode was enough to enable the passage of legislation requiring that vaccine liability claims be filed against the government rather than manufacturers.

31 Harry Schwartz, "Swine Flu Fiasco," *New York Times*, December 21, 1976.

32 Robert H. Kupperman, Richard H. Wilcox, and Harvey A. Smith, "Crisis Management: Some Opportunities," *Science* 187, no. 4175 (1975): 406.

33 Jay Forrester, quoted in Thomas Hughes, *Res-cuing Prometheus* (New York: Pantheon Books, 1998), 141.

34 Ibid., 142.

35 CSIS Science and Technical Committee and Panel on Crisis Management, *America's Hidden Vulnerabilities: Crisis Management in a Society of Networks* (Washington, DC: Center for Stra-tegic and International Studies, Georgetown University, 1984), 2.

36 See, for example, Andrew C. Goldberg et al., *Leaders and Crisis: The CSIS Crisis Simulations* (Washington, DC: Center for Strategic and International Studies, 1987).

37 CSIS, *America's Hidden Vulnerabilities*, 16.

38 "Cooperative action during a crisis requires coordinated preparation beforehand with responsibilities clear for resolving differences concerning both the measures to be taken and the accounts to be charged." Ibid., 17.

39 Two years later he founded the Field Epide-miological Survey Team to track this strain of malaria in the midst of the war. See Norma Mohr, *Malaria: The Evolution of a Killer* (Seattle: Sevil & Pixil, 2001).

40 Llewellyn Letgers, Linda H. Brink, and Ernest T. Takafuji, "Are We Prepared for a Viral Epidemic Emergency?" in *Emerging Viruses*, ed. Stephen

S. Morse (New York: Oxford University Press, 1993), 277.

41 Laurie Garrett, "A Medical War Game," *Newsday*, January 23, 1990.

42 Laurie Garrett, "Searching for Solutions: Preparedness, Surveillance, and the New Understanding," in *The Coming Plague: Newly Emerging Diseases in a World Out of Balance* (New York: Farrar, Straus and Giroux, 1994), 594.

43 As Nicholas King has shown, this vision quickly found prominent adherents in medicine, the life sciences, and journalism; King, "Security, Disease, Commerce." One important report was Institute of Medicine, *Emerging Infections: Microbial Threats to Health in the United States* (Washington, DC: National Academies Press, 1992). Garrett's *The Coming Plague* and Richard Preston's *The Hot Zone* (New York: Random House, 1994) both appeared in the same year. Also see Lyle Fearnley, "'From Chaos to Controlled Disorder': Syndromic Surveillance, Bioweapons, and the Pathological Future," ARC Working Paper #5, Anthropology of the Contemporary Research Collaboratory, March 25, 2005.

44 Stephen S. Morse, ed., *Emerging Viruses* (New York: Oxford University Press, 1993).

45 D. A. Henderson, "Surveillance Systems," ibid., 284; 287. See Fearnley, "'From Chaos,'" for a detailed analysis.

46 Garrett, *The Coming Plague*, 609.

47 The program was described by one of its leaders, Ken Alibek, in *Biohazard: The Chilling True Story of the Largest Covert Biological Weapons Program in the World, Told from Inside by the Man Who Ran It* (New York: Random House, 1999) and by Judith Miller and her colleagues in *Germs: Biological Weapons and America's Secret War* (New York: Simon & Schuster, 2001).

48 Tara O'Toole, Testimony to House Committee on Government Affairs, *Hearing on FEMA's Role in Managing Bioterrorist Attacks and the Impact of Public Health Concerns on Bioterrorism Preparedness*, July 23, 2001.

49 A third organization, the ANSER Institute—run by a former Air Force colonel and specializing in scenario development—lent its technical expertise.

50 A critical question, for example, was the transmission rate assumed. The smallpox transmission rate fluctuates widely based on multiple contextual factors. To determine the rate for the exercise, the developers analyzed thirty-four European cases of smallpox between 1958 and 1973—and chose the example of an outbreak in Yugoslavia as their model. Tara O'Toole, Michael Mair, and Thomas V. Inglesby, "Shining Light on 'Dark Winter,'" *Clinical Infectious Diseases* 34 (2002): 972–83. For a critique, see Ronald Barrett, "Dark Winter and the Spring of 1972: Deflecting the Social Lessons of Smallpox," *Medical Anthropology* 25, no. 2 (June 2006): 171–91.

51 Final script, *Dark Winter Exercise* (Johns Hopkins Center for Civilian Biodefense, Center for Strategic and International Studies, ANSER, Memorial Institute for the Prevention of Terrorism), 24.

52 John Hamre, Testimony before the U.S. House Government Reform Committee, Subcommittee on National Security, Veterans Affairs and International Relations, *Hearing on Combating Terrorism: Federal Response to a Biological Weapons Attack*, July 23, 2001.

53 Ibid.

54 Ibid.

55 Ibid.

56 O'Toole et al., "Shining Light," 980.

57 O'Toole et al., "Shining Light," 982.

58 Sam Nunn, Testimony before the U.S. House Government Reform Committee, Subcommittee on National Security, Veterans Affairs and

International Relations, *Hearing on Combating Terrorism: Federal Response to a Biological Weapons Attack,* July 23, 2001.

59 Jerome Hauer, Testimony before the U.S. House Government Reform Committee, Subcommittee on National Security, Veterans Affairs and International Relations, *Hearing on Combating Terrorism: Federal Response to a Biological Weapons Attack,* July 23, 2001.

60 John Hamre, Testimony before the U.S. House Government Reform Committee, Subcommittee on National Security, Veterans Affairs and International Relations, *Hearing on Combating Terrorism: Federal Response to a Biological Weapons Attack,* July 23, 2001.

61 Monica Schoch-Spana, "Post-Katrina, Pre-Pandemic America," *Anthropology News* 47, no. 1 (2006): 32–36.

62 House Committee on Homeland Security, Subcommittee on Prevention of Nuclear and Biological Attack, Subcommittee on Emergency Preparedness, Science and Technology, *Hearing on Protecting the Homeland: Fighting Pandemic Flu from the Front Lines,* February 8, 2006.

63 U.S. Senate Committee on Health Education, Labor and Pensions, Subcommittee on Bioterrorism and Public Health Preparedness, *Hearing on Public Health Preparedness in the 21st Century,* March 28, 2006.

64 House of Representatives, Committee on Government Reform, *Hearing on Working through an Outbreak,* May 11, 2006.

65 Falkenrath, U.S. Senate Committee on Health, Education, Labor and Pensions, *Hearing on Enhancing Public Health and Medical Preparedness,* March 16, 2006.

66 House Committee on Homeland Security, *Hearing on Protecting the Homeland,* February 8, 2006.

67 U.S. Senate Committee on Health Education, Labor and Pensions, *Hearing on Public Health Preparedness,* March 28, 2006.

68 House Committee on Homeland Security, *Hearing on Protecting the Homeland,* February 8, 2006.

69 U.S. Senate Committee on Health Education, Labor and Pensions, *Hearing on Public Health Preparedness,* March 28, 2006.

70 Ibid.

71 Michael Mair, Beth Maldin, and Brad Smith, "Passage of S. 3678: The Pandemic and All-Hazards Preparedness Act," UPMC, Center for Biosecurity, prepared statement, December 20, 2006.

72 Of course, the situation was not the same—in part because in 2006, awareness of the pandemic threat was due to a vastly increased global surveillance capacity. What is important to note is the predominance in 2006 of preparedness measures—including disease surveillance—that did not exist in 1976.

CHAPTER THREE

Redesigning Syndromic Surveillance for Biosecurity

Lyle Fearnley

During the 1990s, amid proliferating fears of new diseases and bioterrorism, United States defense planners conceptualized public health infrastructure as a bulwark of national security. In an exemplary formulation, global security analyst Christopher Chyba argued that the developing threat of bioterrorism demanded a national "strategy of public health surveillance."[1] The apparent proliferation of biological weapons among nonstate groups and individuals rendered traditional policies of counterproliferation and deterrence ineffective. Chyba and others argued that novel surveillance systems—operating within public health infrastructure—must detect outbreaks, coordinate ameliorative responses, and geographically locate release points for law enforcement.[2] Moreover, this was a "dual-use" strategy: a strategy in which, as historian Nicholas King describes it, "preparations for a biological attack may serve the 'dual use' of enhancing other public health activities."[3]

The effort to turn this strategy of security into a functional apparatus focused on an experimental technology known as syndromic surveillance. Local health departments developed the first syndromic surveillance systems in the mid-1990s to detect unexpected or unusual outbreaks of diseases. These innovative surveillance systems monitored nonspecific data sources—including emergency calls to 911, pharmaceutical sales, and emergency room (ER) triage counts—rather than physician or laboratory diagnoses. This nonspecificity provided health departments with possible early warning of outbreaks, even if the cause of illness was unknown.

By 1999, the U.S. military and the federal Centers for Disease Control (CDC) began adapting syndromic surveillance for bioterrorism preparedness. However, when federal agencies began to incorporate local systems into a national infrastructure, they encountered broad opposition from local epidemiologists and officials. This chapter focuses on the contested development of BioSense, a syndromic system designed and managed by the CDC. As management of syndromic data shifted to federal experts, local public health practitioners declared the national system ineffective and troubling. They argued that a centralized national system disregarded the federalist geography of U.S. public health, in which most health infrastructure is funded and operated at a municipal or state level. Put simply, while the national system detected epidemics, local institutions and epidemiologists undertook all subsequent costs in terms of investigation and intervention. The critique focused on technical and institutional problems, yet it reveals a normative dilemma. The technical reconfiguration of syndromic surveillance for national bioterrorism preparedness pushed it to the limit of public health practice.

Syndromic Detection:
A Problem Both Technical and Normative

The critique of BioSense began with a problem inherent to syndromic surveillance: How does one detect an epidemic in a field of nondiagnostic data? What are the boundaries of an epidemic if not actual cases of disease? Syndromic surveillance does not provide accurate data about disease incidence; rather, it aims to show unexpected changes in the number or distribution of certain syndromes in a population. Syndromes are standard symptom groups, such as *respiratory* or *gastrointestinal*. When ER triage data are collected, for example, the complaints of patients are translated into one of these syndrome categories and geographically tagged by zip code. Spatial aberration detection utilizes geographic clustering methods to locate unusual patterns of syndrome density.[4] Temporal analysis looks for significant increases in syndrome counts across time.[5]

Detecting aberration first of all requires a calculation of the normal rate of syndromes for the population, since syndrome-based health data have not typically been collected. Historical data is analyzed for normal trends, adjusted for seasonal, day-of-week, and environmental patterns so that every day has an "expected" syndrome count. Finally, computer-based detection algorithms interpret the relation between observed and expected counts. These algorithms generate an automatic signal when observed counts are significantly aberrant.[6]

The task of determining what is a *significant* aberration—an aberration that merits investigation—is at once a statistical and normative problem. A variety of statistical operations can be applied to the data inputs in order to rank their likelihood (where the less likely is more significant).[7] Yet setting optimal thresholds ultimately faces a fundamental dilemma. As Arthur Reingold of the University of California, Berkeley, School of Public Health puts it, "increases in the sensitivity of epidemic detection will come at the cost of decreases in specificity, and vice versa."[8] When an algorithmic threshold is lowered, epidemics are detected faster and more frequently. However, the specificity of detection—the rate at which statistical signals refer to actual epidemics—decreases. The "detection" of an epidemic that does not exist is known as a false alarm. Researchers at the University of Pittsburgh elaborate,

> The optimal level of sensitivity relative to specificity depends on the consequences of false alarms and the benefits of true alarms. These consequences are not fundamental properties of the detection method itself, but are specific to the use to which the detection method is applied.[9]

In other words, setting a threshold is an operation guided by norms or values; a threshold's position depends on desired ends. When federal agencies began adapting syndromic surveillance for bioterrorism, syndromic surveillance systems seemed caught between two sets of norms. An example from the first Syndromic Surveillance Conference held in September 2002 is illustrative. The conference began with a pair of linked presentations that showed how syndromic surveillance could be put into two distinct normative "contexts": public health and national preparedness.[10] The purpose of this pairing, undoubtedly, was to validate the claim that a single technique could be equally useful for both objectives: the principle of dual use. In their critique of BioSense, however, local public health workers questioned the compatibility of public health and national preparedness logics. Significantly, while describing their own practice as public health[11] they argued that BioSense did not meet the evaluative standards of public health surveillance.

What are the norms of public health? In a recent debate on the meaning of public health science, D. A. Savitz, C. Poole, and W. C. Miller argued that "public health may be defined solely by its goal: improving the health of human populations."[12] This is a thoroughly modern approach to the problem of disease. Historian of medicine William Coleman points out that the English-language term *public health* became "the most appropriate global expression for the emerging ensemble of thought and action regarding sanitation" only in the 1830s or 1840s.[13] In both France and England, historians have identified the 1830s as the period when disease was first understood as a *social* problem.[14] As modern cities grew, early public health investigators applied rudimentary statistical methods to this new urban mass. The fundamental object of their research was the differential mortality of the population. The regularities they discovered were not what they expected: first climate and weather, then topography (distance from rivers, altitude, etc.), and atmospheric conditions were ruled inconsequential. Ultimately, statistical reports identified "living conditions" as the fundamental factor in excess mortality. The mode of public health redefined the relationship between "population" and "epidemic." No longer a periodic or cyclical element of the natural environment, disease in a population was understood as the effect of a complex interaction of biological and social factors.[15] Contemporary public health practice aims to maximize the health of a population. Both maximization and population are understood in statistical terms: for example, a health department may attempt to reduce cases of malaria to a rate considered normal for a specific population.[16]

Techniques of preparedness developed in reference to a different set of problems and different norms of practice. Preparedness is a product of twentieth-century concerns about the vulnerability of modern infrastructure. Cold War-era civil defense planners developed detailed strategies against the potential impact of firebombing or nuclear weapons on modern, interdependent systems such as electricity, water, and transportation. Part of a larger strategic framework that Stephen J. Collier and Andrew Lakoff call "vital systems security," preparedness secures against dangers that are no longer statistically calculable. Rather, these events are unpredictable and potentially catastrophic. It does not take the population (and its risks and regularities) as its fundamental object, but infrastructure and its vulnerabilities. In the context of surveillance systems, the key preparedness norm is not the maximization of beneficial regularities but the "early warning" of potential events.[17]

Local public health workers have resisted certain aspects of the preparedness framework built into BioSense. Specifically, they argued that a focus on catastrophic but unlikely futures masks the difficult problems of resource allocation faced by underfunded health departments in the present. While CDC officials hoped to rapidly expand BioSense into a federally managed, real-time medical database, local officials developed a critical perspective that favored demonstrated utility.

The disjuncture between preparedness and public health strategies is exacerbated by the federalist geography of health in the United States. Public health is historically and legally a responsibility of state and local government. Federal agencies like the CDC have no authority to mandate disease reporting or unilaterally intervene in epidemic outbreaks. The designers of a national syndromic surveillance infrastructure face two problems of calibration: calibrating automatic epidemic detection with human epidemiological response; and calibrating the geography of surveillance data with the infrastructure of disease control. *How* to calibrate this infrastructure is as much a normative as a technical problem, for ultimately in question is what syndromic surveillance should do.

From Modern Public Health to Syndromics: Uncertainty Comes under Surveillance

In nineteenth-century America, the practice of public health began as a municipal and state government function. Disease was initially considered an urban problem and city governments made the initial interventions, including quarantine and hygienic reform. New York City, for example, legally defined the government's public health duties through the Metropolitan Health Bill of 1866. During the next decades, states like Massachusetts, California, and Virginia formed boards of health with similar responsibilities.[18]

City and state health boards soon began to collect disease reports. In 1874, the Massachusetts Board of Health asked physicians to report on the weekly occurrence of fourteen infectious diseases. This was the first government collection of active disease incidence; previously, health authorities had gained information about disease from death registers. Michigan introduced a similar system two years later, and in 1873 made the immediate notification of certain dangerous diseases—including smallpox, cholera, diphtheria, and scarlet fever—mandatory.

Meanwhile, federal government involvement in disease problems was limited to protecting borders and ports from epidemics of foreign origin. In 1878, Congress authorized the newly organized Marine Hospital Service (MHS) to collect reports from overseas consuls on the incidence of cholera, smallpox, plague, and yellow fever in their host countries. These reports helped the MHS determine when and where to institute quarantines. Not until 1893 did MHS gain access to weekly reports from state and municipal governments. Even then, some states opposed the expansion of federal interest in domestic disease problems, and in particular questioned who had authority to intervene in population health. In 1900, for example, California denied the appearance of plague in the state, hampering the control efforts of MHS workers.[19]

In 1902, the U.S. Congress called for a standardization of reporting and increased cooperation between state and federal health officials. Over the next fifty years, disease reports became more accurate, more comprehensive, and more consistent. Yet it was not until 1950 that disease reporting became a fundamental component of federal health governance through the efforts of the recently formed health agency, the Communicable Disease Center (predecessor of today's Centers for Disease Control). In collaboration with state and local health officers, CDC organized the National Notifiable Disease Surveillance System (NNDSS), a system that collected disease reports for a fixed list of around fifty diseases.

Like previous disease reporting systems, physician or laboratory diagnoses of notifiable diseases were reported to state and city health departments and then to the CDC. However, describing the NNDSS as a simple expansion or consolidation of national disease reporting is inaccurate. S. Thacker and R. Berkelman describe the NNDSS as *functionally* transforming the collection of disease reports from an "archival function prior to 1950 to one in which there is a timely analysis of data and appropriate response."[20] The NNDSS marked a shift from using morbidity reports to inform general policy to a mechanism of disease surveillance in which epidemic events prompted immediate responses. Using the NNDSS, CDC epidemiologists could establish thresholds of reports to define the appropriate time for federal involvement: to quote CDC Director of Epidemiology Alexander Langmuir, to determine when an outbreak of disease was "of national importance."[21] An epidemic of disease would be followed closely until its scale or severity called for federal involvement. For example, in a 1950s campaign against malaria, CDC epidemiologists began investigations when the NNDSS detected two or more cases of malaria in epidemiological relation.[22]

By the early 1990s, the NNDSS—and this federalist consensus—were widely considered to be in crisis. A complex confluence of forces, from increasing antibiotic resistance to budget cutbacks to encroachments on microbial reservoirs, unleashed a series of previously unknown diseases.[23] Some of these microbes are truly new, like HIV; others have mutated into more deadly forms, like avian influenza; still others have simply reappeared after many years, like polio in the United States. Expert organizations such as the Institute of Medicine brought these diverse disease events together under a single framework that Nicholas King calls the "emerging infections worldview."[24] One standard doctrine of this worldview is that a surveillance system dependent on categorical disease reports—lists of known and expected diseases—can only poorly or belatedly detect outbreaks of emerging infections. Other critiques of the NNDSS emerged as well. A CDC–commissioned report described infectious diseases reporting as "incomplete and untimely,"[25] while another report described how cutbacks to state and local health departments left "skeletal staff" and consequently limited follow-up of reported cases.[26]

Two large outbreaks in 1993 confirmed the weaknesses of the NNDSS and directly inspired the development of syndromic surveillance. In January, an outbreak of *E. coli* O157:H7 spread across western states. In one state, "of the fifty-eight retrospectively identified cases of bloody diarrhea and acute kidney failure, none had been accurately diagnosed or reported to the health department."[27] That spring in Milwaukee, a sand filter broke down allowing *Cryptosporidium* parasites to contaminate the municipal water supply. Over four hundred thousand fell ill and thousands were hospitalized. Yet, remarkably, neither the Milwaukee or Wisconsin Departments of Health nor the CDC realized that an epidemic was taking place. They took no action until a pharmacist reported on the local news that his store had completely sold out of antidiarrhea medication. According to Ronald Glasser, the Milwaukee outbreak was widely seen as "a clear sign that our infectious-disease and medical surveillance and prevention programs were no longer working."[28]

The reports that described the failures of disease surveillance and the threats of emerging infections also cited new surveillance systems as a vital and necessary improvement.[29] The CDC's report *Preventing Emerging Infectious Diseases* was particularly influential in subsequent surveillance development.[30] The report focused almost entirely on enhancing surveillance, targeted in four areas: first, strengthening notifiable disease surveillance (NNDSS); second, establishing physician-based sentinel surveillance networks; third, initiating special surveillance of certain susceptible populations (immunocompromised; pregnant women and newborns; travelers, immigrants and refugees); and fourth, increasing global surveillance.

The plan provided technical tools, training, and money to state and local governments, and encouraged "developing innovative systems for early detection and investigation of outbreaks." In New York City, the health department began experimenting with a new form of real-time surveillance—which would become known as syndromic surveillance—in 1995. With the Milwaukee outbreak in mind, the system was designed to detect a large-scale gastrointestinal epidemic in its early stages. Rather than heightening the sensitivity of clinician-based surveillance, this early syndromic system monitored three data sources—cases of diarrhea illness at sentinel nursing homes; cases of diarrheal stool submissions at labs; and sales of over-the-counter antidiarrheal drugs. Traditional disease surveillance systems relied on physicians or laboratories to diagnose specific diseases (such as cryptosporidiosis) and report diagnoses if the disease was notifiable. New York City was now able to monitor for the symptom "diarrhea" itself. While the health department wouldn't immediately know whether *E. coli* or *Cryptosporidium* caused an outbreak, the system alerted and spatially directed epidemiologists towards potential epidemics.[31]

Local health departments developed early syndromic surveillance systems as a direct response to the new conditions and new problems of the emerging infections worldview. Previously unknown diseases and aging health infrastructure posed problems for traditional techniques of public health. Specifically, New York City health officials worried about the water distribution system and inconsistent disease reporting. Yet these health departments did not design syndromic surveillance to completely replace traditional public health practices. They hoped syndromic surveillance could provide a generic awareness: an ability to identify when and where outbreaks take place beyond the scope of traditional disease reporting. This is no substitute for epidemiology itself: in fact, a syndromic signal was clearly understood to be meaningless without follow-up investigation. As New York's syndromic developers described in a later paper, syndromic surveillance is like a "smoke detector" and "should be viewed as an adjunct to, not a replacement of, traditional disease surveillance." In New York, therefore, "the operational, response, and research components are integrated within a health department. The staff members who analyze data are the same as or work closely with those who perform signal investigations."[32]

Military Health, Bioterrorism Scenarios and the Rise of "Dual-Use" Syndromics

By the late 1990s, the U.S. military—with support from other branches of the federal government—began to examine syndromic surveillance as one component of a bioterrorism preparedness strategy. Military involvement in the sciences of health and disease is long and noteworthy, including such important work as screening for chronic conditions among World War I enlistees, efforts to control the spread of the 1918 influenza at military bases, and the discovery of the mechanism behind yellow fever transmission.[33] Typically military science focused on protecting the health of the soldier, though knowledge, technologies, and even institutions which sometimes migrated to the civilian population.[34]

Although for many years the Defense Department played a major role in worldwide research and response to infectious diseases, growing public concern about emerging infections led to a formal and institutional acknowledgement of disease as a threat to national security in 1998. In Presidential Decision Directive NSTC-7, President Clinton wrote that he had "determined that the national and international system of infectious disease surveillance, prevention, and response is inadequate to protect the health of United States citizens from emerging infectious diseases." Along with a number of measures aimed at traditional public health and medical agencies, Clinton wrote that "the mission of DoD will be expanded to include support of global surveillance, training research, and response to emerging infectious disease threats."[35] To implement these goals, DoD formed the Global Emerging Infections Surveillance and Response System (GEIS). GEIS aimed to develop techniques and institutions to fight disease in order to maintain the "medical readiness" of the force, but also the health and security of the national population.[36]

Notably, both Clinton's directive and the DoD–GEIS foundational text, *Addressing Emerging Infectious Disease Threats,* include biological terrorism as a comparable threat to natural infectious disease. In *Addressing Emerging Infectious Disease Threats,* the authors outline the widespread popularity of "dual-use" biosecurity strategies. They write, "Recently it has become common to view diseases resulting from biowarfare/bioterrorism as different from the above emerging infections only with respect to their unnatural origin."[37]

Specifically, both emerging infections and bioterrorism were understood as emergent or *unexpected* outbreaks of disease.[38] An outbreak of an emerging infection would be unexpected because the causative pathogen was either unknown, mutated, or believed to be eradicated from the United States. A bioterrorism-related epidemic would be unexpected because "the most likely and most destructive scenario would be a covert, unannounced attack."[39] Depending on the incubation period of the pathogen, the attack might not be detected until large numbers of infected people appeared at emergency rooms days or weeks later. Moreover, the pathogens likely to be used in a bioterrorist attack are uncommon in the United States (or even genetically altered) and could be misdiagnosed by physicians.

The need to detect unexpected outbreaks inspired widespread calls for novel surveillance systems highly sensitive to any aberration in population health. Rather than specific disease surveillance, these systems needed to be sufficiently generic to detect unknown or unlikely diseases.

Within a year of its foundation, DoD–GEIS developed the first federally managed syndromic surveillance system in an effort to acquire such early detection capability. In comments at the 2006 Syndromic Surveillance Conference, director of GEIS, Patrick Kelley, stated that DoD had experimented with syndrome-based monitoring since the early 1990s, including for Gulf War Syndrome (GWS) during the first Iraq invasion. However, surveillance for GWS focused on a specific, pre-defined syndrome. In 1999, DoD–GEIS designed a surveillance system to monitor nonspecific syndromes in order to gain early warning of unexpected outbreaks.[40] According to Kelley, the program was "heavily inspired" by the technical work of the New York City health department.[41]

Called the Electronic Surveillance System for the Early Notification of Community-Based Epidemics, or ESSENCE, the prototype began monitoring data from the Washington, DC, area. Under the military's medical system, every patient encounter produces an electronic record that describes all medical procedures as well as preliminary diagnoses entered as ICD-9 codes, standard diagnostic codes developed by the CDC. These electronic patient records are linked with patient demographic data, including geographic codes for residence and workplace. Data is collected at a central healthcare server. ESSENCE takes data from this server and groups preliminary diagnostic codes into nine syndromes.[42] Aberration detection algorithms are run on each syndrome group. These algorithms predict syndrome counts and look for differences between actual counts and estimates.[43]

While people involved in the design of ESSENCE equated emerging infections with bioterrorism as similar events, they differentiated the protocols for response. A response to a natural outbreak of disease involves public health personnel and public health methods, from epidemiologic investigation to isolation to prophylaxis. A bioterrorist attack may require a similar public health response but also involves other branches of government, particularly law enforcement and the military. In a 2004 directive on biodefense, President Bush argued that disease surveillance must ensure two objectives: attack warning and attribution. Bush wrote:

> Deterrence is the historical cornerstone of our defense, and attribution—the identification of the perpetrator as well as method of attack—forms the foundation upon which deterrence rests. Biological weapons, however, lend themselves to covert or clandestine attacks that could permit the perpetrator to remain anonymous. We are enhancing our deterrence posture by improving attribution capabilities.[44]

Since the responses would be different, designers began to examine how a natural disease outbreak could be distinguished from a bioterrorist attack. In an article on the "Epidemiology of Bioterrorism," Julie Pavlin of the Walter Reed Army Institute of Research argued that epidemiologic tools must be utilized to provide a differential diagnosis of every outbreak detected. For Pavlin, the first step of any epidemiologic response is to determine whether an epidemic is "a spontaneous outbreak of a known endemic disease, a spontaneous outbreak of a new or reemerging disease, a laboratory accident, or an intentional attack with a biological agent."[45] Pavlin suggested developing an epidemic curve: a chart of infected cases across time. Whereas the number of cases in a natural outbreak is likely to increase gradually,

> a bioterrorism attack is most likely to be caused by a point source, with everyone coming into contact with the agent at approximately the same time. The epidemic curve in this case would be compressed, with a peak in a matter of days or even hours, even with physiologic and exposure differences.[46]

Other differential characteristics of bioterrorist attacks, Pavlin noted, include large size of epidemic, unusual geography or season for a certain pathogen, unusual strains of antimicrobial resistance, or higher attack rates in confined areas.

While public health departments used syndromic surveillance in accordance with longstanding protocols of epidemiological response, the designers of bioterrorism-oriented surveillance systems had no clear framework for determining what bioterrorism-oriented surveillance should do. On the one hand, they turned to past events involving accidental or intentional releases of pathogens. For example, Christopher Chyba cited the anthrax epidemic that took place in the Soviet city of Sverdlosk in 1979, in which hundreds died from an accidental release of weaponized anthrax.[47] From these examples, analysts and designers asked: What kind of surveillance system could detect such an outbreak?

Beyond historical examples, planners turned to scenarios and simulations.[48] In 1993, for example, the Congressional Office of Technology Assessment estimated that a release of 100 kilograms of anthrax over a major city could result in up to three million deaths, depending on wind conditions.[49] Along with the Sverdlosk outbreak, this estimation quickly became a standard example for subsequent discussions of potential attacks.[50] In May 2000, officials from state and federal government participated in a full-scale simulation exercise that included a mock bioterrorist attack. Known as TOPOFF, because of the participation of "top officials" of the U.S. government, the exercise simulated the release of air-borne plague in Denver, Colorado. In subsequently published comments, TOPOFF participants offered vital hints about what they believed might constitute an effective bioterrorism detection system.

In general, they confirmed that the response to a bioterrorist attack would be distinct from the response to a natural outbreak. One participant complained:

> Some from the CDC, state, and local health agencies tried to look at this as a standard epidemiological investigation. In absolutely no way would this [scenario allow] a normal epidemiological investigation.[51]

Other participants complained about what they described as the "democratic processes and consensus building" typical of public health decision making.[52]

More specifically, many participants emphasized lack of information as a pivotal problem; it was considered "unlikely that most health departments would have had the information systems in place to be able to say with speed and accuracy how many confirmed or even suspected cases of plague were believed to be present in hospitals or other healthcare facilities."[53] One official identified the need for information systems that could "deliver real-time data showing the number and location of persons with specific illness in the affected area [and that] allow rapid collection and analysis of patient epidemiological information to determine source(s) of exposure."[54]

Also in May 2000, DoD–GEIS organized a workshop to examine prototype syndromic surveillance systems. The workshop brought together epidemiologists from local health departments like New York City with military disease experts like Pavlin and Kelley. In a summary of the workshop, the participants wrote that the "lessons learned" from TOPOFF provided new "imperatives" for public health surveillance: timeliness, flexibility, and sensitivity.[55] These imperatives clarified how the norms of an early warning system for bioterrorism differed from traditional public health surveillance. The workshop participants wrote:

> Early warning systems for infectious disease outbreaks will rank timeliness first, with acceptability, flexibility, sensitivity, and representativeness following closely thereafter. Data quality and positive predictive value [the ability to predict the

number of "real" cases based on surveillance data], while still important, will be less important than in the case of specific reportable disease surveillance.[56]

The workshop participants wanted syndromic surveillance to remain "an adjunct tool to traditional systems" and emphasized that "the public health practitioners who use these systems must be allocated the necessary resources to launch an appropriate response."[57] However, the workshop concluded with proposals for a national syndromic surveillance plan that seemed to move beyond so-called traditional systems of public health. The participants suggested that "the ideal situation would be a single organization in charge of a 'virtual' data warehouse where all collected data are compiled, integrated, and analyzed."[58] Such plans for a national syndromic infrastructure would in the coming years raise questions about the position of syndromic surveillance within public health practice.

In the aftermath of the attacks of September 11 and the anthrax mailings, DoD–GEIS positioned ESSENCE as a "test bed" (or operational model) for this national syndromic surveillance infrastructure.[59] Initially, ESSENCE was designed to detect outbreaks among military populations in order to maximize the medical readiness of the fighting force. In addition, ESSENCE was implemented during special events, including the 1999 World Trade Organization meetings in Seattle and the 2000 presidential conventions. After September 11, DoD–GEIS expanded ESSENCE to include all military treatment facilities worldwide.

As Patrick Kelley later pointed out, the global expansion of ESSENCE placed the largest population under surveillance of any comparable syndromic system.[60] The military health system generates on average ninety-eight thousand medical records every day.[61] Additionally, the military population is distributed throughout the United States and around the world, though unevenly. Through ESSENCE, the military became a sentinel population for the health of the nation. That is, detected outbreaks within the military could prompt public health interventions in the national population at large.

Military-managed disease surveillance provides an interesting contrast to the United States public health infrastructure. Although civilian governance is federalist and disease reporting to federal agencies voluntary, all military medical care is "responsive to a single command-and-control focal point."[62] In addition, the military manages an electronic medical record system that collects all data (personal identifiers and diagnoses) in a single server. This data is then available for centralized electronic surveillance through ESSENCE. This bears resemblance to centralized healthcare systems, like the British National Health Service, in which medical care and public health are united in a single system. Yet while the military population is granted comprehensive coverage, military-based surveillance can only provide a sentinel warning—and no medical response at all—to the national population at large.

As early as 1999, the military attempted to expand its field of surveillance to the civilian population. In a pilot program called ESSENCE II, surveillance began with a focus on the Washington, DC, area referred to as the National Capital Region (NCR). Data was collected through collaboration between the health departments of Maryland, Delaware, and Virginia, the District of Columbia, and the U.S. military. ESSENCE II has been described as an effort to provide "an integrated view of NCR military and civilian health department data."[63]

This integrated view aimed to bypass a specific weakness of federalist disease surveillance. Typically, health data is collected by states or municipalities and reported upwards to the federal government. Information about disease is therefore geographically constrained by the political boundaries separating states. An outbreak of disease along a jurisdictional border may not be rapidly detected because cases would be spread between two or more health departments. In the overlapping jurisdictions of the NCR, sharing of health data between states and municipalities is particularly important. Military health data, collected from a population of soldiers that is not divided by state jurisdictions, provided a unique view of regional health.

Just as importantly, ESSENCE II began to shift epidemic detection from local to federal—and in this case military—authorities. Data is collected at four "nodes" representing the state and DC health departments. At these nodes, data is (wherever possible) linked to personal identifiers that might later facilitate outbreak investigation, isolation, and quarantine. After arriving at these local archives, de-identified data is transferred to a fifth, regional node managed by the military technicians. There it is integrated with military data from the National Capital Region, a single population that itself crosses state boundaries. At the regional node, data is grouped into syndrome categories for analysis. Temporal aberration algorithms and GIS spatial clustering methods are applied to the data in order to detect possible regional outbreaks.

The ESSENCE system provided a unique model of national syndromic surveillance. Unlike the federalist reporting hierarchy, ESSENCE organized a sentinel military population—integrated with select civilian populations—that could be monitored for unexpected changes in health. Yet bypassing the federalist geography of health raised troubling questions as well. In fall 2003, DoD assigned $420 million to expand ESSENCE II into four major U.S. cities in a program called the Biodefense Initiative. However, the program was located within Admiral John Poindexter's Information Awareness Office, whose other surveillance activities had recently come under public scrutiny. Faced with questions about proprietary data access and information privacy, the DoD curtailed the expansion.[64] Today, ESSENCE maintains surveillance of military populations only.

As DoD–GEIS abandoned plans for expanding ESSENCE, civilian public health officials at CDC took responsibility for national syndromic surveillance. Their initial effort was an eight-city program similar to the military's ESSENCE.[65] However, within months CDC shifted towards a system called BioSense. The BioSense system adapted syndromic surveillance to the existing federalist reporting architecture, although some data from ESSENCE provided integrated views of multiple jurisdictions. Yet despite its federalist form, BioSense would ultimately face questions about federal access to data and the transfer of epidemic detection to federal authorities.

BioSense: Sensitivity or Response-Ability?

In 2003, the U.S. Congress funded a three-part biodefense program, providing funds for BioWatch (environmental pathogen detectors), BioShield (pharmaceutical and vaccine production), and BioSense. The BioSense component was meant to transform the many local syndromic surveillance systems into a coherent national picture. At the time, over one hundred states and municipalities operated some sort of syndromic surveillance.[66] While syndromic programs were often supported by CDC funds, most departments developed systems individuated for local rather than national requirements. Data management and outbreak detection took place at the local and state level. Only detected events, not raw data, were reported to the CDC. Additionally, these reports followed preexisting pathways—the reporting architecture of the NNDSS—from city to state to federal government.

In its earliest incarnation, BioSense was a CDC–designed software application made available to state and local health departments. Data was collected from national sources, including military treatment centers, sales data from a large pharmaceutical chain, and test submissions to Labcorp, a private laboratory service. However, analysis and outbreak detection did not take place on a national field. Instead, data was broken down for analysis by state, certain metropolitan regions, and zip code.[67]

BioSense data was distributed to states and municipalities for analysis. At least in principle, data interpretation—and epidemic detection—remained under local control. In fact, CDC did not interpret BioSense data at all. Yet because syndromic surveillance systems utilize algorithms to automatically analyze data inputs, human interpretation is highly structured by the design of the system. For example, Bio-Sense data inputs were automatically assigned to syndrome groups determined by CDC to be "indicative of the clinical presentation of critical biologic-terrorism associated conditions."[68] In contrast, many early syndromic surveillance systems created syndrome groups similar to the clinical presentation of common or emerging natural diseases.[69]

More significantly, BioSense data was analyzed by a temporal algorithm designed by CDC technicians. The algorithm detects aberrant patterns in the syndromic data and *automatically* generates alerts when aberrations are detected.[70] In addition, CDC technicians designed the visual display of the data.[71] Typically, a local epidemiologist monitoring BioSense would first see alerts indicating possible epidemics rather than raw data scores. Because of these automatic signals, the detection of epidemics lay as much with CDC designers as with local data monitors.

Still, it was soon obvious that health departments were using BioSense at their own discretion, if at all. One paper called state and local monitoring of BioSense "varied," ranging from zero minutes using the application in many states to up to eight hours elsewhere.[72] In a government study, local officials argued that they would prefer to receive data in a raw rather than analyzed form.[73]

In 2004, the CDC acknowledged problems with BioSense and overhauled the system. Yet rather than increasing the distribution of raw data, the CDC centralized data interpretation in its federal office. Supported by $22 million in new funds appropriated for national biosurveillance, the CDC developed a BioIntelligence Center for analyzing BioSense data at the national level.[74] At the center, CDC epidemiologists assist local departments in their interpretation of algorithm-generated alerts. CDC assistance includes computer-based investigation and tracking of data aberrations, an interpretive authority previously the responsibility of local health officials.[75] Moreover, while local departments see BioSense data from their jurisdiction alone, CDC analysts have access to the complete national database.

The federal appropriation of data interpretation functions fueled debate over the way BioSense detects epidemics. At the September 2005 Syndromic Surveillance Conference, local health departments mounted a widespread critique of BioSense that focused on the design of detection algorithms. One technical, if rhetorically neutral, critique demonstrated that BioSense was plagued by false positive detections. The BioSense algorithm scored lowest for specificity in comparison with four other widely used detection algorithms.[76]

Algorithms are important sites of critique because they set thresholds that distinguish normal from epidemic states. These thresholds—based on relations between expected numbers and observed numbers—automatically produce alerts when observed syndrome counts are significantly unusual. Each one of these alerts requires detailed investigations by epidemiologists—including examination of data inputs, phone calls to emergency rooms, and even personal follow-up with potential cases—in order to verify whether a detected event is an actual epidemic or a false positive. A more sensitive system is therefore more costly in terms of investigative hours, many of these hours spent investigating epidemics that don't exist.

At the conclusion of the 2005 conference, Marc Paladini of the New York City health department made a forceful critique of the BioSense detection algorithm. In a presentation entitled "BioSense in Public Health Practice: Perspective and Comments from a Local Health Department," Paladini discussed the implementation and evaluation of BioSense in New York City. Daily monitoring of BioSense data began in New York in August 2004 as part of the preparations for the Republican National Convention. Paladini investigated each of the twenty sentinel infection alerts and 184 algorithm-generated statistical signals during the two-month period of investigation. According to Paladini, none of these were of any "public health importance." New York undertook preliminary investigations into BioSense signals over two hundred times without discovering any actual epidemic.[77]

Local public health workers decry the costs (both economic and operational) of investigating false syndromic alerts. By linking the algorithmic technique of detection with the practice of epidemiological response, they demonstrate that algorithm design must be evaluated in terms of norms of practice. These public health workers do not desire to limit health interventions per se, but rather to accommodate interventions to the actual health problems of the population. The goal of public health is to maximize the health of a specific population within a field of possibility, structured by limited resources, limited time, limited knowledge, and the biological properties of pathogens and hosts. Because of resource limitations, in particular, new technical interventions must be evaluated according to a statistical ratio of costs to benefits. Sensitivity and specificity must be kept within an acceptable balance, this level of acceptability being ultimately a normative decision.

The critique laid out at the conference articulates what I call a norm of response-ability. First, local health departments have a responsibility (legally defined) for the health of their jurisdictional population. For example, in many states and cities, public health charters grant the authority to conduct surveillance on the condition that appropriate responses are made to detected events.[78] The New York City Health Code clearly demonstrates this duality:

> An outbreak or suspected outbreak of any disease or condition, of known or unknown etiology, which may be a danger to public health, occurring in three or more persons, or any unusual manifestations of disease in an individual should be reported to the Department immediately.... The Department shall conduct such investigation as may be necessary to ascertain sources or causes of infection, to discover contacts and unreported cases, and shall take such steps as may be necessary to prevent morbidity and mortality.[79]

Additionally, public health departments must make tough decisions in the present in order to maximize the health of the population against a full range of problems. For example, would resources be best directed towards pandemic flu planning or school nutrition initiatives? For local health departments, careful evaluations are needed to determine how effectively specific interventions accomplish defined goals.

Second, local health workers emphasized that they must be *able* to *respond*. Farzad Mostashari, director of epidemiology in New York City and an early developer of syndromic methods, argued that

> "You can't make up for a lack of local capacity by making a national analysis system.... We have 80 percent of the nation covered but we really have nothing covered, because signals come and go, and an e-mail maybe is sent out, and there's no local capacity."[80]

In the United States, public health is historically a state and local responsibility. State and local health departments today manage most surveillance systems and undertake the vast majority of epidemiological investigations. Meanwhile, federal public health funds (a significant source for many states) continue to dry up, including an overall FY2006 cut of over $1 billion.[81] While some additional funds are distributed for bioterrorism preparedness, these funds are themselves the subject of controversy because they are categorically restricted to preparedness activities, often forcing cutbacks to other basic programs.[82]

Under BioSense, a signal generated at the federal level requires epidemiological investigation by local officials. Therefore the sensitivity of the system has a direct impact on the amount of epidemiological work undertaken by local departments. Frequent false positives both reduce the ability of the health department to accomplish its other responsibilities and decrease responsiveness to future BioSense signals. New York City officials put it bluntly: "For many, if not all, state and local health departments, the emphasis of bioterrorism preparedness should be on hiring well-trained public health professionals with responsibilities beyond bioterrorism."[83]

Technical Infrastructure and Social Infrastructure

Paladini's evaluation of BioSense noted that none of the detected events were of any "public health importance." This is in no small part because BioSense was designed according to norms of preparedness and not public health. Rather than the careful evaluations described by Paladini and others, the construction of BioSense was guided by the results of scenario-based enactments of bioterrorism attacks. As early as the first TOPOFF exercise in 2000 and the "Dark Winter" scenario in 2001, simulations of bioterror attacks had directly guided federal priorities for syndromic surveillance. At the 2005 conference, I heard the CDC's Lynn Steele describe how the TOPOFF-3 exercises conducted by Homeland Security that year prompted the CDC to shift the focus of BioSense towards what they call "situational awareness."[84]

In practice, two projects were undertaken. The first was integration with Bio-Watch, the national network of environmental sensors designed to detect airborne pathogens. Managed by Homeland Security, BioWatch is located in approximately thirty cities nationwide. These sites are chosen according to risk of bioterrorism attack, not likelihood of natural disease outbreak. Second, to facilitate this integration, CDC began collecting real-time medical data from sentinel hospitals in ten BioWatch cities.

Known as BioSense Real-Time, this system aimed to place HL7 routers in sentinel hospitals. HL7 is a standard coding system for all medical information used at hospitals—chief complaints at triage stations, clinical encounter data, place of work, residence, tests taken, radiology, discharge diagnostics, pharmaceuticals, nurse notes. The BioSense routers would translate this into their own code and literally "route" it to CDC headquarters for potential analysis every fifteen minutes.

Yet the utility of most of this data had never been examined, let alone substantiated. And according to CDC this was not a pilot program and there would be no pilot runs. Some local epidemiologists worried that databases of medical information could be used for a range of non-public health purposes. When lots of cross-referenced information is combined, originally de-identified data may become personally identifiable. Or information could be used to guide controversial policies, for example funding cutbacks to hospitals that provide abortion services. Above all, however, the lack of protocols for analysis and response left local epidemiologists without a framework for incorporating BioSense Real-Time into their public health practice.

The resistance of state and local health workers has had tangible impact. In particular within the newly formed American Health Information Community (AHIC) charged with developing national standards for electronic health information, some city and state health commissioners spoke out against BioSense. Within the working group on biosurveillance, four out of eighteen members represent city or state health departments. Through this forum they put pressure on the CDC to slow down data acquisition. Steele announced at the 2006 Syndromic Surveillance Conference that BioSense would cap its "rich data" connections at sixty-five hospitals. Meanwhile, over thirty-five hundred hospitals would have "foundational data" connections: information like the ER chief-complaint data that has been thoroughly studied by a number of local health departments.

Steele was certainly hyperconscious of the conflicts that had consumed BioSense. She spoke often of a desire to "listen" and perhaps most importantly outlined a research and evaluation agenda for the future. She hinted, however, that CDC felt caught in the middle: between public health experts at local and state health departments and biodefense specialists in other federal agencies and elected government. The persistence of a preparedness logic within the federal government was clear in the opening talk at the 2006 conference given by Rajeev Venkayya, Director of Biodefense for the President's Office of Homeland Security. He argued that the syndromic surveillance infrastructure must be built before detection algorithms have been suitably evaluated (in his view a pseudoutopia that he called "the perfect"). Because of the assumed urgency of the threat (catastrophic bioterrorism) and the peculiar temporality of preparedness (imagined future in the present), interventions must come before technologies are evaluated, holistic risks are understood, or potential threats are actualized.[85]

However, Venkayya's limited definition of infrastructure is particularly troubling. He explicitly and exclusively spoke of linking clinical care data with public health departments through surveillance networks like BioSense. After he concluded, however, an audience member commented that all the data is useless if you have overworked and underfunded health departments at the local and state level. Venkayya acknowledged him, responding, "The notion that you can take a strapped public health department and ask [it] to tackle huge amounts of data seems a bit naïve." But arguing that the current problems with syndromic infrastructure can be solved through technological development alone disregards the fact that every infrastructure is social; that wires and pipes can't function without individual operators, organizational networks, and social norms.[86] By speaking of computer networks as "the infrastructure," Venkayya conceals the structural dilemma facing syndromic surveillance today: the continued and severe lack of funding for local and state epidemiology.

New Objects of Surveillance and Security

In late 2004, Congress approved a presidential request of $274 million dollars for an integrated biosurveillance initiative undertaken jointly by the CDC and Homeland Security. The initiative involved communication networks between the agencies that basically combined and subsumed BioSense and BioWatch into a single surveillance system. Anything detected in BioSense is now immediately transferred to Homeland Security for additional analysis.[87] The linchpin of the BioSurveillance Initiative is a new program developed by Homeland Security variously called the National Biosurveillance Integration System (NBIS) or National Biosurveillance Integration Center (NBIC).[88] According to a presentation by Homeland Security official Peter Estacio at the 2004 Syndromic Surveillance Conference, NBIC is an integration point for syndromic health data, environmental data, and threat assessments from intelligence agencies. As a recent DHS audit put it, NBIC "was designed to bring together bio-surveillance data from the various sector-specific systems used for human, animal, and plant health surveillance; environmental monitoring of air, agriculture, water, and food; and intelligence and threat analysis."[89]

Plans for NBIC are ambiguous about the position of surveillance within public health. On the one hand, the Biosurveillance Enhancement Act of 2007 directs the Secretary of DHS to "designate the NBIC as a public health authority" and therefore "as a public health authority with a public health mission, [NBIC] is authorized to collect or receive information, including such information protected under the Health Insurance Portability and Accountability Act, for the purpose of preventing or controlling disease, injury or disability."[90] At the same time, NBIC reorients public health. First, the population is decentered as the object of surveillance and security. Fields of surveillance are multiple (ranging from animal vectors to urban syndromic populations to agricultural products to intelligence reports) but the object of detection is generic: the "biological event." The act is careful to define "biological event" as both "a terrorist act involving biological agents or toxins or a naturally occurring outbreak of infectious disease of potential national significance." Yet the protocol for determining what combination of animal disease outbreaks, emergency room syndrome fluctuations, and intelligence assessments will constitute a significant "biological event" remains opaque. Defining thresholds for intervention is difficult within a localized syndromic surveillance system focused on a single population; the complexity of NBIC poses even greater interpretive problems.

If, as I argued above, public health is fundamentally oriented towards maximizing the health of defined human populations, then generic biosurveillance systems like NBIS may be difficult or impossible to incorporate within public health practice. What sort of intelligence assessment should lead to the mass distribution of antibiotics? Such questions cannot be answered within the normative framework of public health.

Public health may need to modify its norms to respond to new problems, and public health practitioners have heatedly debated new "paradigms" for the science.[91] Syndromic surveillance itself, with its orientation towards unexpected events and nonspecific objects, inevitably moves epidemiology in new directions. Yet the development of new norms of practice—and new norms of security—does not follow in direct parallel to legislation or technological advance. While it may be rhetorically effective to describe biosecurity as an "integration" of public health and national security, the reality is more complicated. During an actual epidemic, public health departments alone have the expertise to contain and control the spread of disease. New biosurveillance systems must account for the procedures of epidemiological response as well as techniques of detection. As one public health participant in TOPOFF emphasized, "contact-tracing" would have been critical in a real epidemic, but was not included (and not possible) in the scenario exercise. The designs of both BioSense and NBIC tend to elide the need for such detailed epidemiological work after events are detected.

The contested development of syndromic surveillance also raises broader questions about the role of information in a contemporary security apparatus. Although the demand for more and better information through novel surveillance seems self-evident, in fact it may be elusive. More information means more interpretive work, without certain benefits; and more detected events requires more epidemiological responses, without (at this point) the necessary epidemiological resources to undertake them. Rather than continued calls to extend the collection of health information, care must be given to what form contemporary biosecurity should take.[92]

NOTES

1   Christopher Chyba, "Biological Terrorism, Emerging Diseases, and National Security," Rockefeller Brothers Fund Project on World Security, 1998, http://www.rbf.org/pdf/Chyba_Bioterrorism.pdf.

2   Chyba, "Biological Terrorism"; Richard Danzig and P. Berkowsky, "Why Should We Be Concerned about Biological Warfare?" *JAMA* 278, no. 5 (1997): 431–32; Donald Henderson, "Bioterrorism as a Public Health Threat," *Emerging Infectious Diseases* 4, no. 3 (1998); Julie Pavlin, "Epidemiology of Bioterrorism," *Emerging Infectious Diseases* 5, no. 4 (1999).

3   Nicholas B. King, "The Ethics of Biodefense," *Bioethics* 19, no. 4 (2005): 432–46.

4   Martin Kulldorf, "Prospective Time Periodic Geographical Disease Surveillance Using a Scan Statistic," *Journal of the Royal Statistical Society* A164 (2001): 61–72.

5   Richard Heffernan et al., "Syndromic Surveillance in Public Health Practice, New York City," *Emerging Infectious Diseases* 10, no. 5 (2004): 858–64.

6   L. C. Hutwanger et al., "A Simulation Model for Assessing Aberration Detection Methods used in Public Health Surveillance for Systems with Limited Baselines," *Statistics in Medicine* 24, no. 4 (2005): 543–50.

7   For some examples, see Heffernan et al., "Syndromic Surveillance."

8   Arthur Reingold, "If Syndromic Surveillance Is the Answer, Then What Is the Question?" *Biosecurity and Bioterrorism: Biodefense Strategy, Practice and Science* 1, no. 2 (2003): 77–81.

9   Hutwanger et al., "A Simulation Model."

10 The two talks were by Margaret Hamburg, "Putting Syndromic Surveillance in Context (National Preparedness)"; and Michael T. Osterholm, "Putting Syndromic Surveillance

in Context (Public Health)."

11 Heffernan et al., "Syndromic Surveillance."

12 D. A. Savitz, C. Poole, and W. C. Miller, "Reassessing the Role of Epidemiology in Public Health," *American Journal of Public Health* 89 (1999): 1158.

13 William Coleman, *Death is a Social Disease: Public Health and Political Economy in Early Industrial France* (Madison: University of Wisconsin Press, 1982): 57.

14 Coleman, *Death is a Social Disease*; John M. Eyler, *Victorian Social Medicine: The Ideas and Methods of William Farr* (Baltimore: Johns Hopkins University Press, 1979).

15 Paul Rabinow, *French Modern: Norms and Forms of the Social Environment* (Chicago: University of Chicago Press, 1995).

16 For a theoretical treatment of the relationship between statistics, the government of health, and liberal cost/benefit reasoning, see Michel Foucault, *Security, Territory, Population: Lectures at the Collège de France, 1977–78* (New York: Palgrave Macmillan, 2007).

17 Stephen J. Collier and Andrew Lakoff, "Distributed Preparedness: Notes on the Geneaology of 'Homeland Security,'" *Environment and Planning D: Society and Space* 26, no. 1 (2008): 7–28; Stephen J. Collier and Andrew Lakoff, "The Vulnerability of Vital Systems: How 'Critical Infrastructure' Became a Security Problem," in *The Changing Logics of Risk and Security*, ed. Myriam Dunn (New York: Routledge, forthcoming).

18 Elizabeth Fee, "Public Health and the State: The United States," in *The History of Public Health and the Modern State*, ed. Dorothy Porter (Atlanta: Editions Rodopi, 1994).

19 D. Koo and F. Wetterhall, "History and Current Status of the National Notifiable Disease Surveillance System," *Journal of Public Health*

Management and Practice 2, no. 4 (1996): 4–10.

20 S. Thacker and R. Berkelman, "Public Health Surveillance in the United States," *Epidemiological Reviews* 10 (1988): 174.

21 Alexander Langmuir, "Surveillance of Communicable Diseases of National Importance," *New England Journal of Medicine* 268 (1963): 182–92.

22 J. Andrews, G. Quinby, and A. Langmuir, "Malaria Eradication in the United States," *American Journal of Public Health* 40 (1950): 1405–11.

23 Institute of Medicine, *The Future of Public Health* (Washington, DC: National Academies Press, 1988); Institute of Medicine, *Emerging Infections: Microbial Threats to Health in the United States* (Washington, DC: National Academies Press, 1992).

24 Nicholas B. King, "Security, Disease, Commerce: Ideologies of Postcolonial Public Health," *Social Studies of Science* 32, no. 5–6 (2002): 763–89.

25 R. Baxter et al., *Assessing Core Capacities for Infectious Disease Surveillance: Final Report* (Falls Church, VA: The Lewin Group, 2000).

26 Ruth Berkelman et al., "Infectious Disease Surveillance: A Crumbling Foundation," *Science* 264 (1994): 368.

27 Ibid.

28 Ronald Glasser, "We Are Not Immune: Influenza, SARS, and the Collapse of Public Health," *Harper's* (July 2004).

29 Institute of Medicine, *The Future of Public Health;* Baxter et al., *Assessing Core Capacities;* Centers for Disease Control and Prevention, *Preventing Emerging Infectious Diseases: A Strategy for the 21st Century* (Atlanta: CDC, 1998).

30 CDC, *Preventing Emerging Infectious Disease.*

31 Richard Heffernan et al., "System Descriptions: New York City Syndromic Surveillance Systems," *Morbidity and Mortality Weekly Report* 53, Suppl. (2004): 17–24.

32 Heffernan et al., "Syndromic Surveillance," 863.

33 Fee, "Public Health and the State"; Roger Cooter, Mark Harrison, and Steve Sturdy, eds., *Medicine and Modern Warfare* (Atlanta: Rodopi, 1999); François Delaporte, *The History of Yellow Fever: An Essay on the Birth of Tropical Medicine* (Cambridge, MA: The MIT Press, 1991).

34 Debra Cowen, "Welfare Warriors: Towards a Geneaology of the Soldier Citizen in Canada," *Antipode* 37, no. 4 (2005): 654–78; Elizabeth Etheridge, *Sentinel for Health: A History of the Centers for Disease Control* (Berkeley: University of California Press, 1992).

35 William Jefferson Clinton, "Presidential Decision Directive NSTC-7," Federation of American Scientists, http://www.fas.org/irp/offdocs/direct.htm.

36 Department of Defense, Global Emerging Infections Surveillance and Response System, *Addressing Emerging Infectious Disease Threats* (Washington, DC: Walter Reed Army Institute of Research, 1998).

37 Ibid.

38 Melinda Cooper, "Pre-empting Emergence: The Biological Turn in the War on Terror," *Theory, Culture and Society* 23, no. 4 (2006): 113–35.

39 Tara O'Toole, "Emerging Illness and Bioterrorism: Implications for Public Health," *Journal of Urban Health* 78, no. 2 (2001): 396–402.

40 K. Henning, "What Is Syndromic Surveillance?" *Morbidity and Mortality Weekly Report* 53, Suppl. (2004): 17–24.

41 U.S. Medicine Institute for Health Studies, "Weaving a National Surveillance System: The Role of Federal Health Care," http://www.usminstitute.org/content/March2003_transcript.pdf.

42 Julie Pavlin, "Rapid Detection of Disease Outbreaks," *Army AL&T* (Nov–Dec 2001): 47–48.

43 Joseph Lombardo, H. Burkom, and J. Pavlin,

"ESSENCE II and the Framework for Evaluating Syndromic Surveillance Systems," *Morbidity and Mortality Weekly Report* 53, Suppl. (2004): 159–65.

44 George Walker Bush, "Biodefense for the 21st Century," Homeland Security Presidential Directive–10, April 28, 2004.

45 Pavlin, "Rapid Detection of Disease Outbreaks."

46 Ibid.

47 Chyba, "Biological Terrorism"; see Matthew Meselson et al., "The Sverdlovsk Anthrax Outbreak of 1979," *Science* 266 (1994): 1202–08.

48 However, these scenarios often relied on historical examples for basic data on the spread of disease; see Ronald Barret, "Dark Winter and the Spring of 1972: Deflecting the Social Lessons of Smallpox," *Medical Anthropology* 25, no. 2 (2006) 171–91. For discussion of the use of simulations in preparedness planning, see Collier and Lakoff, "Distributed Preparedness"; and Lakoff's chapter in this volume.

49 O'Toole, "Emerging Illness and Bioterrorism."

50 See, for example, Arnold Kaufmann, Martin Meltzer, and George Schmid, "The Economic Impact of a Bioterrorist Attack: Are Prevention and Postattack Intervention Programs Justifiable?" *Emerging Infectious Diseases* 3, no. 2 (1997): 83–94.

51 Thomas Inglesby et al., "A Plague on Your City: Observations from TOPOFF," *Clinical Infectious Diseases* 32 (2001): 436–45.

52 Ibid.

53 Ibid., 440.

54 Quoted in Julie Pavlin et al., "Innovative Surveillance Methods for Rapid Detection of Disease Outbreaks and Bioterrorism: Results from an Interagency Workshop on Health Indicator Surveillance," *American Journal of Public Health* 93, no. 8 (2003): 1230.

55 Ibid.

56 Ibid.: 1232.

57 Ibid.: 1234.

58 Ibid.: 1232.

59 U.S. Medicine Institute for Health Studies, "Weaving a National Surveillance System."

60 Ibid.

61 Colleen Bradley et al., "BioSense: Implementation of a National Early Event Detection and Situational Awareness System," *Morbidity and Mortality Weekly Report* 54, Suppl. (2005): 12.

62 U.S. Medical Institute for Health Studies, "Weaving a National Surveillance System."

63 Lombardo et al., "ESSENCE II," 163.

64 William J. Broad and Judith Miller, "Health Data Monitored for Bioterror Warning," *New York Times*, January 27, 2003.

65 Ibid.

66 Dan Sosin, "Evaluation Challenges for Syndromic Surveillance: Making Incremental Progress," *Morbidity and Mortality Weekly Report* 52, Suppl. (2004): 125.

67 Colleen Bradley et al., "BioSense," 12.

68 Leslie Z. Sokolow et al., "Deciphering Data Anomalies in BioSense," *Morbidity and Mortality Weekly Report* 54, Suppl. (2005): 134.

69 Heffernan et al., "System Descriptions."

70 Mark Paladini, "BioSense in Public Health Practice: Perspective and Comments from a Local Health Department," 2005 Syndromic Surveillance Conference, http://www.syndromic. org/sscAgenda2005.doc.

71 Sokolow et al., "Deciphering Data Anomalies."

72 Bradley et al., "BioSense," 17.

73 Government Accountability Office, "Information Technology: Federal Agencies Face Challenges in Implementing Initiatives to Improve Public Health Infrastructure," GAO-05-308 (2005).

74 Ari Schuler, "Billions for Biodefense: Federal Agency Biodefense Budgeting, FY2005–FY2006," *Biosecurity and Bioterrorism:*

Biodefense Strategy, Practice and Science 3, no. 2 (2005): 96.

75 Bradley et al., "BioSense," 17.

76 Mike Jackson et al., "Systematic Comparison of Algorithms Used in Syndromic Surveillance," *Advances in Disease Surveillance* 1 (2006): 35.

77 Paladini, "BioSense in Public Health Practice."

78 Claire Broome et al., "Statutory Basis for Public Health Reporting Beyond Specific Diseases," *Journal of Urban Health* 80, no. 2, Suppl. 1 (2003): i14–i22; Wilfredo Lopez, "New York City and State Legal Authorities Related to Syndromic Surveillance," *Journal of Urban Health* 80, no. 2, Suppl. 1 (2003): i23–i24.

79 Quoted in Lopez, "New York City and State Legal Authorities," i23.

80 U.S. Medicine Institute for Health Studies, "Weaving a National Surveillance System."

81 Coalition for Health Funding, "Statement to the House Labor–HHS–Education Appropriations Subcommittee on the FY 2007 Funding Reccomendations for the U.S Public Health Services Agencies and Programs," http://www.aamc.org/advocacy/healthfunding/testimony/start.htm.

82 Victor Sidel, R. Gould, and H. Cohen, "Bioterrorism Preparedness: Cooptation of Public Health?" *Medicine and Global Survival* 7, no. 2 (2002): 82–89; Victor Sidel, "Bioterrorism in the United States: A Balanced Assessment of Risk and Response," *Medicine, Conflict, and Survival* 19 (2003): 318–25.

83 Heffernan et al., "Syndromic Surveillance," 864.

84 Lynn Steele, "Syndromic Surveillance and Situational Awareness: Update on BioSense," 2005 Syndromic Surveillance Conference, http:// www.syndromic.org/conference/2006/agenda.doc.

85 See, for example, the chapter by Dale Rose in this volume.

86 For more on social infrastructure, see Paul N. Edwards, "Infrastructure and Modernity: Force, Time, and Social Organization in the History of Sociotechnical Systems," in *Modernity and Technology*, ed. T. Misa, P. Brey, and A. Feenberg (Cambridge, MA: The MIT Press, 2002), 185–225.

87 Tom Ridge and Thomas Thompson, "Bio-Surveillance Program Initiative Remarks by Secretary of Homeland Security Tom Ridge and Secretary of Health and Human Services Tommy Thompson," Department of Homeland Security, 2004, http://www.dhs.gov/xnews/releases/press_release_0339.shtm.

88 Government Accountability Office, "Information Technology: Federal Agencies Face Challenges."

89 Department of Homeland Security, Office of Inspector General, "Better Management Needed for the National Bio-Surveillance Integration System Program," 2007, www.dhs.gov/xoig/assets/mgmtrpts/OIG_07-61_Jul07.pdf.

90 H.R. 1290, 110th Cong., 1st sess. (2007).

91 S. Schwarz, E. Susser, and M. Susser, "A Future for Epidemiology?" *Annual Review of Public Health* 20 (1999): 15–33; M. Susser and E. Susser, "Choosing a Future for Epidemiology: I. Eras and Paradigms," *American Journal of Public Health* 86, no. 5 (1996): 668–73.

92 On the assemblage of forms with norms, see Paul Rabinow, *French DNA: Trouble in Purgatory* (Chicago: University of Chicago Press, 1999), 174–79.

CHAPTER FOUR

How Did the Smallpox Vaccination Program Come About?

TRACING THE EMERGENCE OF RECENT SMALLPOX VACCINATION THINKING

Dale A. Rose

In December 2002 President George W. Bush, in light of persistent advocacy and a gathering consensus within the public health and national security communities about the dangers of biological threats such as smallpox, announced the enactment of the Smallpox Vaccination Program (SVP).[1] The somber tone of the president's announcement reflected a particularly unwelcome irony: smallpox—the only infectious disease successfully to have been eradicated (some twenty-plus years earlier) on a global scale through purposive, organized human intervention—had begun to reappear, but in a new guise. There were still no cases of smallpox in individuals; instead there came into view a number of trends, developments, and other elements through which smallpox came to be constituted as a *threat*—not only to public and international health, as in previous decades, but very specifically to national and, eventually, homeland security. Such elements included the viral material itself, securely stored in the U.S. and Russia but also perhaps in unfriendly hands, as well as the notion of U.S. vulnerability to terrorism (as evidenced by 9/11 and the anthrax attacks), and the (now) documented activity by the administration to prepare for war abroad.[2] Arranged in a specific configuration, these and additional elements gave the threat of biological agents such as smallpox a kind of plausibility and immediacy. In other words, the problem of smallpox had emerged not as a problem of "actuality," in the sense of observable cases of disease; rather, smallpox had reappeared as an object of "potentiality," of danger in the present by virtue of a series of events and elements suggesting its possible occurrence in the future.

Thinking about disease in this way—that is, without the benefit of counting actual individual cases in the immediate past or present, or predicting such cases in the future—has not been all that common for public health officials, who have tended to orient their attention toward maladies and afflictions of a more visible and calculable character.[3] This is especially the case for infectious diseases, in which the extent to which a given disease poses a problem is often understood through statements about its incidence or prevalence (that is, how many cases are appearing for the first time or already exist in a given period of time, usually per some large number of people, e.g., one hundred thousand). In theory, the greater the rate on either of these registers, the greater the problem from a public health standpoint, and therefore the greater the resources (ostensibly) devoted to its prevention and control. Conversely, extremely rare infectious diseases tend to garner less attention in the context of routine public health activities.

It should be no surprise, then, that an infectious disease with zero incidence—like smallpox—falls into a curious space for public health practitioners and officials. On the one hand, because it does not "exist," it is easy to see why it may not be given much credence as a pressing problem; with highly prevalent diseases and conditions like HIV/AIDS, hepatitis, diabetes, and obesity there is little room left to think about, let alone organize a program around, a disease that no one has. Complexifying things, if a vaccine to prevent such a (nonexistent) disease is itself known to cause occasionally serious side effects, the question whether to vaccinate can prove decidedly problematic. The issue here is that it would be difficult to state just how the vaccine would be beneficial in terms of, for example, numbers of cases prevented (since no one has it in the first place); however, it would be decidedly easier to figure out the number of people who contract certain vaccine-related illnesses or who, importantly, are perceived by the public to have contracted an illness related to the vaccine—whether they did or not.

On the other hand, the extreme unlikelihood that certain diseases will appear is often matched by the extreme harm they can wreak on human bodies and communities—and, of course, states and economies. In the case of smallpox, the fatality rate for the most common type of the disease has historically hovered around 30 percent.[4] So while the disease does not presently exist in the form of actual cases in humans, the notion that it could—and that should it, it may kill or severely harm a great many of its victims—stirs even the most skeptical public health official to think about the issue seriously.

It is with these comments in mind that this chapter sets out to untangle some of the complexities faced by experts in thinking through the problem(s) of smallpox and smallpox vaccination leading to the Smallpox Vaccination Program. The SVP itself was the product of a series of long, occasionally arduous processes, characterized in no small measure by attempts to articulate new relationships and rationalities for public health, national security, and an embryonic, but increasingly distinct, homeland security apparatus. The program was to bring together elements of the nation's vast, if loosely coordinated, public health infrastructure with additional elements historically at some distance from the field of public health, including the U.S. national security and defense apparatus(es), assorted public safety communities, "first responders," disparate health and medical care communities, and disaster/emergency management agencies.

Under the aegis of a nascent *rationality of preparedness,* the SVP was meant ostensibly to reflect new thinking about the ways in which existing elements of the public health and national security apparatuses could and should map onto emerging strategic demands. This emergent logic of preparedness focuses on uncertain future threats—threats that have eluded traditional measures of calculability. To know these threats—for example, the dangers posed by an engineered pathogen—therefore requires knowledge not about likelihoods—that cannot typically be known in a meaningful way—but about the extent to which the realization of those threats would impact the "vital systems" and critical infrastructures of the United States, including the ability of populations and jurisdictions to respond and recover from a potentially catastrophic event. Thus, preparedness has come to be oriented towards vulnerabilities, and the capabilities or capacities needed to act effectively in light of uncertain future situations.[5]

Although a number of interesting pieces have evaluated the SVP from an operational or programmatic perspective, none has looked at it specifically through the lens of the rationales and practices that have guided it and made it possible.[6] Stated another way, although smallpox and bioterrorism preparedness have been the focus of a great deal of discussion, the rationality of preparedness has not. This chapter contributes some insights in this direction through a look at a select set of events, discussions, and key participants tasked with thinking through and articulating the principal public health response to smallpox, namely through vaccination and associated practices. It is oriented largely towards the ways in which experts, situated in an advisory capacity to the Centers for Disease Control (CDC), as well as officials at the CDC and other organizations, came both to problematize smallpox, and to put forward sets of solutions to those problems in the context of an emergent preparedness rationale.

The chapter is organized as follows: The next section provides a brief overview of the planned structure of the SVP. Next, discussion centers on activity at the CDC and the principal organization charged with producing vaccination recommendations in the United States, the Advisory Committee on Immunization Practices (ACIP). The findings in this section were drawn from nearly twenty interviews with officials in both these organizations and from local public health departments, conducted in 2004–2006. Additional data includes ACIP meeting minutes and transcripts of CDC/ACIP "telebriefings" (press conferences).[7] The subsequent section traces back a particular technique and logic related to risk/benefit analysis, focusing specifically on its employment in the context of vaccination recommendations and the ACIP. The chapter concludes with provisional diagnoses regarding the emergence of recent smallpox vaccination thinking and the SVP.

The Planned Structure of the SVP

The SVP contained both military and civilian components.[8] Only the latter will be treated here. The civilian program consisted of two major stages. A third stage, entailing vaccination of members of the public requesting it, was never formally implemented. Stage 1 would consist of the voluntary vaccination of approximately five hundred thousand healthcare providers throughout the United States, to be accomplished—although this was later deemphasized by CDC officials, as was the target number itself—in a thirty-day time period. Individual states were tasked with requesting vaccine from the CDC and distributing it to local agencies. Local jurisdictions were, in turn, placed in charge of administering the vaccine to individuals. They were further assigned the responsibility, as called for in earlier CDC guidance on the subject, of putting together plans for mass vaccination of their local populations.[9]

Ultimately, these half million individuals were to constitute one of two types of Smallpox Response Teams (SRTs). Public health professionals in a number of specialties would constitute discrete response units based in specific geographic locales. These were to be known as Public Health SRTs, and their purpose was to exist as a ready "force" capable of responding to a smallpox outbreak within their respective jurisdictions. A second type of team, Health Care SRTs, consisting of a subset of an area's, or region's, hospital personnel (principally acute care, emergency care, and other relevant specialties), was to be established throughout the United States. Health Care SRTs were to provide local hospitals with a cadre of immunized personnel capable of handling possible smallpox cases in their respective locations. Both types of team were to have the capacity to vaccinate additional individuals, whether healthcare personnel or members of the community.

Stage 2 of the SVP called for a wide-scale expansion of the voluntary program to include up to ten million individuals situated throughout the public health, medical, and public safety establishments. Specifically, vaccines would be offered to "first responders"; that is, those working in fields such as firefighting, emergency medical services, and law enforcement. The principal argument for bringing this population into the fold initially revolved around the notion—not rigorously developed—that such individuals would likely be involved in some organized response to a smallpox incident.

The programmatic elements of the program's first two stages were designed to effect a vaccination strategy with a proven track record against smallpox on the world stage. According to most experts, the most effective strategy to counter a verifiable outbreak of smallpox (even if only one case), is ring vaccination, also known as trace vaccination, or a surveillance and containment strategy.[10] In concert with mass vaccination (i.e., immunization of entire populations), this strategy had been utilized effectively not only to control outbreaks of smallpox when the disease was endemic to many areas of the world (primarily before 1970), but to eradicate the disease itself worldwide.[11] The principal features of ring vaccination include: (a) surveillance for early signs of smallpox-related illness, especially rashes; (b) identification and isolation of "index" (first) cases; (c) contact tracing of the index case (i.e., investigating who the index case came in contact with; often this would include family members, friends, and other community members); (d) pre- and postexposure vaccination of all such individuals; (e) additional vaccination for individuals who may have come in contact with the previous group of presumably exposed individuals, and so on, thereby creating a "ring" of protected individuals around individuals known to be exposed to the pathogen; (f) continued surveillance of vaccinated individuals and their surrounding environs to monitor for additional outbreaks (with a new round of ring vaccinations should it be called for).[12]

In the context of the SVP, stages 1 and 2 were designed to make possible a strategy of ring vaccination. In previous decades, smallpox campaigns were conducted not only with already-immunized vaccinators, but with some semblance of an infrastructure either planned for or in place (trained personnel, a relatively secure supply chain, planning activities, a funding stream, etc.), as well as a global population with a fair degree of native immunity and prior exposure to the pathogen.[13] These conditions proved necessary to allow for the development of the ring vaccination strategy, which otherwise would likely have been ineffective and rather dangerous for unprotected vaccinators. Because the situation in 2002, when these strategies were debated once again, looked much different than thirty years earlier, public health experts found that to incorporate the proven ring vaccination approach would require a kind of preliminary step—that is, the development of an initial "pre-" strategy so that the "actual" strategy, the desired, primary strategy of ring vaccination, could be carried out if needed. This pre-strategy was actualized, at least in part, with the implementation of the first stage of the SVP.

The implementation of the SVP did not go smoothly. State and local jurisdictions, not to mention healthcare professionals themselves, were not uniformly convinced about the need to vaccinate various occupational groups. Moreover, problems familiar to large-scale vaccination efforts, including issues around liability and vaccine-related injury compensation, quickly materialized as the program got underway and intensified as side effects of the vaccine were reported in the professional literature and the media. Only six months after the program was announced by President Bush, it had for all intents and purposes come to a standstill. In some states, the number of individuals receiving vaccine could be counted on one hand.

Why did the SVP fail? With respect to program implementation, a number of compelling reasons have been given.[14] In the next section, I address this question not through an assessment of the program itself, but rather through an examination of the steps taken by the advisory body tasked with thinking about and making recommendations for this large-scale national vaccination program. Insights into some of the techniques employed by this body to think about the very problem of smallpox and smallpox vaccination can provide a better sense of the precarious foundation upon which the SVP was built.

Chronologies, Actors, and Debates in Smallpox Vaccination Thinking and Policy

Vaccination policy in the United States is messy and not easily defined. It would not be entirely inaccurate to state that a coherent national vaccination policy does not exist now, nor has it in the past. Rather, much of what constitutes vaccination policy in effect is a set of regularly issued recommendations by the ACIP, a committee convened by the CDC every three years under the auspices of the Federal Advisory Committee Act. The ACIP consists of fifteen members specializing in public health, infectious diseases, and related fields, who meet to consider revisions or new proposals for the administration of vaccines to the public. Deliberations tend to focus on routine childhood vaccines as well as vaccines for adult and specific at-risk populations. It is significant that the ACIP issues only advisory recommendations and that, as an independent body of experts, it is linked organizationally to the agency to which it provides its advice: the CDC.

The year 2001 marked the publication, in June, of the first revision to the official recommendations for smallpox vaccination in ten years. These new recommendations covered new strains of *vaccinia* then being studied, and incorporated updated knowledge related to the genus Orthopox generated since 1991. They also kept in place the target population for smallpox vaccination: laboratory workers handling viral cultures. The stated reason for taking up the issue of smallpox vaccination, according to the ACIP, was vague, having been afforded two sentences in a twenty-five-page recommendation. The committee noted:

> Currently, international concern is heightened regarding the potential use of smallpox (variola) virus as a bioterrorism agent. Because of these concerns, ACIP

has developed recommendations for vaccinia (smallpox) vaccine regarding the potential use of smallpox virus as a biological weapon.[15]

More notable, in a later section, was the recommendation's treatment of the risk of (exposure to) smallpox. The committee began by remarking that an intentional smallpox release was unlikely; other biological weapons were considered more likely to be utilized—it is not clear by whom—owing to their availability.[16] The ACIP indicated a certain sense of unease regarding this small likelihood of the appearance of smallpox. It was uneasy in part because quantifiable estimates were unavailable in the public domain, although the language used by the committee to describe this lack of needed information was open to a variety of interpretations. The committee wrote: "The risk of smallpox occurring as a result of a deliberate release by terrorists is considered low, and the population at risk for such an exposure cannot be determined."[17] This statement is telling: it is not clear whether the committee could not, through the scientific and technical means available to it, come up with such estimates on its own—or whether such information could not be provided to them by others with such information at their disposal.

The resulting recommendations were understandably cautious. Having virtually no quantifiable information regarding risks of outbreak or exposure, the committee recommended a no-vaccination policy (other than for laboratory workers) during what it called the prerelease/preexposure stage. Such a "stage," of course, described the state of the world at that point, as it does today. Holding to the view that a positive recommendation for vaccination could only follow from identifiable increases in (quantifiable) risks or (qualitative) threats, the ACIP did indicate its willingness to reconsider its position. However, in articulating this contingency its language was vague and imprecise: "If the potential for an intentional release of smallpox virus increases later, preexposure vaccination might become indicated for selected groups (e.g., medical and public health personnel or laboratorians) who would have an identified higher risk for exposure because of work-related contact with smallpox patients or infectious materials."[18]

In the event of an intentional release—in other words, shifting now to a postevent/postexposure context—the ACIP essentially laid out two recommendations. First, it provided its first indication to the public that the vaccination strategy most appropriate in such an instance would be the tried-and-true ring vaccination approach. Second, the committee recognized that, in addition to vaccinating the contacts around infected individuals, a whole host of people in all sorts of occupational groups related to and supporting healthcare and emergency response functions would probably have to be vaccinated as well. "Probably" because the committee only equivocally indicated vaccination for certain groups, including "law enforcement, emergency response, or military personnel."[19]

These early recommendations are notable for a few reasons. First, absent from them is any mention—yet—of a strategy, or the conditions necessitating a strategy, for universal vaccination. This may largely be explained by the limited availability of vaccine at the time (approximately fifteen million doses), which precluded the possibility of physically vaccinating the entire vaccine-eligible population of the United States. In fact, the available supply of vaccine strongly constrained the options the ACIP and government officials were initially to consider. However, because plans for the procurement of additional vaccine were already in effect, and pressure to produce even more was reaching the higher echelons of the Department of Health and Human Services (HHS), it is still reasonable to ask how it came to be that universal vaccination received very little serious discussion—let alone an actual recommendation—in ACIP meetings between 2001 and 2002. Second, although bioterrorism preparedness efforts had gained traction and funding in the years preceding 2001, such developments had little to do with the ACIP.[20] Consequently, this advisory body was neither directly influenced by nor beholden to such a strategy, especially in the middle of 2001. No reference was made to "preparedness" of any type—bioterrorism, smallpox, public health—in the June 2001 recommendations.

The June 2001 recommendations seem eventually to have been considered insufficient by the administration, especially as the aftershocks of 9/11 rumbled through Washington and anthrax spread through the mail. Although the recommendations explicitly referred to the need to protect various personnel "if the potential for an intentional release of smallpox virus increases," the specific details of what a vaccination program should look like in just such an instance were held back in favor of general indications describing which populations might need to be vaccinated. Clearly the ACIP was not itself sure of the specifics of such a plan; it would, however, get a chance to reconsider these issues within a year's time.

In October 2001, anthrax spores were dispersed through the United States Postal Service. A number of commentators were quick to heap scorn on HHS and the CDC both for failing to respond to the threat in an appropriate manner, and for ensuring that their press conferences produced as many worrisome questions as comforting answers. It was a rough time at the CDC, by the director's own admission.[21]

Undoubtedly the anthrax attacks, coming on the heels of 9/11, constituted a catalyst for immediate action on the part of federal health authorities and the legislature. The vastness of the effort and the speed with which changes occurred were extraordinary by virtually any measure, and arguably unique in modern U.S. history.[22] Unfortunately, there is little documentary evidence describing how the White House and HHS came to the conclusion that the CDC, and ultimately ACIP, should reexamine smallpox and possible vaccination options...again. For most healthcare practitioners and public health experts, it was not obvious that, by virtue of the release of *anthrax* through the mail—let alone the events of 9/11—the risk of *smallpox* (i.e, through an intentional release) had increased, necessitating updated recommendations. Even at the tail-end of the anthrax events in November 2001, the CDC saw no pressing need to consider vaccinating local public health officials, front-line medical personnel, or first responders.[23]

As for *cabinet-level* deliberations on the matter of biological threats, there is little in the public record documenting the ways in which smallpox or other biological agents were considered by the administration during this time. Interviews with public health officials at the CDC and ACIP, on the other hand, suggest quite strongly that, within the executive branch, concerns about smallpox were broached in the context of concerns about Iraq: respondents consistently reported that the threat of smallpox, in a general sense, was linked to specific information about the possibility that Iraq might have or use biological weapons in what was beginning to look like a likely war in the fairly near term.

In February 2002, the ACIP took up the issue of smallpox vaccination once again.[24] From interviews with several CDC officials, it is clear the administration had already decided to institute some kind of smallpox vaccination program, and apparently had some sense about the scope of it; the idea, then, seemed to be to involve ACIP as a conduit for public input into the already-decided-upon program—without, however, indicating to the public that such a program was definitively in the works and essentially inevitable. The following statement by a senior CDC official interviewed during this study is informative in this regard.

> When the committee was engaged around smallpox in terms of a smallpox program, I mean there's I don't think any secret about the fact that that was brought before the committee by [HHS] on behalf of the administration. I mean, you know, a decision had been made at the highest levels of government that we were going to have a smallpox vaccination program [in early 2002]. So, at that point, the parameters became pretty clear, and the committee handled it as well as they could. They recognized that there was a determination by the commander-in-chief, the president of the United States, and his closest advisors, that they wanted to have a smallpox vaccination program based on whatever intelligence they had. And consequently, what we advised, and the administration followed it, was "Okay, maybe you want to have a program and maybe it should be as large as you're talking about, but how about going ahead and using your standard immunization advisory committee to consider the issues, and put it through the regular channels with public meetings and opportunities for public discussion.[25]

A cynical read of this statement would be that the ACIP was asked to rubber stamp a public health intervention desired by the White House on the basis of national security considerations. A conclusion of this nature is speculative, but is supported by the growing unease felt by many ACIP members that the U.S. commander-in-chief was appearing to will into existence a national public health program. Moreover, as one former ACIP official noted in an interview, to some extent the ACIP is constituted precisely to validate the overseeing agency's (i.e., CDC's) "agenda," suggesting, in the context of smallpox, that this occurred to some degree.

The minutes of the ACIP meeting, held June 19–20, 2002, in Atlanta, provide two sets of rationales for revisiting, once again, the smallpox issue. The document notes that "[t]here is no indication the threat has increased since the September 11 attacks, but the perception of risk has [increased], and it is known that the United States is vulnerable to enemies with such an attack capability." The committee's remark about increased perceptions of risk is curious, in part because the committee does not articulate who these perceivers of risk are, and in part because it is the committee that typically makes such determinations. Whatever the risks were, it is clear the ACIP was frustrated that it did not have the means to "know" them.

> To make...decisions, the ACIP needs data. Those on vaccine efficacy and safety are in hand, but not for the risk of disease.... Without it, should the ACIP even make this decision without that information? Doctor Modlin stated, according to the best information published, presented at meetings, and discussed by Doctor [D. A.] Henderson and others, that ACIP was unlikely to have better estimates of risk than it now had. A higher-level briefing arranged for committee members may be possible, but he thought that such would be unlikely to alter any decision reached on this day.... Some information inappropriate to share in a public forum could be provided, but the bottom line would be the same as the message being received here today. *The CDC Director would not place on this committee the burden of making a risk assessment.* The members were informed as best as possible under the circumstances that the risk is not zero but is perceived to be low.[26]

The second rationale indicated by the committee is equally telling. For some years, experts had begun formulating the dangers of bioterrorism and other "non-conventional" threats employing a conceptual schematic other than risk. Utilizing techniques such as scenarios and exercises, the dangers of these agents were linked, conceptually, to the capacities and capabilities of the very public health infrastructure that was expected to detect, track, and respond to them. In June 2001, a key exercise called "Dark Winter" called attention to precisely these capacities and capabilities—or the lack thereof. Sponsored by a central player in bioterrorism preparedness circles, the Center for Civilian Biodefense Strategies at Johns Hopkins University, the scenario was intentionally grim: a smallpox epidemic caused by release of the agent in three shopping malls across the country.[27] The fictitious outcome of the exercise was disastrous: the United States faced utter catastrophe given its public health infrastructure. The *real* result of the exercise, however, was that public health *vulnerabilities* became widely publicized, both among national security types and throughout the public health establishment. As the ACIP came to consider the next round of smallpox vaccination options, the stage had therefore been set to construct a problematic of bioterrorism in which *vulnerability* had guided the logic of response as much as any specific, identifiable *threats*.

The ACIP's June 2002 deliberations were oriented around three main questions: (1) Should the general population be vaccinated? (2) Which occupational groups should be vaccinated? and (3) Is ring vaccination the most desirable post-event strategy? From the outset, debates about appropriate vaccination strategies were centered on a precarious policy equation: What is the appropriate balance between the benefit derived from vaccination and the risks of vaccination? "Equation" is the precise terminology here as the committee's decisions were largely oriented around what was ultimately a cost-benefit analysis—a technique brought to bear on problems of vaccination several decades earlier. Under this decision-making structure, a number of assumptions had first to be determined in order to generate any kind of workable policy model. These included: initial attack size (how many individuals initially infected); the "reproductive rate" (how many additional persons infected from the initially infected case; additional rates possible for later "generations" of infected individuals); vaccine efficacy rate; vaccine-induced mortality rate; and various probabilities of release and of exposure (for certain models). Given the absence of observable, current data in the real world, the committee resorted to expert opinion and a review of the literature on smallpox (looking at transmission, mortality, etc.) on which to base its assumptions. With some exceptions, the committee's understanding of how a future outbreak of smallpox would "behave" was heavily informed by the disease's behavior in populations historically. Generally dismissed by most smallpox experts were viewpoints that espoused more extreme assumptions, such as the possibility of very high initial attack sizes.[28] Once the models were in place, the committee had a concrete set of options from which to work.

The minutes of the June 2002 ACIP meetings indicate that a strategy of universal vaccination was never seriously entertained as a possibility by a critical mass of decision makers in either a pre- or postevent context. The former was ruled out entirely, a telling point given that it arguably would have proven the best deterrent against a nonengineered smallpox strain; the latter was understood to be conceivable as an option only in the direst of circumstances. However, in contrast to its recommendations a year earlier, the ACIP's conservative inclinations (i.e., its reticence in recommending smallpox vaccine) were called into question by its decision to recommend the vaccination of members of occupational groups other than laboratory workers already handling orthopox viruses. Which groups was a matter of some debate. Some argued that "predesignated" healthcare providers in relevant occupational and professional groups should be considered for vaccination; it would be such individuals, after all, who would respond and therefore be exposed during an outbreak. Others suggested that a variety of "responders" of all stripes should be given consideration, beyond an emphasis on designated smallpox response teams specifically, or (specified) healthcare providers more generally. Cogent arguments were made all around, and debate at times was passionate. Ultimately (for the June 2002 meetings), the ACIP honed in on members of outbreak response teams at national, state, and local levels, as well as some hospital healthcare providers (at predesignated smallpox receiving hospitals), to receive the vaccine.

Around this time, the first salvos in a war of numbers erupted, specifically over how many individuals were to make up the two broad groups of professionals for whom the vaccine was recommended. In a press conference announcing the ACIP's recommendations, Chairman John Modlin noted that somewhere between ten to twenty thousand individuals would be vaccinated.[29] A few weeks later, two administration officials made estimates well over an order of magnitude higher than that. Respected smallpox expert D. A. Henderson, and Jerome Hauer, at the time both senior officials at HHS, mentioned a number—five hundred thousand—around which an inordinate amount of debate would subsequently revolve.[30] It seems clear from this alone that the advisory committee and the administration had two very different views about what a smallpox vaccination program should look like. Information elicited from various officials supports this interpretation.[31] The administration made no secret over its disappointment with the ACIP's June recommendations, at least in private. In public there was simply respectful disagreement and eventually the usual glossing over, but no one involved had any illusions about the extent of ACIP's reach: it was an advisory committee only, and its recommendations went to the CDC, which could choose to forward them to the cabinet...or not.

The main source of disagreement voiced publicly had largely to do with which hospital healthcare providers should be vaccinated. The ACIP had based its recommendations on the notion that infected individuals or suspected cases would report to state-designated receiving hospitals. In effect, only a small percentage of hospitals in any given region were expected to be so designated; consequently, a figure of between ten and twenty thousand was aired as the number of healthcare providers likely to be called upon to be vaccinated (voluntarily, of course). Importantly, such assumptions were based upon projected vaccination rates vastly higher than what would ultimately be the case.

Critics of the recommendations pointed to what were felt to be flawed assumptions about how potentially infected individuals were expected to behave in an emergent crisis. Specifically, it was noted, with supporting evidence provided by the events of 9/11, that sick individuals tended to go to the nearest hospital. The implication was that every hospital was vulnerable precisely because the entire population was, in effect, vulnerable as well (both in the sense of being immunologically naïve and because smallpox could appear and reappear anywhere in the country). The ensuing logic is not difficult to follow: select healthcare workers at *every* hospital in the United States should be vaccinated because *any* hospital could receive smallpox victims. Hence, the five hundred thousand number.

Although this number followed an internally consistent logic, it is remarkable that there is little evidence in the ACIP transcript record indicating that anywhere near that number would actually agree to, or demand, vaccination. To the extent that this issue was discussed in public deliberations, it was heavily moderated by concerns (especially among physicians and other healthcare providers) about the conditions under which such vaccination should take place. In interviews, CDC officials noted that adequate discussions regarding "the public," including which groups were presumed to constitute this public and which among these were envisioned to be willing vaccine recipients, had been largely understudied and underdiscussed during the bulk of CDC/ACIP work on vaccination strategies and recommendations.[32] Although studies would later indicate a general willingness among specific healthcare providers to be vaccinated,[33] post–SVP surveys found this not to be the case at all: rates of *actual* vaccination were substantially lower than *expressions of willingness* to be vaccinated.[34]

As word got to the ACIP that the administration was honing in on five hundred thousand vaccinees, some committee members became very nervous.[35] The decades-old Dryvax vaccine had known side effects, and estimates of illness and injury associated with the vaccine had been well documented in the medical literature for decades. One source of unease on the part of some ACIP members and CDC officials had to do with what was seen as the inevitability of injury from the vaccine alone—without a single case of smallpox in the population.[36] Although few, if any, explicitly invoked the language of medical ethics in working through such a vaccination strategy, it is clear that the risk/benefit calculus adhered to by members of the public health and health policy communities was governed by an ethics that tolerated vaccine-induced illness only in certain contexts, none of which included zero-incidence of disease in the population—let alone the world.

It was in light of these debates that in October 2002 the ACIP, in an unusual move, again amended its smallpox vaccination recommendations.[37] Having decided that *all* hospitals were at some risk of smallpox exposure (because all individuals were at some risk), it recommended that up to two "teams" of healthcare personnel at each hospital should receive the vaccine. Other modifications to the recommendations focused on which occupational groups should constitute a hospital response team; contraindications for individuals with skin problems and immunocompromised states; and various other clinical and procedural issues.

The October recommendations provided the first indication that the ACIP had begun to align its thinking towards some kind of "preparedness" rationale. The kind of preparedness the committee seemed to have in mind focused on building out capacity to respond at a national level; that is, on laying a foundation across the nation, irrespective of greater or lesser risks to any one region or city, aimed at establishing an in-place infrastructure of trained, already-vaccinated personnel.[38] This formulation did not, notably, hone in on specific numbers; at least, officials did not wish it to *appear* that numbers were what was important. The by-then-famous five hundred thousand number was deemphasized as a nationwide standard to be met; rather, that number was viewed as something of a best case should a certain number of healthcare providers, say one hundred per acute-care hospital in the United States, be vaccinated. The following comments by the ACIP chair and the director of the CDC's National Immunization Program, Dr. Walt Orenstein, illustrated these tensions in a telebriefing to the press.

> *Dr. Modlin:* [T]he objective of our recommendations is to assure that there are an adequate number of healthcare workers to provide care for the first wave of smallpox victims and that we are not focusing on a specific number, a target number of individuals to be immunized, but rather the objective is to identify and to suggest that there be a sufficient number of healthcare workers in

different categories that we've just talked about to provide care in many, if not most, of the acute-care hospitals in this country. It turns out there, there are approximately 5,100 acute-care hospitals in the United States, and if—a big if—all of them were to take part in this program, we would estimate that there might be roughly, and I want to emphasize very roughly approximately 100 healthcare workers in those hospitals that might be needed to be vaccinated in order to meet that objective, and so if you do the math, that number comes up to about 500,000 healthcare workers.

Dr. Orenstein: I just want to emphasize, again, the goal is a cadre of people who could care for the first several patients in the first seven to ten days on a 24-hour basis. Hospitals have a lot of experience with figuring out what staff they need to care for patients who would be in isolation rooms with negative pressure, and so that's why we're a little uncomfortable with trying to name an actual number for you; that, in fact, the number will come from the hospitals if they decide what staff are needed to cover these patients.[39]

Officials at HHS must not have been all that pleased with a joint announcement that numbers were *not* what was important in putting together a smallpox vaccination/preparedness program. Only a few weeks previous a number in the neighborhood of ten million had been floated in the context of discussions about the wide array of "first responders" envisioned to take part in a vaccination program (this would correspond with Stage 2 of the actual SVP). Although this was an issue substantively separate from the issue of hospital providers, the contradictory nature of the message (it's not about numbers vs. here's a concrete number) was not helping to clarify policy. Clearly, the basic question of what should constitute preparedness had not been resolved; too many divergences still existed between those espousing a conservative, incremental approach based on a limited vaccination program, and those pushing for something much bigger. Despite claims to the contrary, the fight over preparedness was, at this stage at least, a fight over numbers. How else, after all, could the effectiveness of a vaccination program be measured given no incidence of disease?[40]

Additional conflicts and ambiguities arose in other areas as well. A number of CDC and ACIP officials interviewed for this project suggested in more or less unambiguous terms that deterrence—what one official described as taking the disease "off the table"[41]—lay at the heart of the administration's push to get smallpox vaccination up and running. With anthrax already "out there," a war with Iraq in the works,[42] and a realization (which could be parlayed into an opportunity) that smallpox was one of the few Category A agents about which federal and local public health authorities could actually do anything in an organized and concerted way, the line coming from the White House (directed more to government officials than to the public) was that a vaccination program was not only prudent as a protective measure, but as a strategic deterrent as well.

For public health officials tasked with building out some kind of smallpox vaccination program, deterrence was wholly unfamiliar as a rationale for public health activity. In no way, according to respondents, was deterrence analogous to disease prevention, owing to the crucial difference that smallpox vaccination—and hence a logic of deterrence—was sure to harm a small number of people while providing no quantifiable benefit recognizable as such by officials traditionally tasked with implementing public health programs. This outcome was unpalatable for a few senior and other CDC officials, who quietly resigned or were otherwise reassigned to non-smallpox-related tasks.

Despite some reshuffling in the ranks and a degree of disquiet among the rank and file dealing with the issue, the senior leadership of the CDC presented the October 2002 recommendations to HHS in late 2002. With some modifications, these recommendations were endorsed by the agency. The Smallpox Vaccination Program had been formulated.

Vaccination Recommendations, the ACIP, and the Risk/Benefit Balance

One way to understand how the SVP came about—and hence, what contributed to its troubles—is to focus on the practices and techniques that made possible contemporary (expert) thinking about smallpox vaccination. This section focuses on the emergence of vaccination recommendations and a specific technique around which virtually all recommendations are formulated: the risk or cost-benefit calculation.

The U.S. public health apparatus circa the early to mid-twentieth century, having oriented itself towards communicable disease in previous decades, found itself in a good strategic position to incorporate mass immunization—that is, vaccination of entire populations, subpopulations, and/or cohorts—as a technique appropriate for its evolving mission. This, coupled with innovative public health efforts in a number of localities, opened up a space for those properly positioned to adjudicate its benefits, leading ultimately to a form of deliberation that would produce recommendations about which vaccines should be given, which kinds of techniques and practices should be used, and under which kind of schedule(s).

Although its emergence across the land was uneven, mass vaccination came fairly quickly to be accompanied by a need to survey formally the extent to which certain communicable diseases were an "actual" problem, for example in a geographic area such as a municipality or a state.[43] Most vaccination efforts had initially been assessed empirically through a kind of trial-and-error method, typically as observed and reported by private physicians administering vaccines who, especially in the early mass vaccination campaigns of the twentieth century (for example, utilizing diphtheria antitoxin), were relatively few in number and largely suspicious of public health and state medicine on the one hand, and rather revolutionary technologies on the other.[44] Although by the early 1900s statistical methods were already being applied to problems of health and illness with both vigor and some consistency, studies of the effects of immunization on populations grew increasingly amenable to statistical analyses as these techniques gained an even stronger hold, and as something resembling a "national" public health apparatus began to emerge. Although these trends probably did little to alter the likelihood that controversy or debate would accompany any given vaccine—the legacy of anti-vaccination movements still resonated among some parents, and physician-skeptics of vaccination were still vocal—it did change the character and the setting of these debates. Most notably, debates had begun to be cast as issues of effectiveness and later, efficacy.

By the mid-twentieth century, the issue of *safety* had become an object of intense scrutiny as a matter of public health and immunization practice. Because the incidence of many childhood diseases had by this time begun to wane substantially, just after mid-century newer vaccines—in particular the Sabin oral polio vaccine (OPV)—generated intense controversy as experts, clinicians, policy makers, and the public began to wonder whether reducing and eventually eliminating disease through vaccination was worth the cost of actively inducing it in some small number of otherwise healthy children—especially as compared with proven safer vaccines. As will be seen, the polio case is instructive. As very few cases of "wild" polio (as the naturally occurring disease is known) appeared each year, the case was being put forward that recommending continued use of OPV was poor medical practice and, in fact, unethical. The chief tension in the decision calculus was: Should a vaccine continue to be recommended for an entire cohort when (a) the disease in question was extremely rare; (b) the vaccine being used unquestionably *caused* not just illness, but, in this case, *actual paralytic polio in more individuals* than those acquiring the "wild" type, and (c) a safer (albeit slightly less efficacious) vaccine existed, which did not cause the disease?

The main point in illustrating this tension is to highlight the kinds of thinking to which the ACIP would orient itself in the coming years and decades. Although the committee was formed (in 1964) notably *after* many of the debates around polio vaccine had already been resolved, the stage had in some sense been set for it to operate around a new kind of problematic—one involving the techniques, knowledge, and ethical positions associated with risk-benefit calculations. Although notions (and calculations) of risk and benefit were not, at this time, new,[45] their solidification in relation to each other as both technical and ethical problems in the domain of public health was a novel development. Since the committee's formation, its uptake of vaccine-related issues has hinged largely on the extent of disease in a population—and, crucially, the extent of disease projected for a population without vaccination. In other words, a fundamental variable—disease incidence—in the form of concrete numbers, or ranges thereof, formed the basis for generating calculations that experts then compared with alternative future possibilities, or scenarios: disease incidence without vaccine, numbers of likely side effects, and so on. Knowledge about disease incidence, potential disease incidence with and without vaccination, and likely side effects formed a "grid of intelligibility," which tended to boil down to a numbers game: the most favorable numbers usually dictated the policy.[46] The experts, in other words, were convened to produce (or solicit the production of), and then scrutinize, the numbers.

It is a matter of the utmost importance, then, in doubling back on this genea-logical tracing—back to the problem of smallpox in 2002–2003—that by virtually every account in the public record, there was no meaningful numeric estimate of the possibility of a smallpox release. To state it a different way, within the frame-work of understanding to which health experts were accustomed, namely, through practices of risk assessment and other epidemiological techniques, making sense of this specific danger through the meaningful production of (knowledge about) risk was impossible.[47] "The risk is not zero, but appears to be low" constituted a chal-lenging presentation of risk; when coupled with not a single instance of disease, ACIP and public health officials were confronted with a situation with which they had little familiarity and virtually no expertise.

Diagnoses

The task of this chapter has been to present a select overview of the ways in which certain smallpox vaccination options became "thinkable" and "actionable," ulti-mately culminating in the Smallpox Vaccination Program. What remains is to make some sense of the observations presented, although not as matter of adding yet another pronouncement on top of the impressively large list of previous pro-nouncements, which, as far as they go, consist of reasonably plausible explanations as to why the SVP was implemented with such difficulty.[48] What follows, then, are a set of provisional diagnoses out of which additional, explicitly policy-relevant interventions can be generated.

DIAGNOSIS 1

The previous sections have shown that specific practices related to vaccination and vaccine recommendation lay at the center of experts' capacities to formulate smallpox and smallpox vaccination as workable problems. Within the domain of public health, risk assessments and risk/cost-benefit evaluations are employed in such a manner as to estimate the likelihood and magnitude of future outcomes, as well as the extent to which proposed interventions would be favorable relative to their costs. This orientation towards what Lee Clarke has called "probabilistic thinking" has served a clear function in these and many other domains, namely, as a mechanism to inform the allocation of scarce resources "rationally" to a variety of competing needs.[49]

As noted in the introduction to this chapter, much of what constitutes public health is built on this model, particularly as regards infectious diseases. As the risk of disease increases for a given population, various interventions are increasingly considered (possible), their costs and benefits weighed. If the likelihood of a disease outbreak rises, so too does the risk of not doing anything, according to the logic of the model just presented. In just such a case, benefits will tend to outweigh risks. Conversely, as potentially dangerous objects are transformed by these mechanisms of calculability and understood to be increasingly *less* likely, the costs associated with interventions tend to go up, often dramatically, while benefits—understood as averted or treated cases—are either few and/or appear less likely.

For a host of reasons, the formulation of smallpox as a biological threat constituted a problem of a particularly challenging type. It was, after all, a disease that had been eradicated some twenty years earlier. Its ontological basis—that is, the conditions that facilitated its constitution through thought as a real object, let alone a real threat—was therefore grounded in a variety of elements apart from actual observation of cases of disease. It came to exist as real by virtue of sets of (other kinds of) observations from which could be deduced its very possibility, not only as an object, but as a dangerous one at that. A crucial step in this process, it seems, lay in its transformation from a thinkable (dangerous) object, to one in which something like a "knowable" risk was attached. By knowable, I refer to that which understands a thing by virtue of its potential to be, typically in terms of its quantifiable/quantified likelihood or probability. In this case, of course, the extent to which the risk of smallpox was quantified posed particular problems. Low, but not zero—the official public estimate of risk—came to take on a peculiar significance, and required a level of interpretation not typically found in most other systemic public health assessments. Such a risk was open to a number of interpretations. What is one to do—what is one supposed to do—with that kind of information? These are very separate questions, and the latter in particular—as a kind of ethical inquiry—seems not to have been central to vaccination deliberations. As a matter of policy analysis and policy making, one might therefore feasibly hypothesize the utility of incorporating such a question into early decision-making activities.

A cottage industry of risk analysts, disaster preparedness experts, psychologists, and others have produced an array of theoretical work around the issue of low probability–high consequence events.[50] The concept did not appear with smallpox. Nevertheless, it appears that part of what came to constitute smallpox as a threat to be dealt with had very precisely to do with its formulation in these conceptual terms. Since the risk of smallpox given was extraordinarily, even unquantifiably, low, the conditions for producing any meaningful understanding of the benefits of a public health intervention (i.e., vaccination) became uncomfortably narrow. How could there be any meaningful conceptual grasp of the benefit of vaccination when, according to the very techniques of generating public health knowledge, there existed, by definition, virtually no risk? At its most extreme, and to be fair it was not articulated as such, pre-event vaccination could be construed as all cost and no benefit.[51] As strategizing about smallpox vaccination options got underway, all that was certain was that, given the implementation of a pre-event vaccination program, a small number of individuals was going to get sick from the vaccine, and possibly die, without the benefit of related information about how many cases of smallpox, if any, would be averted or rendered less severe. Clearly, how benefits were to be gauged would become central to the smallpox vaccination process, although solutions to this problem were scarce.

This analysis begs the question: If it was logically difficult to gauge the benefit of a vaccination program according to the standard calculus of risk- or cost-benefit techniques (other than through an understanding of "benefits" as derived via hypothetical models and scenarios), then by what criteria could experts decide that a certain strategy of vaccination was appropriate? And for whom? The first diagnosis therefore begins with the observation that risk assessment and risk/cost-benefit practices are conducted according to a calculus within which what is thought (literally) to be actionable is based on a rational-choice logic, whereby costs and benefits are known according to specific counts of disease or injury. The strong claim here is that knowing a thing in such a manner, and acting according to the most favorable numbers, seems to operate in an uneasy relationship with the normative and technical rationality of preparedness, which by the logic governing it, works outside such calculative practices. Such practices are employed for different purposes, to different ends; they do not seem to articulate with(in) the rationality of preparedness.

DIAGNOSIS 2

In a number of reports issued both during and after the SVP's implementation, the prestigious Institute of Medicine (IOM) noted that the program had somewhat ineffectually linked up actual vaccination efforts with its articulated aims of, at various points, either general bioterrorism preparedness, smallpox preparedness, or both.[52] Had such aims been *clearly articulated,* the reports went on, the program stood a better chance of benefiting from more effective implementation. Moreover (again according to the IOM), had vaccination activities been undertaken in the context of a preparedness program oriented towards the augmentation of *capabilities* to handle a public health emergency—as opposed to specific threats—the overall program may have fared better than it did. Perhaps.

The evidence is fairly convincing that there was a good deal of room for improvement in implementing the SVP. Issues like compensation for vaccine-induced injury (variable between states, but generally low) and program funding (there was no special appropriation by the Congress for several months), were, according to most published accounts and study participants, grossly under-estimated by senior officials in HHS and the administration, and perhaps the CDC as well. Moreover, issues of liability and adverse events seemed to plague program officials since nearly the start of the program. Improvements in all these areas would almost certainly have boosted the number of individuals vaccinated, although it is not by any means clear that this would have led to or correlated with a "higher" state of public health preparedness.

Two related points can be made in light of this, constituting the second and final diagnosis. These points can be summed up in a phrase: "There is preparedness, and there is preparedness." Officials, experts, and policymakers have for several years decried the fact that however preparedness has been defined in principle, it has not been satisfactorily operationalized.[53] The various frameworks and metrics meant to give some definition, some measurability, some sense of knowing what preparedness is and whether one (jurisdiction, state, etc.) is prepared have met with a fair degree of controversy. This case study has illustrated just one of several debates in public health and emergency management circles regarding how to put preparedness into practice. In this case, one issue was that of numbers: Should the number of individuals vaccinated count as a salient preparedness metric, or not?

How about the number of vaccines? The number of hospitals with vaccinated staff? Or plans? Whatever the metric, the point is that all of these kinds of "preparedness" (oriented to specific risks and threats) seem to be partially if not wholly *dis*articulated from the *rationality* of preparedness, which is oriented towards uncertain futures and the unknown.

This is not, of course, to say that these activities are not important or necessary. Naturally, putting (vaccinated) people and infrastructure in place is central to some kind of preparedness enterprise. Still, in developing smallpox vaccination options and in implementing the SVP, there seemed to be a telescopic view of what constituted vulnerabilities to be addressed and capabilities to be enhanced. Vulnerability was understood in a strict sense to mean: an immunologically naïve population's vulnerability to (acquire) smallpox; or in relation to this, a jurisdiction's vulnerability (according to degraded or absent capabilities) in responding to a smallpox outbreak. Capabilities were understood in a strict sense to mean, among other things, the capability to conduct ring or mass vaccination operations; or to surveil a particular population, or run diagnostic tests, and so on. All of these needs were framed largely as a function of whether an adequate number of smallpox vaccinations had been or could be given to appropriate individuals. In other words, vaccination was the preliminary step needed to facilitate necessary (additional) public health measures. While all these are clearly important operational questions utterly germane to the issue of smallpox, it seems that they are not fully congruent with a rationality of preparedness.

To orient towards an unknown future, even if that future is understood with respect to a specific infectious disease like smallpox, is not only to provide, pre-event, for the possibility of a massive organized response through vaccination (and surveillance, detection, laboratory work, communication infrastructure, etc.); rather, the logic of preparedness would demand that *all* of the elements and nodes in a preparedness assemblage be rigorously examined for vulnerabilities, with apparent "blockages" remedied or mitigated as part of configuring the assemblage itself. As experts from the CDC and ACIP adjudicated vaccination options, the mold of preparedness, whatever the type (bioterrorism, smallpox, public health), had already been cast: Preparedness would articulate according to a logic with roots deeply entrenched in previous public health campaigns and longstanding practices.

Risks and benefits would be weighed, contraindications would be determined, dosages would be settled upon, and eligible populations would be established. Other elements and practices having to do with, for example, hospital and clinic staffing, compensation for injury or illness, family issues, or liability were, in the early planning stages, only ancillary to "proper" considerations about smallpox vaccination and preparedness. They became issues to consider or redress largely only after they emerged as operationally problematic.

According to a preparedness rationale, however, these should not be understood as "barriers" to an effective program; they are not objects *external* to preparedness that simply get in the way of its successful implementation. Rather, these issues, and the relationships they reflect between different groups, different levels of government, and different centers of activity, are fundamentally just as central to a preparedness effort as more traditional measures and public health interventions. It is therefore not unreasonable to conclude that the "social organization" of preparedness—since it is ostensibly "aimed" at vulnerabilities—should seek to reconceptualize what constitutes vulnerability and to treat *all* vulnerabilities with equal concern and effective prevention and mitigation techniques.

NOTES

Acknowledgment: The author would like to offer thanks and deep appreciation to the Social Science Research Council, and to Carlo Caduff, Stephen Collier, Andrew Lakoff, Kathleen Vogel, and the participants of the SSRC workshop on biosecurity, held in New York in April 2007. Insightful comments have been plentiful and without exception helpful. Thank you. Additional acknowledgment goes to Paul Rabinow and the Anthropology of the Contemporary Research Collaboratory, who/which in many ways helped facilitate my thinking on this piece; Roger Brent and the Molecular Sciences Institute, who welcomed me with open arms and provided a (beautiful) space in which to write; and to UCSF colleagues Renée Beard, Cassandra Crawford, Carrie Friese, Chris Ganchoff, and Rachel Washburn, who were attentive and thoughtful in their comments on various iterations of this paper. Special thanks also to Ruth Malone, whose guidance throughout this undertaking has been especially helpful. The work on which this piece is based was funded in part by Molecular Sciences Institute Prime Grant Award No. HRO011-05-1-0033, and a grant from the Agency for Healthcare Research and Quality (AHRQ), R36 HS015549-01A1. Thanks to both organizations for their generosity.

1 The announcement in its entirety can be found at http://www.whitehouse.gov/news/releases/2002/12/20021213-7.html.

2 Bob Woodward, *Plan of Attack* (New York: Simon & Schuster, 2004).

3 Never mind that public health officials in the United States have tended not to concern themselves about terrorism!

4 D. A. Henderson et al., "Smallpox as a Biological Weapon: Medical and Public Health Management," *JAMA* 281, no. 22 (1999): 2127–37.

5 A growing body of work has begun to explore preparedness in some depth; see Stephen J. Collier and Andrew Lakoff, "Vital Systems Security," Anthropology of the Contemporary Research Collaboratory, http://anthropos-lab.net/wp/publications/2007/08/workingpaperno2.pdf; Stephen J. Collier, Andrew Lakoff, and Paul Rabinow, "Biosecurity: Proposal for an Anthropology of the Contemporary," *Anthropology Today* 20, no. 5 (2004): 3–7; Andrew Lakoff, "Preparing for the Next Emergency," *Public Culture* 19 (2007): 247–71; Lyle Fearnley, "Pathogens and the Strategy of Preparedness: Disease Surveillance in Civil Defense Planning," Anthropology of the Contemporary Research Collaboratory, http://anthropos-lab.net/wp/publications/2007/08/workingpaperno3.pdf; Stephen J. Collier and Andrew Lakoff, "Distributed Preparedness: Notes on the Genealogy of 'Homeland Security,'" *Environment and Planning D: Society and Space* (forthcoming).

6 Hillel W. Cohen, Robert M. Gould, and Victor W. Sidel, "The Pitfalls of Bioterrorism Preparedness: The Anthrax and Smallpox Experiences," *American Journal of Public Health* 94, no. 10 (2004): 1667–71; Government Accountability Office, "Smallpox Vaccination: Implementation of National Program Faces Challenges" (Washington, DC: U.S. Government Accountability Office, 2003); John D. Grabenstein and William Winkenwerder, "U.S. Military Smallpox Vaccination Program Experience," *JAMA* 289, no. 24 (2003): 3278–82; Institute of Medicine, *The Smallpox Vaccination Program: Public Health in an Age of Terrorism* (Washington, DC: National Academies Press, 2005); Daniel

J. Kuhles and David M. Ackman, "The Federal Smallpox Vaccination Program: Where Do We Go from Here?" *Health Affairs,* Web Exclusive, 2003, http://content.healthaffairs.org/cgi/reprint/hlthaff.w3.503v1; G. A. Poland, J. D. Grabenstein, and J. M. Neff, "The U.S. Smallpox Vaccination Program: A Review of a Large Modern Era Smallpox Vaccination Implementation Program," *Vaccine* 23, no. 17–18 (2005): 2078–81; Cynthia P. Schneider and Michael D. McDonald, "'The King of Terrors' Revisited: The Smallpox Vaccination Campaign and Its Lessons for Future Biopreparedness," *Journal of Law, Medicine & Ethics* 31 (2003): 580–89; Laura Taylor et al., "New Jersey's Smallpox Vaccination Clinic Experiences, 2003," *Journal of Public Health Management and Practice* 11, no. 3 (2005): 216–21; Stephen J. Wilson, "Factors Affecting Implementation of the U.S. Smallpox Vaccination Program, 2003," *Public Health Reports* 120, no. 1 (2005): 3–5.

7 Especially CDC, CDC Telebriefing Transcript, "ACIP Vaccine Meeting Media Briefing," October 17, 2002, http://www.cdc.gov/od/oc/media/transcripts/t021017.htm; CDC Telebriefing Transcript, "Update on Smallpox Vaccination Program," March 25, 2003, http://www.cdc.gov/od/oc/media/transcripts/t030325.htm; CDC Telebriefing Transcript, "Interim Smallpox Response Plan and Guidelines Conference Call," November 26, 2001, http://www.cdc.gov/od/oc/media/transcripts/t011126.htm.

8 In addition to information derived from interviews with several CDC officials, this section is based on the following sources: Government Accountability Office, "Smallpox Vaccination"; Institute of Medicine, *Smallpox Vaccination Program;* Judith A. Johnson, "Smallpox Vaccine Stockpile and Vaccination Policy" (Washington, DC: Congressional Research

Service, 2003); Kuhles and Ackman, "Federal Smallpox Vaccination Program"; Richard Pilch, "Smallpox: Threat, Vaccine, and U.S. Policy" (Monterey, CA: Center for Nonproliferation Studies, 2003); Poland, Grabenstein, and Neff, "U.S. Smallpox Vaccination Program."

9 CDC, "Executive Summary for CDC Interim Smallpox Response Plan and Guidelines," 2001, http://chfs.ky.gov/NR/rdonlyres/2BD78E16-317F-463E-A775-5E3675FC9979/0/janfeb2002.pdf.

10 Henderson et al., "Smallpox as a Biological Weapon."

11 Frank Fenner et al., *Smallpox and Its Eradication* (Geneva: World Health Organization, 1988).

12 An authoritative source regarding the effectiveness of the ring vaccination approach (for smallpox) is Fenner et al., noted above. Other sources discussing the ring vaccination strategy include Samuel A. Bozzette et al., "A Model for Smallpox-Vaccination Policy," *The New England Journal of Medicine* 348, no. 5 (2003): 416–25; Committee on Infectious Diseases, "Smallpox Vaccine," *Pediatrics* 110, no. 4 (2002): 841–45; M. Kretzschmar et al., "Ring Vaccination and Smallpox Control," *Emerging Infectious Diseases* 10, no. 5 (2004): 832–41; T. C. Porco et al., "Logistics of Community Smallpox Control through Contact Tracing and Ring Vaccination: A Stochastic Network Model," *BMC Public Health* 4 (2004): 34; B. Pourbohloul et al., "Modeling Control Strategies of Respiratory Pathogens," *Emerging Infectious Diseases* 11, no. 8 (2005): 1249–56.

13 Public health experts suspect that immunologically "naïve" populations—that is, populations with little or no prior exposure to smallpox—would be particularly susceptible to the disease, both in terms of its acquisition and its severity.

14 See note 7.

15 ACIP, "Vaccinia (Smallpox) Vaccine Recommendations of the Advisory Committee on Immunization Practices," *MMWR* 50, no. RR-10 (2001): 1–25.

16 Such a statement was a remarkable anticipation of the dispersion of anthrax through the U.S. mail only four months later.

17 ACIP, "Vaccinia (Smallpox) Vaccine Recommendations," 18.

18 Ibid.

19 Ibid.

20 On bioterrorism preparedness, see George Avery, "Bioterrorism, Fear, and Public Health Reform: Matching a Policy Solution to the Wrong Window," *Public Administration Review* 64, no. 3 (2004): 275–88; Zarnaaz Bashir et al., "The Impact of Federal Funding on Local Bioterrorism Preparedness," *Journal of Public Health Management and Practice* 10, no. 5 (2004): 475–78; Government Accountability Office, "Bioterrorism: Federal Research and Preparedness Activities" (Washington, DC: General Accounting Office, 2001); Donald A. Henderson, "The Looming Threat of Bioterrorism," *Science* 283 (1999): 1279–82; Jeffrey Koplan, "CDC's Strategic Plan for Bioterrorism Preparedness and Response," *Public Health Reports* 116 (2001): 9–16; Scott Lillibridge, "A Public Health Response to Bioterrorism," *Medicine & Global Survival* 6 (2000): 82–85.

21 Julie Gerberding, notes taken at a speech before the Commonwealth Club, San Francisco, California, June 4, 2003.

22 One important measure of this activity is, of course, funding. Overall spending for civilian biodefense at HHS jumped greater than one order of magnitude in the span of one year (2001–2002), from $271 million to nearly $3 billion. Ari Schuler, "Billions for Biodefense: Federal Agency Biodefense Budgeting, FY2005–2006," *Biosecurity and Bioterrorism: Biodefense, Strategy, Practice, and Science* 3, no. 2 (2005): 94–101.

23 CDC, "Interim Smallpox Response Plan."

24 Institute of Medicine, "Scientific and Policy Considerations in Developing Smallpox Vaccination Options: A Workshop Report" (Washington, DC: National Academies Press, 2002).

25 Interview with CDC official #1 (conducted 11/17/2005).

26 ACIP, "ACIP Meeting Minutes," June 19–20, 2002, emphasis added.

27 Tara O'Toole, Michael Mair, and Thomas V. Inglesby, "Shining Light On 'Dark Winter,'" *Clinical Infectious Diseases* 34 (2002): 972–83.

28 See, for example, Edward H. Kaplan, David L. Craft, and Lawrence M. Wein, "Emergency Response to a Smallpox Attack: The Case for Mass Vaccination," *Proceedings of the National Academy of Sciences* 99, no. 16 (2002): 935–40.

29 CDC, CDC Telebriefing Transcript, "Smallpox Vaccine," June 20, 2002, http://www.cdc.gov/od/oc/media/transcripts/t020620.htm.

30 CIDRAP News, "Smallpox Vaccination Decision in White House Hands," 2002, http://www.cidrap.umn.edu/cidrap/content/bt/smallpox/news/decision.html.

31 Interviews with CDC officials #3 (conducted 11/18/2005), #6 (conducted 4/21/2006) and #8 (conducted 5/3/2006); and ACIP member #1 (conducted 1/23 and 1/27/2006).

32 Interviews with CDC officials #1 (conducted 11/17/2005), #3 (conducted 11/18/2005), and #8 (conducted 5/3/2006).

33 W. K. Yih et al., "Attitudes of Healthcare Workers in U.S. Hospitals Regarding Smallpox Vaccination," *BMC Public Health* 3 (2003): 20.

34 Government Accountability Office, "Smallpox Vaccination"; Alex R. Kemper et al., "Hospital

Decision-Making Regarding the Smallpox Pre-Event Vaccination Program," *Biosecurity and Bioterrorism: Biodefense, Strategy, Practice, and Science* 3, no. 1 (2005): 23–30; Taylor et al., "New Jersey's Smallpox Vaccination Clinic"; Wilson, "Factors Affecting Implementation."

35 Interview with ACIP official #1 (conducted 1/23 and 1/27/2006).

36 Interview with CDC official #8 (conducted 5/3/2006).

37 The October recommendations are no longer available online. A summary of them can be found at http://www.immunize.org/acip/acip1021.pdf.

38 CDC, "ACIP Vaccine Meeting."

39 Ibid.

40 This is precisely the question public health officials were grappling with at the time.

41 Interview with CDC official #8 (conducted 5/3/2006).

42 Woodward, *Plan of Attack*.

43 On these matters, a number of sources are informative: Jeffrey Paul Brosco, "The Early History of the Infant Mortality Rate in America: 'A Reflection Upon the Past and a Prophecy of the Future,'" *Pediatrics* 103, no. 2 (1999): 478–85; R. A. Meckel, *"Save the Babies": American Public Health Reform and the Prevention of Infant Mortality, 1850–1929*, Henry E. Sigerist Series in the History of Medicine (Baltimore: Johns Hopkins University Press, 1990); William G. Rothstein, *Public Health and the Risk Factor: A History of an Uneven Medical Revolution*, Rochester Studies in Medical History (Rochester, NY: University of Rochester Press, 2003); Andrea A. Rusnock, *Vital Accounts: Quantifying Health and Population in Eighteenth-Century England and France*, Cambridge Studies in the History of Medicine (Cambridge, UK: Cambridge University Press, 2002). In addi-

tion, classic references include: George Rosen, *A History of Public Health* (Baltimore: Johns Hopkins University Press, 1993); and Paul Starr, *The Social Transformation of American Medicine* (New York: Basic Books, 1982).

44 Evelynn Maxine Hammonds, *Childhood's Deadly Scourge: The Campaign to Control Diphtheria in New York City, 1880–1930* (Baltimore: Johns Hopkins University Press, 1999).

45 Theodore M. Porter, *Trust in Numbers: The Pursuit of Objectivity in Science and Public Life* (Princeton, NJ: Princeton University Press, 1995).

46 This is, of course, an ethical position as well as a strictly expert "technique." On the grid of intelligibility, see Hubert L. Dreyfus and Paul Rabinow, *Michel Foucault, Beyond Structuralism and Hermeneutics* (Chicago: University of Chicago Press, 1982).

47 Although, to be sure, security experts had been accustomed to working through extreme assumptions as well—especially in the context of a nuclear weapons exchange. My thanks to Andrew Lakoff for pointing this out.

48 Government Accountability Office, "Smallpox Vaccination"; Institute of Medicine, *Smallpox Vaccination Program*; Kuhles and Ackman, "Federal Smallpox Vaccination Program"; Wilson, "Factors Affecting Implementation."

49 Lee Clarke, *Worst Cases: Terror and Catastrophe in the Popular Imagination* (Chicago: University of Chicago Press, 2006).

50 See, for example, Howard Kunreuther, "A Conceptual Framework for Managing Low-Probability Events," in *Social Theories of Risk*, ed. Sheldon Krimsky and Dominic Golding (Westport, CT: Praeger, 1992), for an informative primer on the topic.

51 By virtue of the lack of any meaningful risk estimates, experts had to rely on an additional

set of techniques to orient their thinking. As discussed above, this included the generation of possible scenarios and models of smallpox attacks. These models were based on a variety of assumptions—too great to list here (but see Institute of Medicine, "Scientific and Policy Considerations")—as well as widely varying ranges of risk estimates. With these models and those of the CDC, the ACIP and other experts were provided with necessary information to evaluate cost/benefit analyses. By "necessary" I refer to the form that the information took, namely, quantified (albeit guesstimated) data.

52 Institute of Medicine, *Smallpox Vaccination Program*.

53 Sarah A. Lister, "An Overview of the U.S. Public Health System in the Context of Emergency Preparedness," Congressional Research Service, 2005, http://www.ncseonline.org/nle/crsreports/05mar/RL31719.pdf; Nicole Lurie et al., "Public Health Preparedness in California: Lessons Learned from Seven Health Jurisdictions," RAND Health, 2004, http://www.rand.org/pubs/technical_reports/2005/RAND_TR181.pdf; Nicole Lurie et al., "Local Variation in Public Health Preparedness: Lessons from California," *Health Affairs* Web Exclusive, June 2, 2004, http://content.healthaffairs.org/cgi/reprint/hlthaff.w3.503v1; TFAH, "Ready or Not? Protecting the Public's Health in the Age of Bioterrorism 2003," Trust for America's Health, 2003, http://healthyamericans.org/state/bioterror/.

CHAPTER FIVE

Disease as Security Threat

CRITICAL REFLECTIONS ON THE GLOBAL TB EMERGENCY

Erin Koch

Once believed to be under medical control, tuberculosis is currently one of the primary infectious causes of adult deaths worldwide. In 1993, in an unprecedented move, the World Health Organization (WHO) declared a Global Tuberculosis Emergency. This international alert was issued to raise concern about the dramatic rise of tuberculosis and multidrug-resistant TB (MDR-TB) in the late 1980s and early 1990s worldwide, and to urge public health officials at local, regional and national levels to put tuberculosis back on the map.[1]

In response to the emergency, the WHO first recommended a program of short-course chemotherapy that evolved into a highly standardized protocol branded Directly Observed Treatment, Short-Course (DOTS). This tactic proved to be an effective political strategy that brought renewed resources to public health budgets that had been the target of massive cuts in previous years. Establishing strict guidelines for diagnosing, treating and surveying tuberculosis both responded to the need for greater economic efficiency in TB control, and provided a packaged approach that presumably would function in any setting, thus rapidly cutting the chain of infection and curing individual cases. In networks of international public health, DOTS is marketed as the most modern and efficient method for combating the rise and spread of tuberculosis and drug-resistant strains globally and in specific locales.

This chapter draws on ethnographic material about the implementation of DOTS in post-Soviet Georgia to analyze the cultural aspects of standardization, and the public health implications of a clash between the DOTS protocol and local forms of knowledge and expertise that standardization engenders.[2] I show that the mobile, presumably value-free technical elements of the DOTS protocol in fact limit its effectiveness in Georgia; "proper administration" runs up against a local environment for the implementation which is refractory in terms of both cultural and technological factors. My analysis does not claim that DOTS is unnecessary, or the "wrong" approach. Rather, I argue that promoted as a primarily technical intervention, the rigidity of the protocol undermines its fundamental public health goals because the standard procedures for locating, treating, and monitoring patients are often incommensurable with local forms of medical expertise and health service delivery on the ground.[3]

The ethnographic material intersects laboratory, clinical and administrative domains to provide a cautionary tale about how top-down implementation of DOTS—an exemplary global disease-management protocol designed to keep microbial threats at bay—creates barriers for the success of the protocol through the mechanisms that frame it as a purely "technical intervention." We see these effects in Georgia's post-Soviet context. The former Soviet region is a current "hot spot" for tuberculosis and other infectious diseases. The WHO recently reported that rates of drug-resistant tuberculosis in that region "have reached the highest levels ever recorded globally."[4] Moreover, negligent governments are diagnosed as the primary causal agent of these rates, due to insufficient and ineffective adherence to the DOTS protocol.[5] Perhaps it is not surprising, then, that Georgia and other countries in the region are also hot spots for the interventions of international organizations which provide aid for weakened health infrastructures. The issue at stake in this analysis is not whether such assistance is warranted. Rather, my analysis demonstrates that the DOTS protocol is not a value-free technical intervention, but a prescriptive apparatus that is mobilized for governing the behavior of healthcare providers, diagnosticians, and patients, often with unintended consequences.[6]

Global TB Emergency

The declaration of a Global Tuberculosis Emergency demonstrates a shift toward the framing of infectious diseases as security threats, rather than merely as threats to public health, within an international policy discourse of human security that emerged after the end of the Cold War. Tuberculosis and the standardized, global response to it highlight new understandings of biosecurity and its impact on initiatives focused on disease and population management across borders. Approaching infectious diseases as threats to human security creates a heightened sense of urgency about tuberculosis, and emphasizes the global significance of local outbreaks. The framework of human security "attempts to broaden security thinking from 'national security' and the military defense of political boundaries to a 'people-centered' approach of anticipating and coping with the multiple threats faced by ordinary people in an increasingly globalizing world."[7] Here, threats are no longer calculated in terms of weaponry; an emphasis is placed on "human life and dignity."[8]

Under the rubric of human security, infectious diseases have been identified as in particular need of new management strategies that would facilitate effective public policy interventions. Because infectious diseases are caused by microbes, the pathogenic agents are conceived of as naturally occurring entities that could potentially pose threats to security at local, national, and international levels. In 2003 the RAND Corporation published a landmark report about the security threats posed by infectious diseases. In the introduction to the report, the authors emphasize that

> the threats emanating from contemporary gray area influences are far more ambiguous in their patterns, processes, and effects. In many cases, this obfuscates the perceived need for rapid policy responses. Action is typically initiated only after a major crisis destabilizing stage has been reached within the state(s) concerned. Making sense of these changes will require a holistic, nonlinear approach to security...traditional spatial notions of security, of national stability defined purely in terms of territorial sovereignty and integrity...simply do not work in today's more complex geostrategic environment.[9]

From this perspective, infectious diseases—and the global spread of pathogens in particular—are seen as dangerous enemies posing threats to nations and persons within them: "As adversaries, microbial pathogens have particular advantages in terms of invisibility, mobility, adaptability, and silent incubation periods that render national borders meaningless."[10] In the face of escalating concerns about contagion in a globalizing arena, neoliberal technologies of governance—such as DOTS—are designed to combat them.[11]

Notions of danger, risk and warfare are not unique to emergent security-oriented ways of framing and responding to communicable diseases, nor to international efforts to control the spread of pathogens beyond national boundaries.[12] The shift in aligning infectious disease with biosecurity issues recalls older notions of interstate conflict, and the need to develop strategies through transnational collaboration to overcome them.[13] What is novel about the contemporary tuberculosis "emergency" are unprecedented levels of antimicrobial resistance by pathogenic agents; the role of philanthropy in responding to global health crises; and the extent of standardization of the DOTS protocol.

Overconfidence in public health and the assumption that tuberculosis was basically eradicated masked the fact that the illness had never actually disappeared from vulnerable populations.[14] In the 1970s and after, the WHO as well as national public health institutions such as the CDC in the U.S. dramatically cut back on their funding for the disease. As a result of such public health neglect, tuberculosis, in new, more virulent and drug-resistant forms, has "re-emerged." Currently, one out of every three individuals worldwide (approximately 2 billion people) is infected with *Mycobacterium tuberculosis,* the bacterial causal agent of TB.[15] The WHO estimates that one individual is newly infected with *Mycobacterium tuberculosis* every second (amounting to at least 8 million new infections annually), and that one person dies from tuberculosis every 20 seconds. According to the most recent data available from the WHO, approximately 1.6 million adult deaths in 2005 resulted from tuberculosis.[16]

The emergence of extensively drug-resistant tuberculosis, or XDR-TB, is perhaps one of the most frightening examples of infectious diseases that endanger not only populations, but also local, national and international health infrastructures, because of the intensive and expensive treatment regimens they demand.[17] According to the most recent global survey of drug-resistant tuberculosis conducted by the WHO, XDR-TB has been reported in 45 countries (meaning at least one case has been reported per country). The most recent WHO report emphasizes that "MDR-TB cases in the [former Soviet] region have more extensive resistance patterns, including some of the highest proportions of XDR-TB."[18] However, global data is incomplete because very few countries have laboratory facilities necessary to test for such high levels of resistance.[19] The spread of XDR-TB has also exposed weaknesses in national and global public health surveillance systems and in primary care diagnostic services, as well as highlighting "the dearth of new tools for tuberculosis control" including new drugs.[20] However, no novel anti-TB medicines have been introduced to the market in forty years. As the prominent TB specialist Dr. Lee Reichman has argued, anti-tuberculosis medicines do not capture the attention of drug companies because "the vast majority of people with TB are young and poor and live in developing countries. Very often, neither the people nor their countries can afford TB drugs."[21] These inequities, along with the "new tuberculosis"—as the epidemic is widely described in public health literature—are fueled by processes of globalization and the neoliberal reforms that exacerbate poverty.[22]

Microbes that travel by air such as *Mycobacterium tuberculosis* are especially dangerous amid contemporary global flows of people and pathogens. Dr. Reichman emphasizes that

> the recent resurgence [of TB] has taught us that we cannot consider TB control as just another 'social problem' explainable or not by underlying poverty and related concerns. We must continue to treat TB control as a *defense* program, which has been fairly successful in combating the resurgence. In defense programs, critical strategies are not abandoned for budgetary reasons prior to winning the last battle.[23]

According to Reichman it is imperative that national and global public health institutions and programs operate in precautionary, absolute terms, rather than through the lens of a cost-benefit analysis. As such, "we" must be *defensive*. But against what and whom? Killer microbes and "superbugs"? "Non-compliant" patients and healthcare workers? Dangerous or "high risk" populations culpable in their own susceptibility and exposure to infectious agents? Pharmaceutical companies reluctant to invest in R&D for new anti-TB drugs because it is not a high-profit disease?

These questions are extremely important in light of the globalization of DOTS. Despite the successful global distribution of DOTS as a standardized protocol for diagnosis, treatment and management, rates of active tuberculosis and antimicrobial resistance remain alarmingly high. This is partially attributable to the fact that TB and HIV/AIDS are opportunistic infections. High rates of TB suggest that the "threat" posed by any microbe, in this case tuberculosis, emerges through interactions between a specific pathogen and the social and political contexts that remain outside the reach of a technical intervention such as the DOTS protocol.

Cultural Politics of DOTS

The DOTS protocol is designed to direct public health resources through a technical intervention. The program is structured around lab-based diagnosis and six- to 8-month[24] periods of ingesting a fixed regimen of first-line antibiotics typically used to treat tuberculosis: rifampicin, isoniazid, ethambutol, and pyrazinamide. The protocol emphasizes diagnosing and treating individuals who have active cases of tuberculosis (and thus, who are spreading tuberculosis within the community), stressing the direct observation of medicine ingestion. Implementing DOTS requires the cooperation and support of local governments, and is geared towards minimizing the length and cost of treatment, as well as ensuring a heightened accuracy of diagnoses based on laboratory tests of sputum (rather than X-rays, which was the focal point of the Soviet model of TB control, a point to which I turn below).

Officials blame the rise and spread of TB and drug-resistant microbes on both national public health programs for prescribing nonstandardized antibiotic drug regimens, and individual patients for not properly following standards. In both cases, an emphasis on institutional and individual noncompliance masks the fact that DOTS is quite difficult to implement and follow in its standardized form.[25] A focus on compliance and noncompliance constitutes a narrow analytic for measuring success or failure in TB control. Such a perspective diverts attention from preexisting forms of knowledge and tuberculosis management that are displaced by the implementation of DOTS, and the ways in which these infrastructural transformations impact access to resources, social stigma related to tuberculosis, and other social relations that contribute to public health risks.

The technical components of DOTS are embedded in cultural and economic assumptions that presuppose a functioning primary healthcare system. These assumptions are visible in the five official components of the protocol: (1) Government commitment to sustained TB control activities; (2) case detection by sputum smear microscopy among symptomatic patients self-reporting to health services; (3) standardized treatment regimen of at least 6 to 8 months for all sputum smear positive cases, with directly observed therapy (DOT) for at least the initial two months; (4) a regular uninterrupted supply of all essential anti-TB drugs; and (5) a standardized recording and reporting system that allows assessment of treatment results for each patient and of the TB control program performance overall.[26]

In this protocol, standard case definitions are necessary because they perform particular functions in organizing services. These include prioritizing treatment for patients who are infectious; systematizing diagnosis through patient registration and case notification; and monitoring case levels and treatment outcomes on local, regional, national and international levels through a shared approach and shared categories. At the same time, the DOTS protocol operates as a neoliberal technology that is primarily concerned with optimization. In Aihwa Ong's terms, it is a biopolitical *"technology of subjectivity* [that relies] on an array of knowledge and expert systems to induce self-animation and self-government"[27] through health management.

Worldwide, DOTS is marketed and distributed as a medical-technical intervention—as a mobile protocol that can be successfully implemented regardless of context. As such, "DOTS is seen as an essentially technical intervention that, in and of itself, is value-neutral. DOTS, it is claimed, provides a 'common language' through which to develop national and local strategies...however, there remains a limited view of the importance of socioeconomic determinants of health."[28] In other words, standards indicate a baseline according to which compliance to "rational" and "efficient" forms of care are measured, without attention to the social, cultural and political matrix in which knowledge about and experiences of illness are produced and articulated.

Technical advisors and donors often imagine that the components of DOTS will accommodate any local context. As Peter, a representative of an international organization involved with DOTS implementation in Georgia explained to me, adopting the protocol should be relatively straightforward. If the National Tuberculosis Program is supported by the government in accordance with DOTS, other social factors that contribute to TB are not major obstacles: "[With DOTS] your TB program works under whatever conditions: in refugee camps, in prison, wherever. If you take your patients' sputum, you diagnose correctly, you get results. That's a good message.... If you do your program you can forget about the big social economic approach."[29] This perspective contributes to the tensions between DOTS as a response to a global health crisis, and the local factors that limit the possibilities of implementing the protocol in its standard form on the ground.[30]

The extent to which the DOTS protocol functions—or misfires—as an intervention into public health and/or biosecurity is also impacted by specific aspects of any setting where the protocol lands on the ground, including health infrastructure, cultural meanings of medical professionalism and training, and disincentives for following the protocol related to stigma and lack of resources among healthcare providers and patients. The DOTS protocol also exemplifies a new assemblage of national governments, donors, and humanitarian organizations that constitute contemporary public health networks, influence what counts as expert knowledge, and advocate health regimes which are more or less likely to receive funding in the competitive market of global health. DOTS is advocated by the WHO, international donor and aid organizations such as the United States Agency for International Development (USAID) and the Gates Foundation, national governments, and the STOP TB Partnership—a global network of governmental and nongovernmental organizations, public and private donors, and international organizations that address matters of public health, collectively working to eliminate tuberculosis as a global health problem. According to the WHO and the Stop TB Partnership, DOTS has been adopted in 187 countries. The stakes in finding a rapid and affordable system for treating and controlling the spread of tuberculosis are especially high throughout the former Soviet Union, an official "hot spot" of the Global TB Emergency, where the number of cases has more than doubled since the mid-1990s.[31] During research that I conducted in 2001, 2003 and 2005, many Georgians spoke with me about the lack of infrastructure and resources for fledgling institutions in their country, and the subsequent influx of attention from Western aid and development agencies for which health is a prime area of focus. Because of this local shift in governmental regimes, as well as the international response of aid organizations, Georgian medical care responses to the TB epidemic increasingly rely on "outside" intervention for resources that the Georgian state is unable to fully provide. The biomedical, scientific and administrative transformations DOTS implementation engenders constitute a privileged site for viewing global power relations in a local context.

Implementing DOTS in Georgia

In Georgia and throughout the former Soviet Union, collisions between incommensurable forms of knowledge and experience are most clearly visible in the dramatic differences between the Soviet model of TB control and DOTS. While a detailed comparison is beyond the scope of this essay, it is worth summarizing here several key components of the Soviet system that DOTS is replacing, and how these health regimes differ in terms of knowledge production and service distribution.

From the period immediately following the October Revolution until the dissolution of the USSR, the Soviet TB control program emphasized mass screening, vaccinations, and long-term hospitalization in sanatoria, as well as mass training of TB specialists.[32] Diagnosis was based primarily on X-ray evaluations, and treatment regimens relied heavily on the professional expertise and knowledge of individual specialized TB doctors. Although treatment generally consisted of surgery combined with anti-TB drugs, there was limited emphasis on standardized case definitions or treatment regimes.[33] Because drug regimens were nonstandardized, TB doctors frequently changed combinations of medicines for individual patients, often treating them in this way for as long as two years. The Soviet model of tuberculosis control, which comprised an important component of the centralized Soviet medical infrastructure, reported success in controlling active tuberculosis within the population.[34]

From the perspective of DOTS and western biomedicine, however, the Soviet system was irrational and inefficient. Many administrators and doctors told me that the system consisted of too many separate facilities for tuberculosis, which were redundant and inefficient in terms of resource allocation, that nonstandardized drug regimens created drug resistance, that the population of TB doctors was too specialized, and that annually screening the entire population by fluorography and X-ray was a waste of money and unnecessarily exposed people to radiation. As one Georgian doctor working for the International Committee of the Red Cross who was trained with a DOTS-oriented approach from the outset of his career explained to me,

> X-rays do not give enough information. An X-ray is just a picture that helps
> to confirm your doubts. But if you have smears or cultures you can see that

it is tuberculosis. Because they [Soviet-trained doctors] relied more heavily on X-rays people were treated unnecessarily for tuberculosis (which creates drug resistance)...after the system collapsed in the Soviet Union and Georgia, it was impossible to follow the Soviet model of treatment because you don't control your spread of infection, your cure rate, or anything.[35]

Georgia's separation from the Soviet Union in 1991 was immediately followed by ethnic civil wars, primarily between Georgia and breakaway regions Abkhazia and South Ossetia. Civil war, political collapse, and corruption have all character-ized Georgia's long-term processes of free-market reform and democratization. Its geopolitical location makes the country at once a strategic point of defense for the U.S. and Europe, as well as a threat to those regions because of the widespread level of infectious disease in the region and the intense rates of migration.

Decentralization, economic collapse, and the protracted civil war left only shattered remnants of the previous healthcare system. With the dismantling of the centralized Soviet health infrastructure there began a difficult period of decen-tralization combined with nation-building. Georgian state institutions inherited, among other things, under-resourced and overburdened medical facilities. Eco-nomic and social conditions worsened, and the country was left without a health-care system or TB infrastructure until 1995, when the National Tuberculosis Program (NTP) was officially launched under the auspices of the Ministry of Health and with the assistance of a range of donor and aid organizations. These include the WHO; the World Bank; the German Technical Co-operation (GTZ), an interna-tional donor organization that began supplying the NTP with all first-line anti-TB medications in 1995; the Atlanta-Tbilisi Healthcare Partnership, a collaborative network of U.S. and Georgian-based medical and educational institutions sup-porting healthcare reform in Georgia since 1992; and the American International Health Alliance.[36]

Despite this, in contemporary Georgia medical services are limited, and as a result of privatization, generally difficult to afford. As such, an all-in-one approach to treating individuals who are afflicted with tuberculosis may offer an important opportunity to improve the public health situation and cut the chain of transmis-sion. From this perspective, and because primary diagnostic and treatment services within DOTS are available free of charge in Georgia, the protocol appears at the outset to "make sense."

The Georgian NTP is managed in accordance with DOTS, a protocol that, in addition to the benefits of standardization, confers legitimacy in international public health networks and secures resources that the Georgian state is unable to provide. Since its inception in 1995, the participants of the NTP have changed. New actors include the International Committee for the Red Cross (ICRC), which oversees the TB program in Georgia's prisons. In 2000 the ICRC also built a new diagnostic laboratory at the NTP in Tbilisi to meet WHO standards. In 2003 the NTP acquired the support of the United States Agency for International Development (USAID), which has provided more than 2.5 million dollars in funds to support the implementation of DOTS around the country, and the Global Fund to Fight AIDS, Tuberculosis and Malaria, which will support DOTS-plus beginning in 2008.[37] Thus a network of local, national and international participants manages the NTP and the DOTS protocol. The network includes administrators, clinicians, nurses, laboratory technicians and scientists, representatives of donor and aid organizations and government officials.

Some analysts argue that the DOTS protocol falls short because of the over-emphasis on the biomedical—on the ingestion of antibiotics—without accounting for or utilizing local systems of knowledge and meanings about illness, treatments, and community and family networks.[38] Further, although the technologies and practices central to DOTS are standardized, many countries such as Georgia simply do not have the parallel "standard" infrastructure necessary to maintain the prescribed program. Moreover, prescribed cures are cumbersome. With drug regimens involving the observed ingestion of four antibiotics daily for six to eight months, DOTS places incredible burdens on ministries of health, healthcare providers, patients and their families.

Many physicians who were trained under the Soviet model point out that the surveillance of the DOTS protocol is, ironically, more stereotypically Stalinist in its implementation than the former system. One summer night in 2001 I attended a dinner organized by an American physician, a major figure in the international health sector in Georgia, and his American medical students who had been conducting research in Georgia. Most guests were Georgian doctors, several of whom had traveled to the U.S. for medical training. After some time discussing my research and the resistance to DOTS I was encountering among TB doctors who had been trained according to the Soviet approach, one of the doctors turned to me and said, "You know Erin, there is [also] a great resistance to DOTS in Russia. Russian doctors think that the system is too rigid, and does not allow any room for doctors to use their expertise in diagnosing and treating tuberculosis." A colleague of his who had overheard chimed in with a joke that Russian doctors reportedly tell about the implementation of DOTS in the post-Soviet context: "There is a joke in Russian that the DOTS protocol is really an invention of the KGB."[39]

This anecdote regrettably captures the ways in which current changes in TB control, not only in Georgia, but throughout the former Soviet Union, are seen as constricting and disciplining, rather than liberating, in relationships between state and medical administration. Digging deeper, the joke also points to criticism and resistance to DOTS as a technical approach to TB control. Implementation entails a loss of professional expertise among clinicians. From their perspective, the shift to a model designed within and for "developing countries" reflects on Georgian expert strata. As is the case throughout the Caucasus region, many physicians express resistance to the DOTS protocol not only because it undermines their expertise, but because the treatment and monitoring standards are impossible to meet in conditions of social upheaval, war, and economic collapse. As I discuss elsewhere,[40] opinions among clinicians I interviewed in Tbilisi vary from unwavering support of DOTS to resistance, because of fear of job loss and status decline in terms of providing medical expertise about tuberculosis. Moreover, many physicians who are being retrained to follow fixed combinations of anti-TB medicines find that the DOTS protocol limits the care patients need and deserve. These doctors tend to follow a clinical rather than epidemiological approach to prescribing medicines, which from their perspective should emphasize individual patient care. The dramatic differences between the cultural logics of the Soviet model of TB control and DOTS in clinical, laboratory and administrative arenas demonstrate that such "technical interventions" must be implemented in ways that are suitable to a local cultural environment.

The attitudes of the NTP toward changing forms of knowledge and knowledge production practices about tuberculosis in Georgia are articulated in terms of casting away the Soviet "old mentality" and implementing "new" standards of TB diagnosis, treatment and management. These changes are enforced through downsizing TB facilities, as well as training clinicians in DOTS methods of diagnosis, treatment, and management of patients through recording and reporting. In the language of the World Bank, the WHO, and supranational organizations governing healthcare reforms and other aspects of democratization in the former Soviet Union, the successful transition to a market-based primary healthcare system requires "rationalization" and "optimization" in infrastructure (re)building. Overwhelmingly, such processes involve adopting standardized protocols. Throughout the former Soviet Union and Eastern Europe, standardization is a key element of postsocialist transition and brings much-needed capital to fledgling economies.[41]

"Changing the old mentality of Georgian TB doctors," explained Revaz, a Georgian physician who held a prominent administrative position in the NTP in Georgia from 1995–2004, engenders massive changes in the culture of knowledge production and service distribution for TB control. He argued that this is because the Soviet model of TB control "was a closed system, there was no ongoing contact with international organizations...this was a classical Soviet institute. No contact with foreigners."[42] From his perspective, closure was a sign of stagnancy, and a contributing factor to the current low status of Soviet medicine, which was excessive in cost and scope. This perspective is shared by local experts who are critical of the legacy of Soviet medicine.

Yet in the current context in Georgia, the DOTS protocol does not make sense. Administrators from the Tbilisi-based NTP face numerous obstacles to conducting routine surveillance and monitoring, especially in mountainous regions that are largely inaccessible to outreach teams. These are not minor impediments but disabling structural conditions that include shortages of staff, of modes of transportation, and of funds to pay for fuel and accommodations.[43] In the rural and mountainous regions of Georgia, DOTS is difficult to administer because patients, nurses and physicians alike lack the funds necessary to travel to one another on a regular basis. Many physicians throughout the region express resistance to the DOTS protocol not only because it undermines their expertise, but because the treatment and monitoring standards are impossible to meet in conditions of social upheaval, war, and economic collapse.[44]

The cultural politics of DOTS implementation are further illuminated through conflicts that arise when questioning what counts as expert knowledge extends to the laboratory. Under the auspices of DOTS standards, the lab takes on a position of authority in the production of reliable knowledge, in explicit contrast to knowledge derived from X-rays, which was central to the Soviet model of TB control. One official WHO manual for DOTS implementation explicitly states that "within the framework of an effective TB control program, the identification and treatment of infectious cases of pulmonary TB is the highest priority. The laboratory is therefore the focal point of the entire program."[45] With DOTS, confirming the presence of *Mycobacterium tuberculosis* is at the heart of definitive diagnosis. Within the DOTS protocol—and the broader picture of security in which contagion is situated—*Mycobacterium tuberculosis* is now discursively constructed as a "political object" that travels in the bodies of infected individuals at unprecedented rates and must be accurately detected, if it is to be combated.[46] In turn, sputum is the primary work-object on which differential diagnostic tests such as microscope analysis, growing microbial cultures, and drug susceptibility tests are performed.

In Georgia, the NTP includes a network of local and regional laboratories that are monitored by and report to the NTP. These laboratories provide training for technicians in specific methods of preparing sputum smears for microscopic analysis, and in reading slides according to diagnostic categories that measure the rate of infection (by counting the number of bacteria in a smear). Many times during my extensive fieldwork in the laboratory, technicians from other regions of the country would undergo training at the NRL as part of their everyday work there.

For laboratory technicians, sputum samples provide a first order source of information that confirms the presence of bacteria with a level of authority that X-ray images no longer hold. As Lamara, who held a prominent administrative position at the NRL explained, this is largely for epidemiological reasons: "For society, someone like this [TB positive] may be very dangerous. It is very important for society because if there are positive cases and we do not know they are spreading the bacteria, they are a threat. So epidemiologically, it is very important to find if it is positive or negative. We cannot tell by X-ray."[47]

Mycobacterium tuberculosis is part of a larger family of what are called acid-fast bacteria (AFB), a type of bacteria that, because of its chemical makeup, takes up the red fuchsine dye that is used in the smearing and staining process, making the microbes visible. The goals of microscopic analysis of smeared sputum are to confirm the presence of AFB and to assess the patient's level of infectiousness. These tests are run not only at the point of initial diagnosis, but also after the first two months of treatment in order to determine the effectiveness of the medications and whether the level of bacteria present in the individual's sputum has changed. According to the WHO diagnosis, smear microscopy is ideal in resource-poor settings because the process is simple, does not require much equipment and diagnosis can be provided relatively quickly.[48]

There are a number of problems with the sputum smear approach, however. Many public health officials, such as Christopher Dye, coordinator of TB monitoring and evaluation at the WHO, argue that the test is outdated and inefficient. Microscopic analysis of smeared sputum has been the standard diagnostic for 100 years.[49] Another issue is that individuals are only given a definitive diagnosis after providing three samples, over three consecutive days.[50] This delays treatment and discourages individuals from visiting facilities, since they do not want others to know that they may have tuberculosis. Moreover, the accuracy of the test is up for debate. Some argue that with an emphasis on smears as the main diagnostic, up to 50 percent of positive cases remain undiagnosed.[51] This is the case, for example, in individuals who are also infected with HIV. In these instances (and others), the bacterium often spreads from the lungs into the bloodstream and other tissues. This reduces the number of bacterium in the sputum smear, often resulting in false negatives. Smears are often supplemented by X-ray; but this is similarly problematic because necessary equipment or expertise may be limited, causing technicians to see signs that the lung is being consumed. The narrow focus on the lungs may miss bacteria that is harboring in other tissues and organs, or that escapes detection because the infection has spread to the bloodstream and there is not enough bacteria present in sputum to produce a positive test result.[52]

Once smears have been read, lab technicians have enough information to know if someone's sputum has tested negative or positive for acid-fast bacteria. However, an accurate reading of a slide does not provide a total picture of health; nor does it establish the risks an individual may pose to family members and society at large. Many samples, especially those from prison, are cultured to confirm the presence of *Mycobacterium tuberculosis*. Because of the lab's limited resources, they use an "older" method of growing culture, which entails preparing egg-based media in test tubes and waiting eight weeks for cultures to grow.

Cultures also provide a large quantity of bacteria necessary to run drug susceptibility tests. However, in Georgia and other resource-poor settings, few, if any, labs are equipped (in terms of material and labor resources) to perform these tests. Moreover, because they cannot afford faster methods for testing drug susceptibility, test results are not available for at least three weeks.[53] These temporal factors bear serious consequences, including delayed diagnosis and treatment, minimal detection of drug resistant strains (that most countries cannot provide medicines for in any case) and thus the spread of resistant strains between individuals and populations.[54]

Among the most salient effects of standardization in the lab are the ways in which different procedures for manipulating sputum as a work object situate the patient in a larger public health picture in terms of severity of illness, curability, and risk posed to others. However, reliance upon support from donor and aid organizations creates a risk of dependency and uncertainty about the long-term availability of resources necessary for maintaining the technical aspects of DOTS. These issues permeate the DOTS network in Georgia, where challenges of securing access to a long-term supply of antibiotics and implementing the crucial "directly observed treatment" component of the protocol reflect further tensions over the implementation of rigid techniques and standards.

Accessing Antibiotics, Accessing Patients

Tuberculosis is understood as a widespread hazard to populations at large; the response of the WHO and other global organizations to the global TB crisis is one of containment and control—particularly control of the spread of contagions—even if it is not explicitly put that way. Such perceptions were expressed to me throughout my research.

During fieldwork in 2001, I met with Grigol, who at the time was the representative for GTZ in Georgia, overseeing the distribution of first-line antibiotics to the NTP in Tbilisi. From his perspective,

Tuberculosis is a danger not only for Georgia, but also for Europe and Germany, and Germany understands this. If we do not assist the Georgian national TB program, then [the TB epidemic] will get worse. The national TB program provides drugs, and drugs initiate resistant cases...therefore GTZ provides drugs, but [GTZ] is also responsible for monitoring drugs...but [monitoring drugs in Georgia] is difficult because there are not enough people to do all of this work, and they do not trust the people at the regional centers."[55]

As much as GTZ provides assistance in the tuberculosis sector, he went on to explain, they "cannot help with the drug-resistant cases, because they are only providing first-line drugs. No one provides second-line drugs in Georgia, because they are too expensive."[56] At that time, the NTP was unable to treat drug resistant tuberculosis, because of the tremendous demands DOTS-plus would place on the NTP and its supporters, as well as patients. However, in his words,

[The NTP] needs [a system for treating MDR-TB] because most chronic cases are drug resistant. However, the state cannot afford to treat this unless they have a TB program that has been in place and successful for several years. Otherwise, from the perspective of the state, concerning epidemiology and finances, the National TB Program does not yet show good results.[57]

This comment about a lack of "good results" referred to high rates of patients defaulting from the DOTS protocol in Georgia: many individuals did not finish the treatment regimen because they faced social stigma or could not access services. Interrupted treatment creates multidrug-resistant cases and suggests, according to my informant, that the NTP was not operating effectively at that time, resulting in a denial of increased support to treat MDR cases. "If a charity would provide second-line drugs, it would be great. However, at the time, no one was because this is a very high level of assistance. There is more assistance coming in at the level of primary healthcare. Multidrug-resistant tuberculosis is too specialized and too high level."[58]

Health professionals and public health advocates have demonstrated the opposite to be the case. For example, in Peru the NTP, U.S.–based Partners in Health, and Peru-based Socios en Salud launched a community-based program to diagnose and treat patients with MDR-TB.[59] By designing a flexible program, tailored to a specific setting and population, this coalition was able to successfully treat patients with MDR-TB. In this regard, they effectively argue that the primary reasons for preventing such measures are political and economic (rather than biomedical), given the high cost of second-line antibiotics used to treat drug-resistant strains, and the high infrastructural demands of administering DOTS or DOTS-plus.

Whether or not there is a reliable supply of antibiotics, cultural factors such as poverty and the social stigma associated with tuberculosis make it difficult for service providers to access patients, and for patients to conform to the protocol. Some of these difficulties arise from the fact that DOTS is tailored for systems organized around a primary health model, in which general practitioners perform initial diagnoses of tuberculosis and then refer patients to pulmonary specialists for DOTS services. In Georgia, however, tuberculosis services remain overwhelmingly specialized and unintegrated. As a result, in both rural and urban Georgia, many individuals who suspect that they have tuberculosis avoid going to specialized TB centers. To overcome some of these obstacles, the British-based organization Medical Relief International (MRLIN) supported a pilot project that integrated DOTS into a primary clinic in the Shida Karlti region of Georgia. During fieldwork in October 2003, I interviewed Catherine, a representative of MRLIN who had been overseeing the project. She confirmed that DOTS remained difficult to fulfill in Georgia because of stigma and access: "People don't want to stay in the hospital and they don't want to take a handful of antibiotics daily for six to nine months, especially once they start feeling better, usually after a couple of weeks."[60]

Because there is such a high number of staff within the healthcare and TB systems, in theory there are more than enough people who could be trained as DOTS nurses. But this is a job that requires the motivation to travel through the regions to get to people, many of whom are not welcoming. Moreover, salaries for DOTS nurses were to be provided through the Ministry of Labor, Health and Social Affairs; in Georgia, during the majority of my fieldwork trips, salaries provided by the state were minimal and rarely paid on time. DOTS nurses would have been required to pay out of pocket for transportation. It was therefore necessary for patients to travel to doctors. Catherine framed her concerns in social and economic terms:

Bear in mind that a pension is seven dollars a month [approximately 14 Georgian Lari at the time of fieldwork], and those who are unemployed don't receive their pension anyway. They're living in the villages, they haven't got any money, they've got food, some of them have food and it costs two Lari [approximately $1 USD] for a return journey into town. Forget it. And while doctors aren't being paid I'd like to think none of the doctors in Gori are asking for [additional] payments [from patients]. But I suspect that they are, and that pride is a factor. So with the cost of transport and with the potential cost of payment patients aren't continuing their treatment and there is a high default rate.[61]

Catherine also pointed to the ways in which stigma hinders the success of DOTS. The emphasis on DOTS makes patient populations highly visible in the community, especially in cases where DOTS nurses visit their homes on a daily basis. As a result, many people interrupt the treatment before they complete the full course of antibiotics, making them "defaulters" in the language of the DOTS protocol. Defaulting demands creativity on the part of the nurses:

We've got a couple of cars that go out each day to follow up with patients. This is terrifying some of the patients who get very angry and say they don't want other people to know that they've got TB. So it's a huge stigma thing. But our aim is really to get through this and cure patients within the community so that they can be seen to be curable. Then some of the stigma will gradually die down. But that is a lot of years ahead and it's a big big big job. We go out hunting to find our patients. Sometimes we get pretty cool receptions...and then there are others who are delighted when we come because they are completely down and they can't afford to get treatment. We are actually paying for bus rides as well to bring them into Gori.... So DOTS in Georgia is somewhat based on self administration by patients. Self administration in Georgia is, I think, is a very very dangerous thing.[62]

These dangers are not reducible to the recalcitrant behavior of "noncompliant" patients or physicians; they highlight the ways in which local forms of knowledge, expertise and everyday life challenge the effectiveness of DOTS as a purely technical intervention. In the capital city of Tbilisi, social stigma is a particularly salient factor in determining the extent to which DOTS is successful. In 2005, with support from USAID, U.S.-based Medical Services Corporation International (MSCI) opened several "DOTS Spots" in five densely populated areas of the city. At the time of fieldwork, these sites of service delivery were housed in general polyclinics—rather than specific TB clinics or hospitals—that patients can visit on their own to ingest the antituberculosis medicines under direct observation of a nurse. The introduction of the DOTS Spots—and the anonymity and flexibility they provide—has proven successful in improving treatment rates and lowering the number of "default" cases. Here, the conditions of success are at once economic and social, demonstrating the public health rewards of tailoring DOTS to work in particular social contexts.

When I visited two of the DOTS Spots in the Gldani region of Tbilisi in June 2005, I learned that in the city, this innovative approach has raised the rates of successful medicine distribution within the DOTS protocol from 22 to 95 percent. As the Georgian doctor who was project coordinator at the time explained to me, each facility is open from 9 o'clock in the morning until 5 o'clock at night, from Monday to Friday. Of the 800 tuberculosis patients registered in Tbilisi as out-patients at the time of writing, 150 are registered at DOTS Spots.[63] However, there remain numerous limitations to service delivery and to reversing widespread social stigma. Obstacles created by the implementation of DOTS in Georgia and broader reforms of "optimization" presuppose chaos and excess. Donors and others who intervene with much-needed aid and technical assistance encounter many barriers to the "optimization" of DOTS or more general health reform.

Diagnosing DOTS

The urgency reflected in the declaration of a global TB emergency, and the resultant global protocol for TB control, shed light both on how infectious diseases have become a problem of security and on possible implications of marshalling public health resources and policy interventions. At an extreme level, it would seem that protecting the "outside" world is one of the main factors motivating international donor and aid organizations to participate in TB control in the former Soviet Union, and that curing individuals is secondary. Using a case study about responses to tuberculosis in post-Soviet Georgia, I have argued that current global standards for TB management and treatment fall short on the ground in part because they do not take into account local cultural and infrastructural conditions.

The assertion that DOTS is purely a technical intervention that can be implemented in any context, which one could argue represents a general worldview shared by many international technical advisors whose work is integral to the institutional context of DOTS, reveals rigidity in "meeting standards" that may undermine the goals of the protocol and the efforts of local and international participants. In Georgia, for example, I have shown that cultural debates about what counts as expert knowledge, access to medicines, and overcoming obstacles such as poverty and social stigma that create barriers between health service providers and patients are particularly salient in the success or failure of DOTS implementation.

To be sure, as a global, standardized response to the TB epidemic, DOTS is urgently needed; and antituberculosis medicines distributed according to the DOTS protocol do provide an effective means of curing infectious cases and halting the spread of infection. Furthermore, Georgia and other former Soviet republics are desperately in need of a wide range of resources, including guidelines for health management and administration, which international aid and donor organizations provide. It is equally imperative that many resources go to establishing the primary healthcare system. My goal here has not been to suggest otherwise. This is evident in the contemporary moment, when (largely donor-sourced) spending and national foreign policy concerns for infectious diseases and global health have increased to unprecedented levels.[64]

Deploying ethnographic tools and perspectives, I have examined the ways in which these standardized protocols, definitions, and modes of knowledge production such as DOTS conflict with a local environment in which the technical aspects of the protocol are in tension with local ecologies of knowledge and experience. Because of these tensions, successful diagnosis and treatment of people living with tuberculosis may be undermined. What remains to be seen is how the urgency of the situation continues to impact the quality and availability of tools and forms of expertise, as well as how the solutions proposed to mitigate crisis and danger sustain or challenge the ways in which certain regions of the world and vulnerable populations bear both the burden and blame of infectious disease.

NOTES

1 MDR-TB refers to strains of *Mycobacterium tuberculosis* that are resistant to at least isoniazid and rifampicin, the two most powerful first-line anti-TB drugs currently in use.

2 Erin Koch, *Free Market Tuberculosis: Georgia and the Management of Disease after the Fall of the Soviet Union* (unpublished book manuscript). The larger study is based on sixteen months of fieldwork that I conducted during the following time periods: 2000 (April); 2001 (March–December); 2002 (May–July); 2003 (October); 2005 (June); and 2007–2008 (December–January). Research consisted of interviews with scientists, healthcare workers, administrators and representatives of international donor and aid organizations. I also conducted participant-observation research with affiliates of Georgia's National Tuberculosis Program (NTP), at the National TB Reference Lab (NRL), in clinics, at training sessions for health professionals, and in the prison sector where tuberculosis cases concentrate. In this essay, I use only first names when I use pseudonyms.

3 Koch, *Free Market Tuberculosis*. Among the general constraints are the ways in which the direct observation aspect of the protocol is experienced as patronizing by healthcare workers and patients and also perpetuates stigma, not to mention the physical side effects of the antibiotics and the economic constraints that the protocol entails.

4 Lawrence K. Altman, "Drug-Resistant TB Rates Soar in Former Soviet Regions," *New York Times* (February 27, 2008). Accessed at http://www.nytimes.com/2008/02/27/health/27tb.html?scp=1&sq=Altman+TB&st=nyt on February 27, 2008.

5 Ibid.

6 Roy R. Chadury and Urmila Thatte, "Beyond DOTS: Avenues Ahead in the Management of Tuberculosis," *National Medical Journal of India* 16, no. 6 (November–December 2003): 321–7; Ziad Obermeyer, Jesse Abbot-Klafter, and Christopher J. L. Murray, "Has the DOTS Strategy Improved Case Finding or Treatment Success? An Empirical Assessment," *PLoS ONE* 3, no. 3 (2008), accessed at e1721.d oi:10.1371/journal.pone.0001721 on March 12, 2008; John Porter, Kelley Lee and Jessica Ogden, "The Globalisation of DOTS: Tuberculosis as a Global Emergency," in *Health Policy in a Globalising World,* ed. K. Lee, K. Buse and S. Fustukian (Cambridge: Cambridge University Press), 181–94.

7 Lincoln Chen and Vasant Narasimhan, "A Human Security Agenda for Global Health," in *Global Health Challenges for Human Security,* ed. L. Chen, J. Leaning and V. Narasimhan (Cambridge, MA: Harvard University Press, 2003), 3–10.

8 Kenji Shibuya, "Health Problems as Security Risks: Global Burden of Disease Assessment" in Chen et al., eds., 209.

9 Jennifer Brower and Peter Chalk, *The Global Threat of New and Reemerging Infectious Diseases: Reconciling U.S. National Security and Public Health Policy* (Los Angeles: The Rand Corporation, 2003), 3.

10 David L. Heyman, "Evolving Infectious Disease Threats to National and Global Security" in Chen et al., *Global Health Challenges,* 106.

11 Ian Harper, "Interconnected and Inter-infected: DOTS and the Stabilisation of the Tuberculosis Programme in Nepal," in *The Aid Effect: Giving and Governing in International Development,* ed. D. Mosse and D. Lewis (London and Ann Arbor: Pluto Press, 2005), 139.

12 Heyman, "Evolving Infectious Disease Threats to National and Global Security," 113.

13 Brower and Chalk, *The Global Threat of New and Reemerging Infectious Diseases,* 7–10. Brower and Chalk outline six ways in which this occurs. While their framework and larger analysis merit lengthier discussion and debate, I only note them here. First, disease is a threat to human life. Second, epidemics may threaten political stability, especially if confidence in the state is called into question. Third, infectious diseases negatively impact the economy and impose financial burdens that may lead to further instability. Fourth, the functioning of state apparati may be compromised. Fifth, political and social instabilities may emerge at a regional level during epidemics. Sixth, microbes may play a significant role in bioweaponry or bioterrorist events.

14 Matthew Gandy and Alimuddin Zumla, "Introduction," in *The Return of the White Plague: Global Poverty and the 'New' Tuberculosis,* ed. M. Gandy and A. Zumla (London and New York: Verso Books, 2003), 7–14.

15 Pranaya Mishra, Ebba H. Hansen, Svend Sabroe, et al., "Socio-economic Status and Adherence to Tuberculosis Treatment: A Case-Control Study in a District of Nepal," *International Journal of Tuberculosis and Lung Disease* 9, no. 10 (October 2005): 1134–1139. Only 5 to 10 percent of those infected will become actively sick, a process that is directly linked to poverty. This percentage does not include individuals who are HIV–positive and much more likely to become actively sick if infected with the TB bacillus.

16 Statistics from the World Health Organization. Accessed at http://www.who.int/mediacentre/factsheets/fs104/en/index.html on March 16, 2008.

17 XDR-TB (extensively drug-resistant TB) are strains that are multidrug-resistant TB (MDR-TB) plus resistance to (i) any fluoroquinolone (a class of antibiotics that inhibit DNA replication and transcription in the microbe), and (ii) at least 1 of 3 injectable second-line drugs capreomycin, kanamycin, amikacin (new definition agreed October 2006), World Health Organization. Accessed at www.who.int/tb on March 16, 2008.

18 World Health Organization, *Anti-Tuberculosis Drug Resistance in the World, Report No. 4* (February 26, 2008): 16. Accessed at http://www.who.int/tb/publications/2008/drs_report4_26feb08.pdf on March 2, 2008.

19 Altman, "Drug-Resistant TB Rates Soar in Former Soviet Regions"; WHO, *Anti-Tuberculosis Drug Resistance in the World, Report No. 4.*

20 Mario C. Raviglione and Ian M. Smith, "XDR Tuberculosis—Implications for Global Public Health," *The New England Journal of Medicine* 356, no. 7 (February 15, 2007): 656–9.

21 Lee B. Reichman with Janice Hopkins Tanne, *Timebomb: The Global Epidemic of Multi-Drug Resistant Tuberculosis* (New York: McGraw Hill, 2001), 176.

22 Jim Y. Kim, Joyce V. Millen, Alec Irwin and John Gershman, eds. *Dying for Growth: Global Inequality and the Health of the Poor* (Monroe, ME: Common Courage Press, 2000).

23 Lee B. Reichman, "Defusing the Global Timebomb," *Journal of Public Health Policy* 26, no. 1 (April 2005): 117 (emphasis in original).

24 In the majority of cases, treatment under DOTS consists of two phases: an intensive phase of two months and a continuation phase of four to six months. During the former, patients take medicines 3–5 days a week until they are no longer contagious. During the latter, the prescription of antibiotics is reduced. If an individual does not convert from positive to negative in sputum smear analysis after 2 months of

intensive treatment, this phase of the regimen may be extended for a third month.

25 For similar analyses see Gene Buckhman, *Reform and Resistance in Post-Soviet Tuberculosis Control,* Doctoral Dissertation, University of Arizona (2001); Harper, "Interconnected and Inter-infected."

26 WHO, *Anti-Tuberculosis Drug Resistance in the World, Report No. 4.* The persistence of TB and various resistant strains, as well as widespread limits of the DOTS protocol (especially in sub-Saharan Africa and Eastern Europe) have encouraged new collaborations in management and R&D for vaccines and treatments. In 2006, a new approach to TB control, the Stop TB Strategy, was adopted by the WHO and the Stop TB Partnership. In this strategy, DOTS expansion and enhancement is one of six components. Nonetheless, the DOTS approach remains the cornerstone of alleviating the global burden of tuberculosis.

27 Aihwa Ong, *Neoliberalism as Exception: Mutations in Citizenship and Sovereignty* (Durham and London: Duke University Press, 2005), 6 (emphasis in original).

28 Porter, Lee and Ogden, "The Globalisation of DOTS," 190–91.

29 Personal communication, Peter (pseudonym), Medical Service Corporation International (MSCI), Tbilisi, Georgia, October 16, 2003.

30 Ian Harper, "Anthropology, DOTS, and Understanding Tuberculosis Control in Nepal," *Journal of Biosocial Science* 38 (2006): 57–67.

31 World Health Organization, *Global Tuberculosis Control: Surveillance, Planning, Financing* (Geneva: WHO, 2008); Paul Farmer and David Walton, "The Social Impact of Multidrug-resistant Tuberculosis: Haiti and Peru," in Gandy and Zumla, eds., 163–177; WHO, *Anti-Tuberculosis Drug Resistance in the World, Report No. 4.* According to WHO estimates for Georgia in

2006 (the most recent data available) there were approximately 50–99 new cases per 100,000 people. This is compared to 0–24 in the United States, 100–299 in Russia, and more than 300 new cases per 100,000 people in Sub-Saharan Africa. With an estimated population of 4.5 million, these numbers in Georgia are comparatively low. However, the actual rates of new cases annually are increasing, while the percentage of case detection is not necessarily improving.

32 Richard Zalesky, Farman Abdullajev, George Khechinashvili, et al., "Tuberculosis Control in the Caucasus: Successes and Constraints in DOTS Implementation," *International Journal of Tuberculosis and Lung Disease* 3, no. 5 (May 1999): 394–401; A. I. Lapina, "The Development of Tuberculosis Control in the USSR," *Bulletin of the International Union Against Tuberculosis* 43 (1970): 188–92.

33 Mikhail I. Perelman, "Tuberculosis in Russia," *International Journal of Tuberculosis and Lung Disease* 4, no. 12 (December 2000): 1097–1103.

34 During interviews I repeatedly heard that it is difficult to know what the rates of tuberculosis were for much of the seventy years of Soviet administration. Under-reporting the number of TB cases during the Soviet regime was common. Doctors who reported actual numbers of cases faced job loss, expulsion from their community, and other punishments, because high rates of tuberculosis reflected badly on the Soviet state and medical infrastructure.

35 Personal communication, Iveri (pseudonym), ICRC, Tbilisi, Georgia, July 17, 2001.

36 David Gzirishvili and Gegi Mataradze, *Healthcare Reform in Georgia* (Tbilisi: UNDP, 1999). At the time of writing, GTZ was still supplying first-line anti-TB drugs to Georgia. This program is administered by GOPA, a German develop-

ment consulting firm, and financed by KfW, a German banking group. They have committed to supplying these antibiotics to the NTP through 2009 (Personal communication, director of NTP Tbilisi, December 25, 2007).

37 Personal communication, Archil Salakaia, National Center for Tuberculosis and Lung Disease, Tbilisi, Georgia, December 25, 2007. DOTS-plus is the protocol designed by the WHO for treating MDR-TB.

38 Salmaan Keshavjee and Mercedes C. Becerra, "Disintegrating Health Services and Resurgent Tuberculosis in Post-Soviet Tajikistan: An Example of Structural Violence," *JAMA* 283, no. 9 (March 2000): 1201.

39 Personal communication, Paata (pseudonym), Betsy's Hotel, Tbilisi, Georgia, 2001.

40 Erin Koch, "Recrafting Georgian Medicine: The Politics of Standardization and Tuberculosis Control in Postsocialist Georgia," in *Caucasus Paradigms: Anthropologies, Histories, and the Making of a World Area,* ed. Bruce Grant and Lale Yalçin-Heckmann, Halle Studies in the Anthropology of Eurasia (Münster: LIT Verlag, 2007), 247–272.

41 Elizabeth Dunn, "Standards and Person-Making in East Central Europe," in *Global Assemblages: Technology, Politics, and Ethics as Anthropological Problems,* ed. Aihwa Ong and Stephen J. Collier (Oxford: Blackwell, 2004), 173–193.

42 Personal communication, Revaz (pseudonym), NTP, Tbilisi, Georgia, March 29, 2001.

43 Several administrators explained this situation to me, emphasizing that it is not possible for them to stay as guests with doctors while conducting supervisory visits. Occupying the role of guest in Georgia, hosted by those they are monitoring, would risk compromising their objective position, as generous hosts might expect a generous evaluation in return.

44 Maryline Bonnet, Vinciane Sizaire, Yared Kebede et al., "Does One Size Fit All? Drug Resistance and Standard Treatments: Results of Six Tuberculosis Programmes in Former Soviet Countries," *International Journal of Tuberculosis and Lung Disease* 9, no. 10 (October 2005): 1147–1154.

45 World Health Organization and the International Committee of the Red Cross, *Guidelines for the Control of Tuberculosis in Prisons* (Geneva: WHO, 2000).

46 Ian Harper, "Interconnected and Interinfected," 137.

47 Personal communication, Lamara (pseudonym), NTP, Tbilisi, Georgia, May 17, 2001.

48 World Health Organization, *Treatment of Tuberculosis: Guidelines for National Programs, Third Edition* (Geneva: WHO, 2003).

49 Quoted in Emma Marris, "From TB Tests, Just a 'Yes or No' Answer, Please," *Nature Medicine* 13, no. 3 (March 2007): 267.

50 Obtaining three separate samples from a single patient over three days is challenging, especially if the individual is stigmatized or cannot afford transportation to the lab, as is the case for many people in Georgia and around the world. For this reason, the WHO has reduced the required number of samples from three to two. At the time of writing, these recommendations have not yet been fully adopted in Georgia.

51 Marris, "From TB Tests, Just a 'Yes or No' Answer, Please," 267.

52 Ibid.

53 At the time of writing the NRL was in the process of adopting a much more rapid method for growing cultures and running drug susceptibility tests. Although these methods provide test results in a fraction of the time they are much more labor-intensive, and stretch the temporal work demands of the laboratory technicians very thin (personal communication,

Tbilisi, Georgia, December 2007 and January 2008).

54 Raviglione and Smith, "XDR Tuberculosis."

55 Personal communication, Grigol (pseudonym), NTP, Tbilisi, Georgia, October 31, 2001.

56 Ibid.

57 Ibid.

58 Ibid.

59 Sonya Shin, Jennifer Furin, Jamie Bayona, et al., "Community-based Treatment of Multi-drug-resistant Tuberculosis in Lima, Peru: 7

Years of Experience," *Social Science and Medicine* 59, no. 7 (July 2004): 1529–1539.

60 Personal communication, Catherine (pseudonym), NTP, Tbilisi, Georgia, October 2003.

61 Ibid.

62 Ibid.

63 Personal communication, Lela (pseudonym), MSCI, Tbilisi, Georgia, June 13, 2005.

64 Laurie Garrett, "The Challenge of Global Health," *Foreign Affairs* 86, no. 1 (January/February 2007).

CHAPTER SIX

Vital Mobility and the Humanitarian Kit

Peter Redfield

"Speed saves lives."
—*MSF fundraising brochure, 2005*

As numerous commentators have noted, graphic moments of human suffering elsewhere play a significant role in contemporary moral and political imagination.[1] Once reported and framed as a humanitarian emergency, disasters worldwide now regularly elicit calls for action, and both the affected communities and those experiencing anguish secondhand through the wonders of global media commonly expect a response. But what might it actually entail to try to protect the well-being of distant populations? What techniques and logics might be involved, in order for the expectation of a response to become a norm? And how might they relate to security concerns focused on matters of life?

In this chapter I approach "biosecurity" from the perspective of medical humanitarianism, particularly the dramatic form featured in contemporary crisis response. Such a vantage point alters the field of assumptions surrounding biological emergencies such as outbreak diseases from those of a defensive model of national public health to a more altruistic, international vision of medical care. Although actively involved in responding to epidemics worldwide, and deploying similar strategies and equipment to those of military and public health authorities, medical humanitarian organizations do not commonly think through the category of "biosecurity." For the humanitarian actor, the problem of securing populations and vital infrastructure is not primarily a matter of self-interest or defensive strategy. Rather, it involves a concern for others, even very distant others, and their continuing welfare. Considering "security" from this perspective may reorient the schema laid out by Stephen Collier and Andrew Lakoff in several ways.[2] First, it shifts the focus one step away from the nation-state, given that intergovernmental and nongovernmental entities play significant roles in defining and enacting humanitarian projects. Second, it also moves concerns about people and things one step closer to the domain of ethics, to the extent that humanitarian conceptions of suffering commonly and overtly mobilize discourses about good, evil, and moral obligation. And finally, if the horizon is truly global, it both enlarges and diminishes the sense of infrastructure involved, amplifying the degree of mobility essential to achieving care from a distance even as it reduces the sense of "life" to a minimal proportion of needs. The populations in question here are generally poor and often displaced, the states weak or fractured, and the material conditions limited and fragile even before any state of emergency. The sense of welfare involved is often that of physical survival, not any social fulfillment. The humanitarian project, at least in this "classic" form, then, constitutes a work of minimalism.

I will try to outline these general points by reference to one story of preparedness: the development and limitations of the humanitarian "kit." The kit is a mobile repository of potentially useful implements. Forms of it feature in the long history of military equipment and logistics, as well as craft production. Humble medical versions are common features of private and public, stored in small boxes found in closets, automobiles, aircraft, schools, and many other nonmedical settings in anticipation of minor emergencies. The humanitarian form is particularly interesting in that it casts the problem of "first aid" at a more global level. As primary protagonist for this story, I will feature the organization I have tracked on and off since 2000: Médecins Sans Frontières, otherwise known as Doctors Without Borders, or MSF.[3] MSF is hardly the only entity to develop or use kits in humanitarian work. However, it offers the advantage of embodying humanitarian ambition in global terms, and doing so in an oppositional, restless, and frequently innovative way. Emerging in response to the older Red Cross movement, MSF both carries forward a longer tradition and marks a break within it. Although the scope of the group's action now extends far wider, emergency response defined its primary technical and ethical ethos, and continues to inflect its public image. Moreover, the bulk of MSF's projects unfold in places that public health describes as "resource-poor settings," places, in other words, without much health infrastructure. Due to its rebellious self-conception, MSF also produces a steady stream of external and internal criticism, commenting on humanitarian shortcomings while also seeking to provide aid. Thus MSF can serve as a barometer of sorts for a wider field. The story of medical logistics outlined here, I suggest, is thus both particular and particularly telling.

Even as humanitarian-inspired operations proliferate, and versions of their associated technologies appear in all manner of agencies, MSF's wider experience also reveals the limits of the kit form itself. Embodying essential techniques of mobility, a standardized package performs well in emergencies and outbreaks, but falters when facing chronic conditions. What works for a rapid health threat like cholera cannot encompass a slower disorder like AIDS, which requires longer-term intervention in a wider social milieu. The point is both obvious and always in danger of being overlooked, particularly by those seeking quick technical solutions. If something like the mobile medical kit didn't already exist, biosecurity advocates with global ambitions would have to invent it. Yet not all health risks come in the form of sudden outbreaks, any more than risk in general spreads evenly across the world's population. The antipolitical political space that humanitarianism claims remains a special case, not a general model for strategic action. As members of MSF well know, the politics and ethics of health extend beyond the seductive and significant metric of "saving lives."

"Populations in Danger"

"Nobody should die from cholera."
—MSF fundraising letter, March 2007

MSF often uses the phrase "populations in danger" to identify its primary object of concern. Appearing across numerous internal and public events and documents (including an occasional book series published since 1992), the expression combines categorical concern for human suffering with a realistic commitment to evaluation.[4] Like the group's related tradition of annually listing the top ten "underreported" crises, MSF's identification of populations in danger claims a degree of authoritative expertise, one motivated by humanitarian principle rather than political interest.

It is, in this sense, a properly medical opinion, cast on a world scale out of human interest, rather than technical curiosity alone. Monitoring the globe as a concerned, independent observer, the group sees dangers to human life and welfare in many directions. The most recent volume in MSF's series brims with potential disaster.[5] Ordinary people can be threatened by warlords (Liberia) or by strong states (U.S. action in Afghanistan and Iraq). They may be hurt by a shortage of international attention (Democratic Republic of Congo) or by the misappropriation of humanitarian aid (North Korea, Sudan). In addition to suffering derived from human conflict and displacement, MSF also worries about potential outbreaks of disease, both exotic and mundane. And it is increasingly concerned about general issues of biomedical infrastructure, including discriminatory policies of pharmaceutical pricing, and the general lack of medicines for unprofitable conditions. In terms of categories like "security, territory and population," then, the frame is strikingly large and the threats quite varied.[6]

Beyond efforts to sway public opinion, MSF also practices "frontline" medicine, mounting projects almost anywhere in the world it deems sufficiently endangered and to which it can gain access. In the case of crisis situations such as sudden population displacements or disease outbreaks, the goal is to arrive on site as quickly as possible, with sufficient equipment to be effective. To quote a line from fundraising material used by MSF–USA, "speed saves lives." Although the slogan made some veteran members of the larger organization wince when I mentioned it to them, it does capture the essential logic of emergency response. Since MSF casts itself as global organization, it needs to travel across all sorts of terrain when pursuing emergency projects. The core technical challenge facing this variety of humanitarian medicine, then, is that of mobility, and the rapid, seamless transfer of enough equipment to operate. Unsurprisingly, the group has developed considerable expertise in logistics. To better frame this logistical tradition, I will sketch elements of the larger organizational history from which it emerged.

The Geopolitics of Suffering, "Sans Frontières"

For all that the Holocaust shadows contemporary conceptions of human suffering and disaster, it is important to remember that Auschwitz was never televised or framed as a "humanitarian crisis" in the manner it might be today.[7] The close of the Second World War may have ushered in a new political configuration, along with categories and institutions for its governance, but its massive relief works transpired in a less visual and instantaneous era of communications. Rather, the conventional demarcation for televised suffering is that of the Biafran war in Nigeria at the end of the 1960s, when satellite broadcast brought starvation into middle-class living rooms worldwide. Whatever the actual causal history of that tragic episode, it provoked reflection and reorganization on the part of a number of existing humanitarian organizations and inspired the formation of others.[8]

By the time of Biafra, the Red Cross movement had been in existence for a century, even if its efforts to transform military medical practice and international law rarely addressed colonial settings.[9] The slow dismantling of empire, however, created a new humanitarian terrain for the second half of the twentieth century. As the United Nations expanded fitfully into an institutional framework for international governance, it enlarged expectations, if not always results. At the same time the development of emergency medicine out of military medicine (institutionalized in the French context by the establishment of a national service known as the Service d'Aide Médicale Urgente [SAMU] in the 1960s), along with the routinization of air travel and rapid transport, extended the scope of potential action.[10] Suffering, whether near or far, could now elicit expectations of response.

MSF itself appeared at the end of 1971 in Paris, when journalists from a medical publication helped bring together a small group of doctors who had volunteered for the French Red Cross in the Biafran conflict in Nigeria and a similar group with a background in Bangladesh. Troubled by their experience of ineffectual and constrained relief work, they sought to establish an independent alternative to the Red Cross, unfettered by the constraints of national and international mandates, and hence free to be daring (and, some hoped, outspoken). At the outset MSF existed largely on paper, but by the end of the decade it had mounted a number of short interventions into areas afflicted by natural disasters and war as well as achieving greater prominence within France by launching a publicity campaign around the slogan, "Two billion people in their waiting room."[11] The ambition of aid now stood grandly global.

Although the ethos of MSF proved thoroughly antiestablishmentarian, and a number of its prominent members had backgrounds of political activism, the organization presented itself as an alternative to both anticolonial and Cold War loyalties. Rejecting all justification for civilian suffering, it would oppose the French intellectual romance of "third worldism" and denounce leftist regimes that proved inhumane. Amid the disillusionment of post-1968 France and the evident excesses of state socialism, MSF offered the prospect of ethical action to defend the life and well-being of ordinary people. A "rebellious" form of humanitarianism would be both nonaligned and thoroughly engaged through the practice of medicine. Bernard Kouchner, the charismatic one-time student activist instrumental in the group's founding, could thus discover both himself and the third world as a physician, practicing "without illusion." Rony Brauman, his most prominent successor within the organization, could similarly trade Maoism for clinical work in Benin and Thailand, redirecting his militant sensibilities from the streets to refugee camps.[12]

Even as MSF found its calling, the geopolitics of the Cold War struggle shifted increasingly in the direction of proxy wars after the end of U.S. involvement in Vietnam.[13] In the paralyzing shadow of nuclear apocalypse, irregular armies fought savagely in settings like Angola, Afghanistan, and Mozambique during the 1970s and 1980s. These confrontations only enhanced the international flow of conventional weaponry, fueling ancillary conflicts and alliances, while prompting the displacement of civilian populations. The number of refugees worldwide grew exponentially during these decades, providing a surplus of humanitarian need well beyond the capacity of UN agencies. A nongovernmental group with a global vision thus had plenty of opportunity to offer medical assistance.

Three early engagements were particularly formative for MSF. First, the exodus of boat people from Vietnam, combined with mass suffering in Cambodia under the Khmer Rouge, set the ground for an ethics of action that prioritized "humanity" over political ideology. As longtime opponents Raymond Aron and Jean Paul Sartre marched together in Paris, young MSF volunteers worked in refugee camps in Thailand, becoming radicalized through encounters with suffering rather than revolution. Even though the group would experience loud squabbles and schisms alongside growth, the different factions continued to share this common perspective. Next, the Soviet invasion of Afghanistan only further confirmed the French humanitarian break with socialism. MSF undertook clandestine missions in the Afghan mountains, experiencing its own romance of third world solidarity alongside the mujahideen. Finally, during the mid-1980s famine in Ethiopia, the original French branch of MSF found itself evicted after denouncing the Derg regime's policy of forced resettlement. The episode, which resonated amid the televised glamour of *Live Aid*, established the group's outspoken reputation and willingness to oppose all political orders that produced suffering. At the same time, MSF faced criticism of its own, suggesting that it was an amateurish organization, long on hot air but short on actual capacity. The charges stung enough that MSF redoubled its efforts to improve its technical abilities.[14] By the end of the decade it had in place both a new logistics system and an epidemiological subsidiary. Soon it would be known not only for taking oppositional positions, but also for fulfilling its rhetorical claims to speed and efficiency.

Limits and Anticipation in Uganda, 1980–1986

What would effective humanitarian action actually entail at a material level? To illustrate the technical problems involved, I will focus briefly on another case from the early 1980s, that of Uganda. Uganda was never a central front in the Cold War, though its post-independence turmoil had deeper colonial and regional roots behind the rise and fall of Idi Amin.[15] Nonetheless, the Ugandan period of crisis occurred at a transitional moment, and holds the comparative advantage of combining a less mythic profile with widely recognized deficiencies.

At the beginning of the 1980s, the Karamoja and West Nile regions of the country experienced extreme famine. The crisis in Karamoja, an arid area bordering Kenya and peopled largely by seminomadic, photogenic cattle herders with a fierce reputation, received a good deal of media attention, and a number of aid agencies responded to the images of starvation by rushing teams and materials into the field. Amid the greater aftermath of the fall of Idi Amin, the general situation in Uganda was, in the words of a UNICEF official of the time, "at best chaotic," and the relief operation quickly encountered a host of problems. Subsequent analysis by a group of scholars and humanitarian workers identified a long list of specific setbacks as well as some general issues: lack of coordination and turf struggles between different organizations (and even branches of the same organization), a greater landscape of need extending beyond the targeted recipients of aid, and the "disaster within a disaster" of food supply and the greater infrastructure of logistics required for its movement and distribution.[16] A former representative of another UN agency observed that many of the people who had been alongside her in Uganda had participated in major relief operations elsewhere over the previous decade, and their discussions identified a repeated pattern of failure: "One of the recurring themes was that time and time again the same problem arose in every disaster situation: logistics."[17] She imagined creating a "strike force" of reservists within the UN system, a cadre of experienced professionals with access to stockpiles of equipment, who would be ready to leave at a moment's notice. The UNICEF official similarly concluded that responses like this must be "quick, rational and experienced" rather than "prolonged, irrational and nonexperienced," but doubted that his own agency, created for long-term activities, would be suitable for the task: "To use a metaphor, such a rapid shift in activities and allocation would amount to demanding a shipping company to turn into an airline overnight."[18]

Included among the many organizations briefly present in both the Karamoja and West Nile crises was MSF. At the time it was not yet ten years old and still a relatively minor, if flamboyant, entity in the world of humanitarian affairs. The missions to Uganda were its first in a famine zone, and not a particular success. As a lead participant dryly noted in an interview with me years later, "in that era we improvised; later we became more efficient."[19] The group's bulletin report at the time summed up the general situation with one graphic image: a bullet-ridden bulldozer sitting useless, its brand new tires stolen by raiders to make sandals.[20] Within a decade, however, MSF had grown into a large and complex organization, fully capable of both technical innovation and logistical efficiency in crisis settings. Its professional system of logistics guidelines and kits embodied the UN administrator's vision of a global humanitarian strike force.

Indeed, MSF already saw its mission in something like those terms. At the time of the Karamoja famine, it had just survived a schism in which a number of its original members, including the future French political figure Bernard Kouchner, lost a power struggle and subsequently established another group known as Médecins du Monde (Doctors of the World, or MDM). There are a number of possible ways to understand this split in terms of personalities and political differences. But the stated ambition of those who now controlled MSF was to make it a more effective organization, favoring greater pragmatism over symbolic protest.[21] This ambition was to prove remarkably productive. Not only would MSF grow from its French base into an international movement, but it would also establish a technical template for expanding humanitarian operations at the end of the Cold War.[22]

Before proceeding to a description and analysis of MSF's technical florescence, however, I will first introduce an additional layer of background. To understand the nature of the apparatus MSF eventually set in place, as well as its spatial significance and temporal politics, it is helpful to return to the Second World War, and the advent of large-scale aerial warfare and the landscape of destruction it produced. Humanitarian logistics has many obvious lines of descent, from military supply lines to industrial food distribution; but the need for a portable medical infrastructure became critically visible amid the rubble of European cities during the 1940s. A key antecedent for this third world story thus appears in the fading centers of empire, newly pulverized by waves of bombers.

A Prototype: *Materia Medica Minimalis*

Amid the devastation of the Second World War, the newly formed Joint Relief Commission of the International Red Cross (JRCIRC) faced a significant technical problem. Created to coordinate the efforts of the Red Cross's mosaic of national societies with those of the Swiss-based International Commission of the Red Cross (ICRC), the commission found itself at a loss in the face of massive aerial bombardments that left civilian populations in urban centers medically bereft:

> "There is a total lack of medical supplies here." It was by a summary appeal of this kind that the Joint Relief Commission of the International Red Cross was asked in the beginning of its activities to send medical relief to a capital which had just undergone an air raid. Such a request, put so tersely, left us somewhat nonplussed. What should be sent? What medicaments would be required by a large city which had been devastated by an air attack? What quantity of each medicament would be required? No statistics were there to enlighten us, no document on the problem was available. We had to improvise.[23]

How best to provision a landscape of total devastation? Most urgently, what medications to provide when the entire health infrastructure was knocked out? The commission first surveyed the national Red Cross societies about the medical requirements of their respective countries. The response was, however, "surprisingly diverse, one might almost say, disconcerting." No simple, uniform agreement could be found. Therefore the commission took it upon itself to quickly marshal medical experience and science, in an effort to determine what was "absolutely indispensable to ensure medical care and to meet the emergency needs of a population which has been deprived of food and medical supplies."[24] Newly sensitized to local culture, the commission also took note of the fact that national preferences and therapeutics both varied across the European continent. The Red Cross, then, needed a document that would be simultaneously encompassing and precise, allowing for regional differences and yet conducive to medical and pharmacological accuracy.

The condensed result was entitled *Materia Medica Minimalis* (*MMM*). Produced in Latin, it was subsequently published in French, German, and English editions. The inherited tongue of Rome served as a convenient means of scientific expression, the collective authors of the text explained, being "a language which does not confine to any frontiers and which unites all minds that have grown up in the culture of the classic world."[25] Balancing this scholarly touch with a quartermaster's eye for practical detail, the authors offered estimated quantities necessary to treat a "population unit" of one hundred thousand persons for six months. They based their estimates on the consumption of medicaments in Switzerland, recognizing that these figures may prove controversial and require alterations. Given the urgent need to be immediately useful, however, they ventured into the messy realm of calculation. Recognizing that "circumstances and difficulties" may affect actual delivery, they further divided the *MMM* into two categories, the first of which should receive the greatest priority. The list itself included only the pharmaceutical end of medical supplies; bandages, cotton and surgical instruments were to be handled in separate consignments.[26] Nonetheless, its content lived up to its name in defining a baseline state of medical infrastructure.

The *MMM* marks a catalytic moment in humanitarian thinking. Although the Red Cross's international meetings had addressed a variety of training activities related to medical techniques in the past, with the *MMM* it was now constructing a mobile template for crisis response around a principle of flexible standardization. The final report of the commission composed after the war mused that "[t]his work, which was called into existence by the needs of the moment, possessed a usefulness which it seemed would outlast the war period," an assessment that would prove prophetic.[27] For although the *MMM* may not have directly become an icon of relief work, its conceptual descendents proliferated in the coming decades. As the zone of crisis recognition shifted beyond Europe, the reconstruction of a minimal bio-medical infrastructure emerged as a central problem for all manner of disasters in resource-poor settings. Effective medical assistance required basic equipment and guidelines, preferably prepared in advance.

Standardization: The Moment of the Kit

When MSF reoriented its logistics system in the middle of the 1980s, it focused on creating modular, standardized kits. The concept of the kit itself has a long military and medical history. The *Oxford English Dictionary* suggests that by the late eighteenth century the English term had expanded from a wooden vessel or container to indicate the collection of articles in a soldier's bag. An equipment case or chest had long been the steady companion of naval surgeons and other mobile healers, and by the early twentieth century groups like the Red Cross assembled first aid kits. MSF's variant would be more comprehensive and ambitious: collections of supplies designed for a particular need and preassembled into a combined package. These packages could then be stockpiled and shipped rapidly to any emergency destination in the world. As an MSF catalogue later summarized the approach: "A kit contains the whole of the needed equipment for filling a given function. Intended for emergency contexts, it is ready to be delivered within a very short time frame."[28] Thus the diffuse problem of acquisition was effectively translated into a concentrated one of transportation, more easily solved from a central office. Essential materials no longer had to be hastily assembled anew in response to every crisis, or uncertainly negotiated on the ground amid fluctuating availability, quality, and price. Moreover, by preassembling materials with a checklist, the kit could function as a form of materialized memory, whereby previous experience extends directly into every new setting without having to be actively recalled. For an organization built around both crisis settings and a constantly shifting workforce of volunteers and temporary employees, such continuity would prove especially valuable.[29]

The kit system was the product of a small number of early MSF masterminds, now receding into organizational legend. Its immediate origin lay in the experience of a French pharmacist responsible for Cambodian refugee camps on the border of Thailand in 1980. Guerilla raids from there led to periodic Vietnamese bombing runs, whereupon the Thai army would seal the camps, preventing access for several days at a time. In due course the MSF teams learned to assemble essential equipment until they had the process down to a system. As the main protagonist recalled, this evolved less from any grand design than the banal practice of packing a bag for a series of weekend trips, and translating the experience into anticipatory habit:

> The kit, it's nothing more than someone who's leaving for the weekend [would take]...who needs his backpack with something to drink, something to eat, something to put on his feet if they get sore. He needs all that. So, how does he do it? The first time he imagines what will happen, and assembles his bag with that imagination. And then after that first experience, he sees that there are things that didn't amount to much and others he was missing. And then after the second, third time, he'll finally have a perfect bundle and he prepares it before the weekend, checks it, and then leaves and it works.[30]

The head of that mission went on to take charge of MSF–France's logistics operation, and, together with a close associate, applied the principle learned in Thailand to analogous problems elsewhere.

A central health concern for displaced people living in crowded conditions is cholera. Anticipating this problem step by step in detail, the MSF logistics team developed a general kit:

> We knew that we were going to have a cholera epidemic there. OK, we get together people who have already worked on cholera, when we get there, there's nothing of what we need to put in place for a cholera epidemic. So, we need a cholera camp, that is to say an isolation tent.... If there are thousands of people, that's too many, so we'll create a unit to treat 500 patients.... What will be necessary? Some tents; OK, how many tents? OK, we'll need a hundred 50-square-meter tents. We'll have

perfusions because we're going to give infusions and on average there are those who have 2–3 liters and then there are those who have up to 20 liters. So we'll say 10 liters on average, OK. Out of 500 patients there are how many who will receive 10 liters; OK, there will be a hundred...when we finish planning, voilà, we have the kit. We try to really make this kit, in order to see how it is, how it fits into boxes, how much it weighs. We physically create this kit, and then we use it in the next cholera epidemic...and then an evaluation. And then we revise it.... It's like that that the kits advanced, succeeded, not so much because of the notion of the kit, which is really something supremely banal [archi-banal], but following many years where we imagined the kits and evaluated them in numerous situations. And then we divided the operations up like sausages [saucissonné], we cut, we sliced. That is to say, there's a cholera epidemic, a measles epidemic, put in place in a dispensary of a refugee camp. In doing all that, all the units like that, then when it's necessary to mount an operation we have all our equipment.[31]

Through this combination of organic practice and assembly-line routine, MSF created a more global, component variation of the Red Cross *MMM*. By the latter part of the decade the concept of the kit became central to the group's emergency work. MSF–France also established a logistics depot in 1986 and worked to standardize its supply chain across the board, constantly adjusting and refining its techniques on the basis of experience.

To provide a sense of the level of detail involved, I will briefly examine Kit 001, designed for refugee camps, although capable of being modified for either rural or urban displaced populations. Built on a unit of 625 treatments, it weighs in at just over 6,000 kilograms and includes an array of drugs (e.g., 6,500 sachets of oral rehydration salts and 10,000 tablets of the broad-spectrum antibiotic doxycycline) as well as materials for taking patient samples (e.g., dissecting forceps and a permanent black marker) and performing basic medical procedures (e.g., surgical gloves, tunics, trousers, and boots of several sizes, ten 500g rolls of cotton wool, 25 arm splints, and catheters and bandages galore). But the kit does not stop there; it also features support items such as well over a hundred buckets and a hundred disposable razors, not to mention logistical articles like notebooks, pens, wire ties, and even two staplers. Simply put, the degree of preparedness contained within this collection of trunks and boxes would put most Boy Scouts to shame.

Alongside the kit system MSF also created a system of guidelines: short, informative instruction books detailing responses to practical problems, and available in several major international languages (English, French, Spanish, some Russian and Arabic). The core subject matter centers on clinical and engineering dilemmas volunteers might encounter in the field, such as how best to conduct minor surgery in a war zone or how to set up a simple water sanitation system. The guideline system acknowledges that even volunteers with established general expertise may possess inadequate technical background for unfamiliar conditions; neither a nurse from Lille nor a logistician from Toronto, for example, are likely to have much training in combating cholera or building a pit latrine.

While the MSF's different sections pursue slightly different logistics strategies, the kit system has greatly expanded within the overall organization. It has also influenced other groups like the ICRC, where several former MSF figures ended up working.[32] Kits are now available for all manner of eventualities. The Toyota Land Cruiser, the workhorse vehicle for MSF like for many other NGOs, comes as a kit (modified for either warm or cold climates); so too does a collection of stickers and flags to mark its affiliation. Members of a mission can order an "emergency library kit" and request items from a field library list that includes such assorted titles as "How to Look after a Refrigerator," "Human Rights in a Nutshell," and "Blood Transfusion in Remote Areas."[33] Governing the overall design are principles of quality, efficiency, and simplicity of maintenance. In some domains a spirit of standardization dictates a particular brand of product (for example, MSF only orders Toyota vehicles, greatly simplifying its parts list), in others a desire for flexibility of procurement allows substitution of any generic equivalent (most articles are listed as "open" rather than brand specific). MSF also has a long tradition of improvisation, and modifying the designs of others to fit its needs, usually working to simplify systems and reduce their cost.[34]

Analysis: Evaluating the Equipment

The first point I wish to stress analytically is that MSF's kit system represents a self-consciously *global* system, mobile and adaptable to "limited-resource environments" worldwide. While parts of it may be flexible in application, the result is not at all fluid in the sense of flowing around community involvement.[35] Indeed, the kit system is the exact opposite of local knowledge in the traditional sense of geographic and cultural specificity in place. Rather, it represents a mobile, transitional variety of limited intervention, modifying and partially reconstructing a local environment around specific artifacts and a set script. While in practice it may require considerable negotiation to enact (in keeping with actor network theory), its very concept strives to streamline that potential negotiation through provisions that reconstitute a minimal operating environment. The cold chain system used in vaccine distribution serves as a useful general analog in this regard.[36] Just as a cold chain extends the essential environment of a vaccine alongside the vaccine itself with different forms of refrigeration, so too the kit system extends the essential environment for biomedicine into the landscape of a disaster. To insure reliability and quality, MSF is willing to ship almost anything anywhere during an emergency.

Deeply invested in a practical logic of standards, the kit system reflects something of Bruno Latour's analysis of circulating inscriptions as "immutable mobiles."[37] MSF's constellation of guidelines and tool kits collect and distill local clinical knowledge into a portable map of frontline medicine. Developed and refined through practice, they connect one outbreak and crisis to another. In this sense the cholera epidemic in Thailand travels to stabilize the cholera epidemic in the Congo. Together, as a vast chain, the kit assemblage standardizes disaster through responding to it worldwide. Such a characterization reveals the degree to which biomedical knowledge and practice depends on infrastructure, and the background work necessary to translate it into a new setting.

Second, I would like to emphasize that the kit system is not the product of either corporate or state need. Rather, it stems from a humanitarian focus on the moral imperative of responding to immediate human suffering. To be sure, the greater logic of standardization has a long history in both military and business settings. Moreover, MSF's tool chests draw from commercial commodities, and its administration maintains plenty of balance sheets. However, the central motivation for its decisions derives from valuing human life rather than profit.[38] And although MSF may find itself in a position of temporary governance relative to a population in crisis, that governance remains ever partial and impermanent and it refuses the responsibility of rule. Thus, although I have initially cast the emergence of the kit system somewhat along the lines of Fordist production, with factory-like processes of centralized control, that analytic comparison should never lose sight of the fact that the kits were designed to respond to situations of *crisis,* social rupture where the goal is temporary stabilization. Moreover, standardization here was never an end unto itself, nor part of an effort to reshape or capture economic terrain.

The defining role of crisis has grown all the more clear as MSF activities extend beyond emergency interventions into an array of other projects targeting specific diseases over a longer term, advocating policy positions and even facilitating pharmaceutical research and production. In these contexts the logic of the kit no longer holds sway, and missions both purchase a greater variety of materials from local sources and place orders for items in bulk rather than in prepackaged assemblies. At the same time MSF's kit system has recently experienced alterations of a more "post-Fordist" nature, with outsourcing and flexibility playing an increased role in their production.[39] Once beyond crisis settings the group's missions reenter a larger world of exchange and circulation, and here autonomous standardization melts away.

To illustrate this last point I return again to Uganda, and the post–Cold War present. Two decades after the initial forays there, several sections of MSF ran a variety of programs in the country. Among them was a workshop to maintain and repair vehicles, and an ambitious project to provide antiretroviral medications for an expanding number of AIDS patients, both of which I visited in 2003 and 2004.[40] Located in Kampala, the workshop was the domain of a veteran French logistician, a taciturn but dedicated man who nursed it as a longer-term venture amid MSF's many short-lived interventions. In addition to servicing the vehicles of MSF–France and MSF–Switzerland in the country, it also cared for some in less stable neighbors like Sudan and the Congo, where parts were unavailable, and undertook contract work for other NGOs. Well equipped with standards, catalogues, and a computerized ordering system connecting it to MSF's depot, the workshop exemplified stabilized humanitarian infrastructure. At the same time, however, its continued existence was under continual threat, not only from the turnover rate of MSF's fluid administration and their varying visions, but also the pressures of competing interests on the part of the local mechanics who labored there. Once trained, they would often leave for a better paying position, and even when on the job they did not always work with the fervor the director expected. As he noted wryly, they were, after all, driven less by humanitarian ideals than a search for their liveli-hoods. The workshop also faced potential competition from commercial garages that threatened to undercut it, and the impatience of field personnel in project sites who wanted to circumvent central control and make purchases directly. "It's a constant battle," he acknowledged, especially since some parts could be found in local markets more cheaply, and quality was improving. Although a firm believer in the value of the kit system, and the advantages of using standard, well-selected materials, he emphasized that MSF's logistics network was really designed for crisis settings. A stable entity like the garage regularly interacted with the local economy, each small transaction pulling it away from the institutional orbit.

Similarly, efforts to address specific diseases and broader health inequities altered MSF's technical circulatory system, exposing its limits in the process. The project in the northern town of Arua was part of an ambitious, worldwide foray into HIV/AIDS medicine. After years of resisting extensive involvement with the disease, the organization threw itself into the movement to demonstrate the fea-sibility of treating poor people in poor places, rolling out a wave of antiretroviral projects in 2001. MSF added Uganda to the list a year later, locating the project in a region where it had extensive prior experience. By 2004, the Arua clinic served over one thousand patients, and was set to expand further. In one sense the AIDS clinic represented a metakit. By combining experience from multiple locations, MSF could create a mobile set of treatment protocols, less dependent on full-scale laboratory support and adapted to shifting personnel. In this way no project would be open to the charge of representing only an anomaly, since the larger chain was clearly replicable. In another sense, however, the AIDS clinic revealed the limits of the kit approach. MSF's initial commitment was to five years of treatment. The therapy provided, however, would need to last a lifetime, since the drugs produced temporary remission rather than a cure. MSF's approach depended on imported materials, personnel, and funding, none easily substitutable in a provincial town. The team worried about these issues, even as they worked frenetically to expand patient rolls in the face of tremendous demand. "It's not an emergency project, but most days we work at this speed," the mission head told me, wondering how it would all keep going. At the same time, as patients improved they began to refocus on the hardships of their everyday life, and seek support and counsel well beyond medical therapy. Finding jobs and forging new relationships were matters of keen interest for members of patient support groups I encountered. Although sympathetic, MSF was poorly equipped to respond to matters of poverty, unemployment, and family expectations. The translation of treatment from rich to poor countries could not alter the structural imbalance between contexts in economic terms. That particular crisis exceeded the boundaries of a shipping container.

MSF's growing involvement in disease-specific work also reconfigured its form of nonaligned humanitarian engagement. Concerned about drug availability and pricing, not only for AIDS, but also less profitable conditions like sleeping sickness, the organization began aggressive advocacy on the issue, and even created a spin-off nonprofit venture for pharmaceutical research and development. This "Campaign for Access to Essential Medicines" produced its own wave of documentation related to patents and trade agreements, featuring titles like "What to Watch for in Free Trade Agreements with the United States."[41] Inscribing MSF's field experience into political and legal struggles around health policy, the effort highlighted everyday implications of economic inequity, not just exceptional episodes of political failure. Nonetheless, the organization retained its historical focus on health and medical action, even while embracing an expanded sense of crisis.

The Suffering Human Amid Security

"In terms of the destruction of human life, what difference is there
between the wartime bombing of a civilian population
and the distribution of ineffective medicines during a pandemic
that is killing millions of people?"
—Jean-Hervé Bradol, President MSF–France

What then to make of humanitarian logistics amid contemporary problems of biosecurity? The field of humanitarian concern is clearly focused on a fluid and expansive conception of vital need, spread beyond the citizen to the figure of the human. To respond to widespread instances of suffering, humanitarian actors have borrowed central techniques from military logistics, as well as commercial supply lines (such as refrigeration cold chains) to achieve mobility through the modular kit. The kit solves the problem of missing infrastructure by transporting a skeletal operating environment for biomedical operation. But it provides only a temporary patch, in the form of minimal infrastructure dislocated from another setting. To maintain such a graft is expensive in every sense. The expanding scope of humanitarian operations reveals a further limit of this modular approach. What works well for rapid forms of epidemic such as cholera, might not work as well for a more sustained medical condition such as HIV/AIDS, let alone psychological trauma. And once any urgent threat has passed, daily struggles of poverty come back into view.

Over the final decades of the twentieth century, humanitarian operations have become a common, indeed normative, part of international affairs. New agencies mushroomed within and around the UN and other international bodies, while NGOs proliferated to champion a range of causes. At the same time personnel involved in aid projects professionalized, following career trajectories that span multiple governmental and nongovernmental agencies, and formal degree programs at universities and specialized institutes.[42] With the circulation of personnel and ideas, practices and technologies standardized. Kits are now common among most organizations that engage in emergency response, and such work has become an increasingly visible part of global health concerns.[43] Although embodying the technical principle of modular mobility, with all attendant possibilities and limitations, the kit is ultimately an open container. Like humanitarianism itself, it remains available for appropriation into a wide range of projects related to global health and well beyond.[44]

MSF's sense of endangered populations is generally broader than that of state institutions, and is positioned as an ethical response to political failure rather than as a political concern for security. That said, just as military and humanitarian traditions intertwine, areas of common concern certainly exist. Although frequently caustic about inflated fears surrounding emerging diseases compared the actual threats of longstanding ones, MSF actively participates in responding to them. When an outbreak of Ebola threatened Gulu, Uganda, in 2000, MSF specialists joined with counterparts from WHO, CDC, and other international and local teams to combat it. Such threats of sudden outbreak fit readily into the humanitarian tradition of vital mobility. The group's logistics catalogue includes a kit for Ebola (also deployed for Marburg in Angola in 2005), and it produced a SARS kit based on its experiences in Vietnam in 2003. Moreover, the wide publicity surrounding these activities also contributes to the organization's medical reputation.[45]

Nonetheless, MSF worries more about mundane threats well within the capacity of biomedicine to treat. Members of the organization like to point out that most people die not from exotic causes, but rather from "stupid things," effectively condemned by a lack of infrastructure and care.[46] The humanitarian project from this point of view remains largely a minimalist endeavor, focused on fostering existence rather than enhancement. Its biopolitics are those of survival. This minimalism, however, offers no clearly defined end. In an essay outlining biosecurity as a problem area for anthropology, Stephen Collier, Andrew Lakoff, and Paul Rabinow echo Foucault in noting that both health and security lack internal principles of limitation, and thus pose inflationary demands.[47] One can never be too healthy, or too secure. Positioned at the intersection of those twin concerns, and facing a species-level landscape of need, humanitarianism offers no exception to this rule. Within a value of life one can never have too much survival.

NOTES

1 See, for example, Luc Boltanski, *Distant Suffering: Morality, Media and Politics* (Cambridge: Cambridge University Press, 1999); and Craig Calhoun, "A World of Emergencies: Fear, Intervention and the Limits of Cosmopolitan Order," *Canadian Review of Sociology and Anthropology* 41, no. 4 (2004): 373–95.

2 Stephen J. Collier and Andrew Lakoff, "Vital Systems Security," Laboratory for the Anthropology of the Contemporary Discussion Paper (2006), http://anthropos-lab.net/wp/publications/2007/01/collier_vital-systems.pdf (accessed August 1, 2007).

3 Although I present it here as a single entity, MSF is actually an assemblage of semiautonomous national sections. For more on the group's general history and profile, see Dan Bortolotti, *Hope In Hell: Inside the World of Doctors Without Borders* (Buffalo, NY: Firefly Books, 2004); Renée Fox, "Medical Humanitarianism and Human Rights: Reflections on Doctors without Borders and Doctors of the World," *Social Science and Medicine* 41, no. 12 (1995): 1607–16; and especially Anne Vallaeys, *Médecins sans frontières: La biographie* (Paris: Fayard, 2004). For elements of this project, see Peter Redfield, "Doctors, Borders and Life in Crisis," *Cultural Anthropology* 20, no. 3 (August 2005): 328–61; and "A Less Modest Witness: Collective Advocacy and Motivated Truth of a Medical Humanitarian Movement," *American Ethnologist* 33, no. 1 (2006): 3–26.

4 "Every November on its International Day for Populations in Danger, Médecins Sans Frontières tries to draw the attention of public opinion to the ten most urgent humanitarian crises in the world." Jacques de Milliano, "Foreword," in *Life, Death and Aid: The Médecins Sans Frontières Report on World Crisis Intervention,* ed.

François Jean (New York: Routledge, 1993), vii. "The 'danger' mentioned in the book's title is the danger of death, the very thing we struggle with on a daily basis." MSF, "Introduction," in François Jean, ed., *Populations in Danger* (London: John Libbey, 1992), 4.

5 Fabrice Weissman, ed., *In the Shadow of "Just Wars": Violence, Politics and Humanitarian Action* (Ithaca, NY: Cornell University Press, 2004).

6 See Michel Foucault, *Security, Territory, Population: Lectures at the Collège de France, 1977–78* (New York: Palgrave Macmillan, 2007). Although MSF clearly occupies a different era, and resists political positioning beyond humanitarianism, it shares general concerns that Foucault outlines for the emergence of European liberalism by conceiving of human groups as populations in relation to milieu and "the nature of things." Thus while not sovereign in any conventional sense, the organization participates in government, or more precisely "nongovernmental government," by addressing the welfare of ordinary people. See Didier Fassin, "Humanitarianism: A Nongovernmental Government," in *Nongovernmental Politics,* ed. Michel Feher, Gaëlle Krikorian, and Yates McKee (New York: Zone Books, 2007), 149–59.

7 Rony Brauman, *Humanitaire, le dilemme* (Paris: Editions Textuel, 1996), 76; and David Rieff, *A Bed for the Night: Humanitarianism in Crisis* (New York: Simon and Schuster, 2002), 75, 86, 166. These authors caustically suggest how little protection this would offer. The apotheosis of the Holocaust as the extreme of evil may well have occurred a generation later in the 1960s; see Paul Rabinow, "Midst Anthropology's Problems," *Cultural Anthropology* 17,

no. 2 (2002): 135–49; and Peter Novick, *The Holocaust in American Life* (Boston: Houghton Mifflin, 1999).

8 Rieff, *A Bed for the Night;* and Alex de Waal, *Famine Crimes: Politics and the Disaster Relief Industry in Africa* (Oxford: James Currey, 1997).

9 Suffering in the colonies was primarily a matter for missionaries or the civil service of empires, and colonial warfare usually operated by different rules. For more on colonial medicine in Africa, see Rita Headrick, *Colonialism, Health and Illness in French Equatorial Africa, 1885–1935,* ed. Daniel Headrick (Atlanta: African Studies Association Press, 1994); and Megan Vaughn, *Curing Their Ills: Colonial Power and African Illness* (Stanford, CA: Stanford University Press, 1991). For a suggestion of the complex colonial history surrounding the term civil society, see John L. Comaroff and Jean Comaroff, eds., *Civil Society and the Political Imagination in Africa: Critical Perspectives* (Chicago: University of Chicago Press, 1999); and for a collection on military logistics, see John A. Lynn, ed., *Feeding Mars: Logistics in Western Warfare from the Middle Ages to the Present* (Boulder, CO: Westview Press, 1993). While the Red Cross focused on civilizing conflicts between "civilized" countries, it helped transform both military medicine and international law. See David Forsythe, *The Humanitarians: The International Committee of the Red Cross* (Cambridge: Cambridge University Press, 2005); and John Hutchinson, *Champions of Charity: War and the Rise of the Red Cross* (Boulder, CO: Westview Press, 1996).

10 MSF–France's former leader and long-time *philosophe,* Rony Brauman, frequently underscores the tie to SAMU, travel, and media technologies when recounting MSF's history, including in my own interview with him; see

Rony Brauman, *Penser dans l'urgence: Parcours critique d'un humanitaire* (Paris: Seuil, 2006), 58; also Joelle Tanguy, "The Médecins Sans Frontières Experience," in *Framework for Survival: Health, Human Rights and Humanitarian Assistance in Conflicts and Disasters,* ed. Kevin M. Cahill (New York: Routledge, 1999), 226–44; and an online variant posted at http://www.doctorswithoutborders.org/volunteer/field/themsfexperience.cfm (accessed July 31, 2007).

11 "Dans leur salle d'attente deux milliards d'hommes." The publicity campaign is outlined in *Bulletin Médecins Sans Frontières* 6 (1977); see Vallaeys, *Médecins sans frontières,* for a more complete history of the group's origins and early squabbles.

12 Bernard Kouchner, *Le malheur des autres* (Paris: Editions Odile Jacob, 1991), 327; Rony Brauman, *Penser dans l'urgence,* 39–70. Following a power struggle in 1979, Kouchner left MSF to found Médecins du Monde (Doctors of the World), and later emerged as a significant political figure in France. For a caustic assessment of his trajectory as a generational icon, see Kristin Ross, *May '68 and Its Afterlives* (Chicago: University of Chicago Press, 2002), esp. 147–69. Although opposed on such matters as a "right to interference" and state humanitarianism, Kouchner and Brauman both define their ethics of engagement around a response to suffering, understood in medical terms. See Tim Allen and David Styan, "A Right to Interfere? Bernard Kouchner and the New Humanitarianism," *Journal of International Development* 12 (2000): 825–42; and Bertrand Taithe, "Reinventing (French) Universalism: Religion, Humanitarianism and the 'French Doctors,'" *Modern and Contemporary France* 12, no. 2 (2004): 147–58.

13 For more on proxy wars and their significance

during the post-Vietnam period, see Odd Arne Westad, *The Global Cold War* (Cambridge: Cambridge University Press, 2007); and Mahmood Mamdani, *Good Muslim, Bad Muslim: America, the Cold War, and the Roots of Terror* (New York: Pantheon, 2004).

14 Vallaeys, *Médecins sans frontières,* and de Waal, *Famine Crimes.*

15 Tim Allen, *Trial Justice: The International Court and the Lord's Resistance Army* (London: Zed Books, 2006); and Mark Leopold, *Inside West Nile: Violence, History and Representation on an African Frontier* (Santa Fe, NM: School of American Research Press, 2005).

16 See the collected papers in Cole P. Dodge and Paul D. Wiebe, eds., *Crisis in Uganda: The Breakdown of Health Services* (Oxford: Pergamon Press, 2005). Karl-Eric Knutsson uses the evocative phrases "at best chaotic" and "disaster within a disaster" in his chapter, "Preparedness for Disaster Operations," in Dodge and Wiebe, *Crisis in Uganda,* 183–89. As a number of the contributors note, the Karamoja famine could be traced not only to drought, but also to a background of social factors, including colonial land management policies in the region, shifting practices of cattle raising, and increased availability of automatic weapons that altered the balance of cattle raids.

17 Melissa Well, "The Relief Operation in Karamoja: What Was Learned and What Needs Improvement," in Dodge and Wiebe, *Crisis in Uganda,* 177–82. The model for Well's strike force was a Swedish government team known as the Swedish Special Unit, whose efficient work in the West Nile region received accolades from several contributors to the volume.

18 Knutsson, "Preparedness for Disaster Operations," 187–88.

19 Interview conducted in Paris by author; field-

notes, June 2003.

20 Rony Brauman, "Karamoja: les difficultés d'un sauvetage," *Bulletin d'information de Médecins Sans Frontierès* 7 (1980): 9–12. Brauman, who would go on to become the longtime leader of MSF–France and one of the forces behind its technical improvement, recalled the chaos of the Ugandan action relative to later interventions in an interview in June 2003. Unlike Oxfam or Action Contre la Faim (Action Against Hunger, or ACF), MSF has never been centrally devoted to nutritional issues. Nonetheless, famine relief has played a significant role in its history, most notably in Ethiopia in 1985.

21 Fox, "Medical Humanitarianism"; Tanguy, "The Médecins Sans Frontières Experience"; and Vallaeys, *Médecins sans frontières.*

22 While there are now nineteen national sections of the larger movement, the central five directing operations remain European: MSF–France (founded 1971), MSF–Belgium (1980), MSF–Switzerland (1980), MSF–Holland (1984), and MSF–Spain (1986). For the purposes of this brief essay I am treating MSF as a single entity, since the sections share a general logistical system if not all particulars. However, the different sections remain effectively autonomous, even if linked by flows of funds and personnel as well as a charter and a loose international association. At times they have experienced moments of extreme acrimony and near civil war, particularly between the largest three (France, Belgium, and Holland).

23 Joint Relief Commission of the International Red Cross, *Materia Medica Minimalis* (Geneva: International Committee of the Red Cross and League of Red Cross Societies, 1944), i.

24 Ibid.

25 Ibid.

26 Ibid., ii.

27 Joint Relief Commission of the International Red Cross, *Report of the Joint Relief Commission of the International Red Cross* (Geneva: ICRC and LRCS, 1948), 245.

28 This and all descriptions refer to the 2003 English edition of the MSF catalogue. The current version is available online at http://www.msfsupply.be/UK/Frame/FramesetUK.htm or http://www.msflogistique.org/public/pub_an/pub_an.htm (both accessed July 31, 2007).

29 Here I should also note that while MSF may remain an association of doctors in nominal terms, only 25% of its overall expatriate volunteers in 2001–2002 fit that category, with another 32% being nurses or paramedical and 43% nonmedical. In addition to the 1,605 field posts that cycle, the organization counted 13,320 "national" staff hired locally; see *MSF Activity Report 2001–2002* (Brussels: MSF International, 2003), 97.

30 This account of the origins of MSF's kit system draws from an interview with Jacques P. conducted in French by Johanna Rankin, December 21, 2004; see Johanna Rankin, "A New Frontier for Humanitarianism?" *Médecins sans frontières* Responds to Neglected Diseases" (honors thesis, Curriculum in International and Area Studies, University of North Carolina at Chapel Hill, 2005). The translation is mine.

31 Ibid.

32 The ICRC also began significant logistics developments in the late 1970s, and established a unit to centralize vehicle purchase and management in 1984; see International Committee of the Red Cross, *Logistics Field Manual* (Geneva: ICRC, 2004), 24. The UN established the United Nations Joint Logistics Center (UNJLC) after the 1996 crisis in eastern Zaire. For a more general account of the larger humanitarian "apparatus," see Emile Cock, *Le dispositif humanitaire: Geopolitique de la générosité* (Paris: L'Harmattan, 2005).

33 MSF Field Library List, as recorded by the author in Brussels, July 2003.

34 Innovations include such items as insect netting on vehicle grilles to simplify maintenance, or experiments to improve a portable system for mixing food used in nutritional therapy. To quote the logistics director of MSF–Belgium when I interviewed him in 2003: "The market usually favors things that are expensive and use a lot of energy. We want to try and find things that are less so, for example solar panels or a bike as an energy source."

35 Marianne de Laet and Annemarie Mol, "The Zimbabwe Bush Pump: Mechanics of a Fluid Technology," *Social Studies of Science* 30, no. 2 (April 2000): 225–63.

36 For an overview of the history of refrigeration, see David Wilson, *The Colder the Better* (New York: Atheneum, 1980).

37 See Bruno Latour, *Science in Action* (Cambridge, MA: Harvard University Press, 1987), 226–27; and *Pandora's Hope: Essays on the Reality of Science Studies* (Cambridge, MA: Harvard University Press, 1999).

38 In recent years MSF has emerged as a relatively wealthy and financially independent NGO, with over 450 million euros in annual income, some 80% of which derives from private sources (MSF, *Manuel des Acteurs de l'Aide* [2007], 113). It thus maintains a high measure of independent capacity, and is not directly dependent on donor agencies or foundations for the bulk of its operations. Although private fundraising through public appeals may have its own pressures of image management, these are not identical to those of private capital.

39 As the kit concept has spread and the humanitarian market expanded, many kits are no longer manufactured in-house at either MSF Logistique in Bordeaux (the primary logis-

tics depot for MSF–France, MSF–Switzerland, and MSF–Spain), or MSF Supply in Brussels (a similar unit for MSF–Belgium, formerly named Transfer). Instead of maintaining a proprietary logistics center at all, MSF–Holland relies on agreements with established suppliers to provide it with materials on a flexible, rapid-response basis (interview notes, Holland, November 2002). For more on Fordist and post-Fordist production, see David Harvey, *The Postmodern Condition* (Oxford: Basil Blackwell 1989). However, the historical comparison only partially applies, given that the spatial ambition of the kit has always differed from the national space and scope of Fordist regulation. I thank Stephen Collier for pointing this out in discussion.

40 Observations and quotations drawn from author's fieldnotes, Kampala, July 2003 and May 2004.

41 See websites for the Campaign for Access to Essential Medicines, http://www.accessmed-msf.org/, and the Drugs for Neglected Diseases Initiative, http://www.dndi.org (both accessed July 31, 2007).

Epigraph: Jean-Hervé Bradol, "The Sacrificial International Order and Humanitarian Action," in *In the Shadow of "Just Wars": Violence, Politics and Humanitarian Action* (Ithaca, NY: Cornell University Press, 2004), 8.

42 For example, the French training institute Bioforce offers programs in management and logistics: http://www.bioforce.asso.fr/english/

english.htm (accessed August 1, 2007).

43 For example the WHO, a policy-oriented entity, now maintains a set of guidelines for "health actions in crises": http://www.who.int/hac/techguidance/en/ (accessed August 1, 2007).

44 On the one hand, see, e.g., Laurie Garrett's "Doc-in-a-Box" project at the Council on Foreign Relations, http://www.cfr.org/project/1247/docinabox_project.html (accessed August 1, 2007); and, on the other, the humanitarian projects of Mandalay International, http://www.humanitarianproducts.com/ (accessed August 1, 2007). I thank Carlo Caduff for alerting me to the former project.

45 MSF press releases issued April 30, 2003; March 24, 2005; May 23, 2005; as well as *MSF Activity Report 2001–2002*, 35.

46 In 2004 MSF–Switzerland was back in Gulu, treating a cholera outbreak as well as running a night shelter for displaced children, complete with counseling for former child soldiers. By the time I visited the cholera project it was already winding down in textbook fashion, a matter of local public health far more than international security.

47 Stephen J. Collier, Andrew Lakoff, and Paul Rabinow, "Biosecurity: Toward an Anthropology of the Contemporary," *Anthropology Today* 20, no. 5 (2004): 7; see also Michel Foucault, "The Risks of Security," in *Power: Essential Works of Foucault, 1954–1984*, vol. 3, ed. Paul Rabinow (New York: The New Press, 2000), 373.

CHAPTER SEVEN

Mapping the Multiplicities of Biosecurity

Nick Bingham and Steve Hinchliffe

Integrating Biosecurity?

Biosecurity has become a familiar term in policymaking circles over the past few years. Its meanings, problems, and practices however have varied significantly. In Europe, for example, biosecurity has emerged primarily in relation to attempts to manage the movement of agricultural pests and diseases. The focus has been on individual farm-based practices, including emergency measures to contain outbreaks and techniques to prevent infection of livestock. In contrast, in Australasia and other places—mainly islands—where the effects of ecological colonization (the importation, often from Europe, of farming systems and species) have been most pronounced, biosecurity has figured mainly with reference to efforts to reduce the effects of so-called invasive species on "indigenous" flora and fauna. Characteristic practices here have included border controls in the form of restrictions on the importation of living (or not-long-since dead) tissues, and the attempted eradication of established but ecologically damaging "pest" species. Finally, in the United States, biosecurity has come to represent a governmental concern with the—either purposeful or inadvertent—spreading of biological agents into the human population, with particular attention given to laboratories that handle potentially hazardous organisms; possible use of pathogens in bioterrorism; and the prospect of animal-borne diseases crossing to humans (zoonoses). This has prompted various high-expenditure, technology-intensive programs (such as Project Bioshield) as well as other practices, such as anticipatory research in molecular sciences, the stockpiling of antiviral drugs, heightened regulation of laboratories, the development of real-time and near–real-time surveillance technologies, scenario planning, and the construction of information and processing centers designed to serve as command and control centers in the event of a positively identified disease event.

Clearly, then, while something called biosecurity has risen to prominence in many locations over a similar period, it has not been exactly the same thing everywhere. This fact has been widely noted in policy dialogue and documents, not least in those international contexts where different understandings of the term could cause confusion. More significant—and the focus of our attention in this chapter—has been the development across domains of a concerted effort to articulate a unified and universal version of biosecurity that could be the basis of a standard, worldwide approach to dealing with "out of place" biological entities of various kinds. From aspirations to see a "harmonization and integration" of approaches to biosecurity within and between the Food and Agriculture Organization of the United Nations (FAO)[1] and the World Health Organization (WHO), through discussions of "dual-use" research in the life sciences,[2] to academic advocates of a "global biosecurity concert,"[3] various attempts at "joined up thinking," all with the aim of bringing the various matters of concern of biosecurity into a single problem space, are gathering momentum. In what follows we will explore the motives for, the building of, and the possible risks involved in this one-size-fits-all culture of biosecurity.

Specifically, we will draw some lessons from a particular moment in this unfolding story, namely the arrival of the H5N1 strain of highly pathogenic avian influenza (hereafter HPAI) in Cairo, Egypt, in 2006. By way of some brief introductory remarks, we might first note that avian influenza is a common enough condition for wild birds, with a large reservoir of such viruses continually circulating in bird populations. In many cases such viral infections produce few clinical effects. However, more pathogenic forms of avian influenza exist that can spread rapidly and approach a lethality rate of close to 100 percent in the birds they infect. All are H5 or H7 subtypes with a distinctive set of amino acids in the cleavage site of hemaglutinin. How avian influenza viruses circulate and how they change is thus a topic of vital concern for bird health. But it is also a matter of concern for many others too, since subtypes of bird flu can jump species, including to humans. Such transspecies crossing of avian influenza viruses have been relatively uncommon and have to date and in the main produced only mild forms of human disease. The exception is the H5N1 strain, which had already crossed to humans in 1997 (in Hong Kong where there were eighteen reported cases) and whose travels have gradually increased in frequency and distribution in subsequent years. Such outbreaks have all occurred when H5N1 has been clinically present in nearby poultry flocks and as yet there have been few if any clear-cut cases of human-to-human transmission, all of which suggests that the current H5N1 viruses are poorly adapted to their human host. This situation has not prevented speculation that HPAI might develop the capacity to move quickly and effectively through human populations, either by gradual adaptive mutation or—more worryingly in the sense that it may give rise to a rapid onset, pandemic strain—by genetic reassortment (where avian and human viruses "exchange" genetic material during a coinfection of a host pig or human).

For many experts, the appearance of HPAI H5N1 in a city like Cairo offers the sort of circumstances that might favor the emergence of just such a human pandemic. A postcolonial, cosmopolitan megacity, Cairo is home to a large concentration of both backyard (or rooftop) and industrially reared poultry, as well as being a major intersection for international bird migrations. The mutability and adaptability of viruses combined with the complexity, density, and intensity of animal-human and human-human interactions in this kind of setting offer obvious causes for concern. In what follows, we offer a roughly chronological account of how HPAI came to be in Cairo and what the preparations for and responses to its arrival entailed. Along the way we will briefly pause at various junctures to extract some general points about the enaction of biosecurity from the particularities of this event.

Preparing for H5N1

On October 17, 2005, an urgent bulletin from the WHO Regional Office for the Eastern Mediterranean (EMRO)—located in Cairo itself—declared that due to the fact that "migratory bird flyways pass through the EMR [Eastern Mediterranean Region] on their way between Asia, Europe, and Africa" and "daily dynamic interaction with other countries in the world (expatriate workers, trade, religious visitors, and tourism) could easily result in the introduction of influenza into the Region," the "EMR is the nearest region to the current focus of unprecedented outbreaks of avian influenza than any other WHO region outside Asia." The same report made it very plain that what is "expected from countries" is to identify "rapidly and appropriately destroy all infected or exposed birds with proper disposal of carcasses," "functional and efficient influenza surveillance hand in hand with focused and timely public health measures," "reasonable stockpiles of Tamiflu," "production of influenza vaccines," and "an efficient communication system" as critical measures to have in place. The release ends with the sentence: "There is no need to panic but to be better prepared."[4]

Clearly, then, Egypt was supposed to be "prepared" for the arrival of HPAI. The text of the bulletin gives a sense of what this should mean in practice, but where did such an expectation come from in the first place? We might trace the beginnings of an answer back to the now-celebrated conference on "Emerging Viruses" that took place in Washington, DC, in May 1989.[5] For it was here—in the collective anxieties expressed about the simultaneous appearance on the world stage of both multifarious new infectious agents (such as HIV and Ebola) and drug-resistant strains of more familiar ones, the changed map of the global landscape of threat that resulted, and the consensus for the need for action—that we find the basis of what historian of medicine Nicholas B. King has termed the "emerging diseases worldview."[6] It was also the moment at which the apparatus into which Egypt found itself being enrolled two decades later began to take shape. After the significantly titled report from the U.S. Institute of Medicine, *Emerging Infections: Microbial Threats to Health in the United States,* helped convince policymakers in that country that its citizens were no longer immune to the effects of diseases previously considered to take place elsewhere in the world, the impetus had arrived for a new way of dealing with matters biological.[7]

This new way of doing things was soon termed "global health governance," and was characterized by a strengthening of and increased coordination between three major international bodies, the WHO, the FAO, and the World Organization for Animal Health (OIE). What this involved began to become evident in the response to the outbreak of Severe Acute Respiratory Syndrome (SARS) in 2002–2003, and was further formalized in the new set of international health regulations (IHR) of 2005 that (among many other provisions) made it a legal requirement that states notify the WHO of any event that may constitute a "public health emergency of international concern." Influenza was an obvious target of this emerging way of managing disease, and four "critical functions" of global influenza governance have been identified: first (and most important), surveillance; second, protection (such as vaccines); third, response (for example drugs such as Tamiflu and regulation of the movement of both goods and people); and, finally, public communication.[8]

Having got a flavor of the developments that shaped what it meant for Egypt to "be prepared" for HPAI (compare the list of critical functions of global influenza governance with that detailing "what was expected" of EMRO countries quoted at the start of this section), we are also in a position to make a first point about biosecurity in general: Regimes of security such as this are perhaps not best thought of simply in terms of a logical response or set of responses to a preexisting threat or set of threats. Rather, they are more usefully considered as problematizations of existing ways of doing things that simultaneously articulate a particular kind of world and a particular kind of intervention appropriate to that world. In this sense, thinking in terms of "worldview" might not be quite adequate to the situation in the sense that it implies a particular perspective on the world rather than the world-making processes that our initial tracings of the emerging global apparatus of biosecurity indicate. We tentatively suggest (drawing strongly on the work of Michel Foucault[9]) that, considered as a world-making problematization, this biosecurity has three significant characteristics. First, it concerns itself with regulating circulations, such that "good" things (e.g., trade) or people (e.g., tourists) can continue or be encouraged to move while "bad" things (e.g., viruses) or people (e.g., terrorists) are stopped or at least slowed down. Second, it proceeds by paying close attention to the material specificities of particular environments insofar as those specificities (from the global distribution of poultry farming to the networks of international travel) represent opportunities or obstacles to the management of the aforementioned circulations. Finally, the biosecurity that we are describing here intervenes not by attempting to totally refashion the spaces in which it operates (imagining, for example, that it might be possible to completely eradicate certain sorts of diseases from the world), but instead by modulating or adjusting existing conditions such that the best possible conditions are in place for ensuring the future maximization of positive circulating elements (being well prepared for what the WHO describes as the "inevitable" influenza pandemic).

We can see all of these characteristics at work in the official etiology of H5N1 HPAI that solidified as the outbreak spread. By the middle of 2005 and following the deaths of more than six thousand migratory birds (mostly bar-headed geese) at the Qinghai Lake nature reserve in central China—"a very unusual and probably unprecedented event"[10]—the WHO (in coordination with the FAO and OIE) had refined its narrative of H5N1 avian influenza transmission and the conditions required for species crossing. According to this updated version of the disease, it was (1) wild birds that act as the reservoir for various strains of bird flu, (2) the mixing of wild birds with poorly controlled domestic bird populations that results in the spread of viruses into poultry, and (3) poorly regulated poultry handling practices where wild and domestic birds exist in close and visceral proximity to pigs and people that exacerbate the risk of highly infectious diseases crossing species barriers.

What this account implies is that the problem of avian influenzas and their likely transformation into viral forms that can spread among humans clearly resides in particular parts of the world (mainly southern and Southeast Asia and parts of Africa) and with particular forms of agriculture (found in those places where large numbers of small, poorly regulated animal husbandry and slaughter practices exist). For the institutions of global health governance, these were the sites of so-called low biosecurity and therefore high danger. Following such straightforward logic, an equally straightforward plan of action emerged. Control is easiest, it was argued, on large commercial farms "with birds housed indoors, usually under strictly controlled sanitary conditions, in large numbers. Control is far more difficult under poultry production conditions in which most birds are raised in small backyard flocks scattered throughout rural or periurban areas."[11] The FAO followed the WHO's lead, reversing its former policy of encouraging small-scale poultry farming (as a means to development, self-sufficiency, and small business promotion) and instead began encouraging secure factory farms.

However, getting this plan to work in practice proved fraught with difficulties, with stark differences between national capacities to meet the standards of preparedness that the comprehensive schemes of the WHO, FAO, OIE, and so on were now both expecting and relying on for success. Egypt was a case in point. On September 29, 2005, David Nabarro—the newly appointed senior United Nations system coordinator for avian and human influenza—publicly warned that an outbreak of avian influenza that crossed the species barrier to humans in such a form that it could be transmitted through the air could kill anywhere between five million and one hundred fifty million people worldwide. By now, cases had been confirmed in Romania, Croatia, and Greece, as well as Turkey, and it was the start of the bird migration season in Egypt. The Egyptian government had to be seen to act and it did, announcing that the bird hunting season was to be banned for the year. The nets strung up to waylay quail and wild ducks were removed and all dealings in both species banned. Imports of poultry from infected countries were also prohibited, while increased border monitoring and testing of migratory flocks were announced. After the EMRO bulletin of October 16, what counted as a responsible response was now clearer than ever and the Egyptian government immediately convened a Supreme National Committee to Combat Bird Flu, with representatives from the ministries of defence, agriculture, and health as well as the WHO. The next day, Egyptian President Hosni Mubarak held a ministerial meeting to discuss the measures to be taken in the event that avian influenza was detected within the country. Dismissing rumors of lack of planning and low stocks of vaccine and Tamiflu, officials assured the public that all possible safety measures had been taken and that Egypt was fully prepared.

As we shall see, making preparations does not necessarily ensure that one is prepared; but first, we want to pause again to draw out a second general point from our case study: There is more than one mode of security at work in the world. Above, we sketched the key features (the management of circulation, the working with material givens, the modulation of conditions) evident in the building of a global regime of biosecurity. Now (again following Foucault but see also Michael Dillon[12]) we have evidence of two more versions of security at play. First, in the promotion of factory farms by the WHO and then FAO, we find an example of a more disciplinary version of security, concerned with making matters safe through the production of totally controlled environments (note the contrast with the previously detailed, less interventionist model). And second, in the list of new border controls introduced by the Egyptian government at the prompting of the institutions of global health governance, we have a classic case of a more territorial version of security, aiming to keep threats at a distance by demarcating and protecting certain spaces (again, note the contrast with the emphasis on circulation in our first example). The mode of security that we first identified, then, is not the only version of security possible. Indeed, the boundary-maintenance based, prophylactic interpretation demonstrated in Egypt's intensified policing of its borders is probably the most intuitively familiar. Neither has the circulation-centric version of security simply replaced previously existing modes, as quite clearly at least three are operating simultaneously in our case study. A number of different ways of doing security coexist in our contemporary moment. In this instance we might be more specific and say that the circulation-regulating version of security is in the dominant position, coordinating the other two toward its own ends. More than that, in the process this hierarchization reorients characteristic features of the nondominant modes such that controlled spaces of the disciplinary version become more like key nodes in a wider system of circulation rather than simply isolated environments, and the borders of the territorial version become more like monitoring mechanisms than hard-and-fast perimeters. As we shall see, however, other relationships between versions of security are also possible.

Culling Avian Influenza

According to the official version of events, H5N1 HPAI eventually reached Egypt in mid-February of 2006. As reported by the "government-friendly" newspaper *Egypt Today*, at 3 o'clock in the morning on February 17, the Health Minister El-Gabali woke Dr. Zuheir El-Halaj to inform him of the discovery. A government statement followed within hours, making Egypt the first country with avian influenza to make the announcement before the WHO. Later that same morning, Prime Minister Ahmed Nazif went on national television to reassure the country that the cabinet would now be putting into place a comprehensive plan of action that had been formulated the previous autumn when the possibility of bird flu in Egypt became apparent.

Despite some indications that the initial outbreaks of avian influenza in Egypt had occurred at least in part on factory farms, public officials began stressing the safety of such "highly controlled environments" and suggested that the vast majority of reported cases were occurring in flocks of home-raised birds. Then, after banning all movement of poultry between the different Egyptian governorates on that day, a further statement was released from the prime minister's office the next day, February 18, announcing a cull of all backyard and rooftop poultry and the banning of live bird markets (where 80 percent of the country's poultry was sold). The faithfulness of the wording of this announcement to the joint WHO/FAO/OIE line on the association between certain farming practices and the prevalence of bird flu was noticeable. Echoing specifically the words of a senior FAO official who had stated that "the fight against bird flu must be waged in the backyard of the world's poor,"[13] the prime minister declared that "the world is moving towards big farms because they can be controlled under veterinarian supervision...the time has come to get rid of the idea of breeding chickens on the roofs of houses."[14]

Such careful alignment could not conceal, however, that the extent of the new measures marked a significant departure from accepted good biosecurity practice as defined by institutions of global health governance. Although culling was widely recommended by the WHO and FAO as "the first line of defence" for containing avian influenza, its suggested use was in the immediate aftermath and in the immediate (3–4 kilometer) vicinity of a confirmed outbreak. The policy put into action by the Egyptian government was something else again. Radically preemptive and precautionary, it targeted areas and activities in which no empirical association let alone detection had yet taken place. For many, the decision to cull was similarly bound up with a need to be seen as modern in various ways, in this case responding (if obliquely) to the prompting of the major international health organizations and associated pressures (notably from the United States whose presence in Cairo through Naval Medical Research Unit number 3 [NAMRU-3] was significant at a number of junctures); the expectations of a sceptical public that the government was taking control of the situation; and an ongoing project of rebranding Cairo as a contemporary world city where one is more likely to find the final of the African Nations Cup (held only a few days—suspiciously few, for some—before the announcement of the presence of H5N1 in Egypt) than chickens in the streets.[15]

As such, it offers an excellent example of our third general point about biosecurity: In a situation in which there are multiple modes of securing at work, they will not always operate according to the sort of clear hierarchy that we noted earlier, where both disciplinary and territory-securing practices were being put to work by a circulation-managing version of security. If we consider culling as another disciplinary security technique in the sense that it is seeking to produce a fully controlled environment, we can see how in Cairo it shifted from being another available tool brought to bear by a global health governance approach in order to ensure future circulations (like the promotion of factory farms), to much more than that as it became entangled with the purifying schemes of the Egyptian elite of "experts." Exceeding its original role and generating new things from public panic to new opportunities for the spread of the disease, this was a case of modes of security (and other kinds of orderings) interfering with each other in unforeseen and unpredictable ways.[16]

The endeavor to cull poultry in Cairo swung swiftly into action, led by teams of officials from the ministries of health, agriculture, and environment but enforced by the security forces. The process was far from clean and smooth with confusion following their every move. Panic and a run on bottled water and soft drinks ensued almost immediately, after emails and texts were circulated declaring that the water supply was unsafe because diseased bird carcasses were being thrown into the Nile. In some parts of the city terrified citizens were more than happy to report their neighbors to the government information center for failing to dispose of or admit to their rooftop or backyard flock. Elsewhere, householders sceptical of the government's promises or level of compensation (although the fines for keeping birds were clear, the reparations for handing them in were not) successfully hid their birds, unwilling to let such valuable possessions be needlessly culled. Others did not know whom to believe and called on the normally reliable NGOs for a response. Meanwhile the Cairo zoo had been closed after an outbreak there, and several of the slaughterhouses designated by officials as the only places where poultry could be legally killed turned out not to be usable, having been closed down due to little demand under normal conditions (most killing of poultry usually takes place in other, less industrial conditions). The sense of chaos was further exacerbated by the uncertainties and rumors surrounding human health, especially after the first fatality in the country was announced in March. Such practical difficulties in managing the disease in terms of urban food provision, public health, employment, and economies were exacerbated outside the capital city. Poor information, noncompliance, and a lack of personnel made the cull completely unenforceable in practice in twenty of Egypt's twenty-six governorates where bird flu had been detected. Authorities in Cairo, attempting to govern a crisis at a distance, then had to declare that backyard flocks could be kept as long as they were healthy and caged.

This is our fourth general point: We do not find security perfectly implemented according to a singular internal logic. Rather, security consists of attempts at ordering that involve disparate and often desperate measures (of which the cull of poultry in Cairo is only a particularly stark example). As a result we prefer to speak of biosecurings rather than biosecurity to give a sense of more or less trial-and-error, more or less partial, more or less successful attempts to make matters safe.[17]

Nevertheless, despite all this messiness, the mass killing of birds seemingly reduced the problem. New infections had declined by early summer and for all intents and purposes the country was thought to be free from the disease by mid-2006. According to the vice-head of the poultry union, however, this success was not due to the preventative measures taken by the government but simply to the extermination of an estimated thirty-four million birds in the cull. In a few weeks, "Egypt lost 75 percent of its egg-laying flocks and 50 percent of all fowl. Since there is almost no poultry in the country, infection rates of bird flu are decreasing."[18]

Farming Avian Influenza

When the Egyptian government announced the cull on backyard and rooftop birds, they would have been fully aware that such a move represented a hugely significant intervention into Cairo's urban ecology. Historically, poultry has been one of the major areas of livestock production in Egypt, the rapid reproduction and quick response to feeding of chickens and ducks offering a flexible source of protein and/or revenue with no need for land ownership or large capital investment (and all the more important in a predominantly Muslim country where keeping pigs is not socially acceptable). So widespread is this practice that the FAO reported that prior to the 2006 outbreak of HPAI virtually all women in rural areas of Egypt who did not have another occupation would have been rearing birds at home. In urban areas too this was far from an unusual situation, one estimate putting the proportion of Cairo households that kept animals of some sort (but mainly poultry) at well over 25 percent if one includes the informal settlements and former villages.[19]

Subsistence husbandry is thus well established in both Egypt and Cairo. It is not however an ecological relic in terms of capitalist relations in those spaces. The existence and patterns of household poultry raising today is deeply implicated in (though not reducible to) a set of other practices that together mark the emergence of Egyptian capitalism in the twentieth and twenty-first centuries.[20] Parts of the poultry industry underwent huge restructuring in the 1970s. Large factory production developed in the north, subsidized with International Monetary Fund loans and supplied with non-market-priced feed grain imported from the United States. At the same time, Egyptian agriculture abandoned 1950s nationalist land reform and the U.S. Office for International Development encouraged a shift in food production to nonstaple foodstuffs (replacing staples with surplus U.S. grain imports). In the 1980s the latter supply was cut as part of the World Bank–led program of agricultural price reforms, making bread, other food, and grain-fed poultry extremely expensive.

Simultaneously, import restrictions on frozen poultry from abroad were relaxed, and the combination of cheaper imports of chicken products and high grain prices led to a collapse in the Egyptian poultry industry with only the larger companies surviving. These companies formed a cartel, acting to control prices and poultry supplies. Add to this food price increases resulting from reduced retail subsidies, a newly privatized food retail and distribution system, a huge increase in landless and urbanizing poor (itself related to the lack of land reform), and the result is a large increase in urban, periurban, and rural subsistence animal production and small-scale husbandry, most of it undertaken by women. Despite the rhetoric of free market rationalization and privatization it is worth noting, after Mitchell, that it was largely nonmarket practices related to U.S. surpluses, military provisioning, cartels, and political power that produced the new food situation in Egypt. As Gertel and Samir put it, "animal husbandry...does not take place in isolation from the wider economy, but is rather embedded and intertwined in a variety of ways within the local community and broader development processes."[21] Keeping poultry is thus an interwoven part of capitalism in Egypt; and any attempt to claim that rooftop agriculture is premodern, archaic, and antithetical to the modernization of Cairo and Egypt's economy might well look at the very modern causes of this political ecology. However, that is exactly what was claimed; the sights, smells, noises, and now diseases of poultry were all officially unwanted elements of a modernized Cairo.

Though the city's citizens were by now well used to the banning of certain activities like book- or clothes-selling in particular areas as highly purified and segregated zoning took hold, they had never experienced anything like this new policy. For while official government policy did not recognize let alone support urban agriculture, in practice the authorities had always turned a blind eye.[22] It is hardly surprising, then, especially coming from a government not exactly renowned among its citizens for its transparency, that the announcement of the cull generated fear, suspicion, and confusion. Many were faced with a stark choice between complying with an externally imposed version of biosecurity and the certainty that they would go hungry if they got rid of their home-reared birds.

As the government initiative proceeded, many millions of birds were culled by officials in Cairo. But many were hidden. Others were rushed to the live markets to generate much-needed income. Still others again—possibly subclinical—were killed for food or exchange ("rescuing" them, as it became known). Even when chickens were given up to the cull, many households kept their ducks as these seemed to stay healthy (but ducks are good at staying healthy even while they host HPAI). All sorts of birds, then, some infectious and some not, entered the food chain. In addition, the suddenness and severity of the cull led to food shortages, particularly among the poor. The formal as well as the informal poultry industry quickly found itself near collapse. Once responsible for exporting one hundred eighty million day-old chicks and five hundred thousand mature fowl per year, worth around EGP (Egyptian Pounds) 17 million and employing (directly and indirectly) nearly three million people, as soon as the internal and external market for the birds collapsed, prices dropped, up to a million workers were laid off, 35 percent of the poultry farms closed down, investors pulled out, and the industry was losing EGP 10 million per day. At the same time, the price of fish and nonbird meat had risen 40 percent as Cairo consumers—already constrained by the lack of home-reared poultry—looked elsewhere for their protein. When the government sought to import chickens to make up the shortfall, poultry breeders and workers held demonstrations in the streets to protest the effect on what was left of their businesses.

In the aftermath of the cull and in this climate of huge food insecurity, bio-security practices pulled avian influenza in yet another direction as a massive pro-gram got underway to restock Egyptian poultry flocks. Restocking was distributed in a certain way, favoring those places where, according to the official WHO and gov-ernment narratives, HPAI was less likely to be found. Thus, with 35 percent of com-mercial poultry farms closed down, and vast numbers of householders having lost their source of additional food and income, others like the Cairo Poultry Company (CPC) had actually increased its capital by the summer of 2006, paid out dividends, and announced plans to build a new EGP 100 million slaughterhouse in Noubaria. The new facility would increase the company's output by 350 percent from eighty thousand chickens slaughtered per day to two hundred eighty thousand, and the company hoped to supply 10 percent of the country's poultry consumption. More broadly, an associated shift from selling fresh to selling frozen poultry seemed to suit both large firms like CPC and the government, with a spokesman for the Egyptian Ministry of Health and Population quoted as saying that "despite financial losses, this is a good chance to restructure Egypt's poultry industry and place it on the right track...gradually transforming the market from eating livestock chicken into consuming frozen chicken like the rest of the world."[23]

Here we can make our fifth general point: As well as relating in various ways to other modes of securing (from simple hierarchies to more complicated interfer-ences, as we have already noted), different modes of securing also interact with other, already existing and not primarily security-based ecologies of practice.[24] These will, as both the preceding two agricultural examples illustrate very well, have their own objects of concern, be organized through their own apparatuses, and be justified by their own logics, meaning that the degree to which they lend themselves to security orderings is likely to be partial at best. Nevertheless, as between modes of securing, such encounters can take a variety of forms. The shape of Cairo's post-HPAI poultry keeping offers two extremes. On one hand we have a cityscape radically altered by the destruction of many of the chickens and ducks, and the smallholdings and markets that previously populated it, a change born of the incommensurability between the imperatives and methods of officially sanctioned biosecurity and popular practices of smallholding and food provisioning. On the other hand, we have the landscape of opportunity generated by the operational and ideological cross-fertilizations and cross-subsidies between the securing by culling of Cairo's "at risk" rooftop and backyard birds and the commercial Egyptian and international practitioners of a very different version of poultry farming. However, if contradiction and complementarity are two of the easier kinds of relationships between modes of securing and other practices, we might also briefly point to others, such as resonance (between the externally imposed need for biosecurity and the Egyptian government's longstanding and ongoing attempts to "clean up" Cairo), confusion (between the implementation of the cull and public information about the same), concession (when the Egyptian government was forced to rein in the extent of the cull after being faced with lack of resources and widespread resistance in rural areas), and adaptation (as when the government had to manipulate the market and bend some of its own biosecurity rules in order to provide cheap poultry in the run-up to Ramadan in 2006).

Remapping Avian Influenza

In the middle of 2006 a report was published by a parliamentary committee asked to assess the Egyptian government's handling of the avian influenza situation. It did not make for flattering reading, as it criticized the authorities on a number of grounds including a lack of consultation with civil society groups at the planning stage, poor public information, the rash announcement of the cull which led to the spreading of disease after infected birds were left on the streets and riverbanks, the absence of measures to protect the livelihoods of dealers with infected birds, unhygienic transport of culled bird carcasses to often unsuitable burial sites, and a confusing vaccination policy (exacerbated by the fact that after the supplies eventually arrived from China, their distribution seemed to accelerate rather than protect against the rate of bird death). Finally, the committee also reported that—contra the WHO etiology—they had found no scientific evidence that migrating birds brought the virus to Egypt. This was not the only place in which questions were being asked about what had become the official version of the distribution and transmission of HPAI H5N1. In fact, almost every aspect of the story of how avian influenza moves and is moved was being problematized as researchers all over the world gained access to the data on which that narrative was based as well as some that had not been taken into account.

First, the confident identification of migrating wild birds as a primary vector for bird flu has been reexamined. A comprehensive "critical review" of the "recent expansion of highly pathogenic avian influenza H5N1" pointed out that if migratory birds were indeed a key agent of the dispersal of H5N1 then the pattern of infection worldwide would almost certainly have been very different from that which has in fact thus far been the case.[25] The same article also notes work that suggests that the wild mortality event at Qinghai, which was key for claims regarding the role of migratory birds in spreading HPAI, was radically misinterpreted. According to some, the wild birds arrived in breeding areas that were already infected with the virus. Since Qinghai Lake is surrounded by intensive poultry farms and the manure generated by the birds is used as feed on the many fish farms that exist on the lake and as fertilizer on the fields around the lake (and it is well known that bird flu viruses can survive for over a month in cold temperatures), it is possible that the wild birds acquired the disease from the commercial poultry and not the other way around.

Such theses about alternative pathways for the cycling of H5N1 between wild and farmed birds are controversial. But, what is significant about them in this context is their very existence and the challenge they are beginning to pose to the widely circulating narrative of the disease and the regime of biosecurity that is being built around it. Another example of such reconsideration of the etiology of avian influenza can be found in increasingly prevalent suggestions that the international mass movements of birds and bird products from factories that have made the chicken the most mobile bird on the planet are deeply implicated in the disease network.[26] It has been argued that both historical comparison and epidemiological mapping of the current outbreak support the hypothesis that human movements of domestic poultry have been the main agent of human dispersal of the virus to date.[27] Poultry smuggling in particular—until recently regarded mostly as an economic nuisance but now being acknowledged as a huge and previously overlooked business, perhaps second only to drugs in terms of international contraband—is increasingly being pointed to as a previously overlooked and underresearched vector of transmission. A senior veterinarian at the FAO is quoted as saying, "I would love to have a map of illegal trade—but I'm embarrassed to say we don't have a good handle on it."[28] Nonetheless another FAO official has said that illegal trade could "easily" have introduced avian influenza into Egypt, as producers there frequently import day-old chicks because it is easier to buy them than to become practiced in the tricky techniques of hatching.

Finally, in terms of the current remapping of avian influenza, we can return to Egypt and specifically the growing prevalence of large, single-produce farms with tens of thousands of birds kept together in a handful of buildings. As we have already noted, these sorts of arrangements are not implicated in avian flu according to the WHO, FAO, and OIE. Indeed, they are envisaged as the cure and not the source of disease. However, according to some commentators (Mike Davis has been a particularly prominent example[29]), such facilities are the problem and not the solution. In this version, the density of populations; the systematic use of antibiotics and the resultant production of drug-resistant strains; the long-distance movement of livestock, livestock products, and dead stock; the uniformity of the gene pool; the known stresses that industrially raised animals suffer—all these ecologies of production contribute to an increasing prevalence of species-specific and zoonotic viruses, with the probabilities for further viral mutation.

Although highly contentious, the notion that factory farms are effectively breeding grounds for certain kinds of diseases allows us to make our sixth and final general point about biosecurity: There are reasons to doubt that a worldwide culture of safety can be engineered that is adequate to a form of organization that neces-sarily exists on the edge of breakdown. If not doubts, we at least raise questions as to what such a worldwide culture of safety would mean for the sorts of global systems—like the international poultry industry—which involve vast distances (between producers and consumers), tightly coupled processes and procedures (to facilitate the rapid and continuous flow of all sorts of things from birds to trucks), and highly complex relationships between multiple sets of logics and practices (commercial and security, for example, to say nothing of the differences between various versions of security). According to some, such systems are prone to "normal accidents,"[30] the ramifications of which tend to be rapid in their spread, unpredict-able in their direction, and potentially devastating in their scope. Whether the fermenting of zoonoses in the contemporary global poultry industry might be an example of such a "normal accident," as Davis and others seem to be suggesting, is an unanswerable question at this moment. But that is not really the point. With the past experiences of mad cow disease and foot-and-mouth disease in Britain, we have just two examples of how the presumption that systems involving an incredible variety of lively things (animals, technologies, people, currency, microorganisms, documents, etc.) can be reliably secured now and in the future is a risky one.

The Risks of Biosecurity

In this chapter we have drawn six key lessons from a case study of the arrival of HPAI H5N1 in Egypt during 2006. To briefly review: We suggest that (a) biosecurity can be best thought of as a specific problematization of conventional ways of dealing with living matters of concern; (b) the apparatus emerging from this problematization involves various different versions of security; (c) modes of security do not always operate in a neatly organized hierarchy but can also interfere with each other; (d) in practice, any version of security will only ever be an imperfect attempt at keeping things safe; (e) such attempts at securing always exist alongside and are entangled with various other sets of practices; and (f) the global systems that have resulted from this sort of entanglement might be more precarious and prone to breakdown than we usually credit.

Taken together, what do these propositions and the complex landscape they describe imply for the contemporary project of worldwide integration and harmonization of biosecurity measures that we identified in the introduction? To put it bluntly, it is fraught with risks, however appealing it might sound. One response to our account of the multiplication of, interactions between, and complications arising from the modes of biosecuring through which avian influenza was enacted in Cairo in 2006 would be to argue that it was the imposition of order that ultimately saved the day, even if the methods and practice were messy; and that more order and less diversity and divergence in the way HPAI is managed (of the sort proposed by global health governance) would have saved the day sooner and better.

This seems reasonable as a conclusion, but it misses two points. The first is the simple empirical fact that H5N1 has not been eradicated from Egypt: far from it, in fact, with over three thousand suspected human cases and fifteen confirmed deaths between February 2006 and the time of writing (late 2007), and growing fears that the disease is becoming endemic in the country after returning in the middle of 2006. But more than this, our argument is not simply that things do not always work out the way they were planned (although that is part of it), or even that global approaches to biosecurity need to be tailored to local circumstances (the distinction between the two having been problematized by our method). Rather it is that in practice, biosecurity always involves more than it knows or can possibly deal with. A full world does not mean a fully integrated world. More than that, perhaps, a full world means a world that can never be fully integrated.

So perhaps order did not win out after all, and perhaps that is at least in part because it could not or did not take seriously the heterogeneity either of the world it was trying to make safe, or of the practices of securing (which are of course part of that world). All of which raises for us the possibility that the metaphors and practices of integration and harmonization that are guiding current developments in biosecurity might not be quite right. Perhaps we should be thinking more in terms of articulation, partial connections, coordination at best when considering how to relate modes of biosecurings: images, in other words, that better fit with what we have learnt both about biosecurity and the world in which it operates. What that means in turn is that we might need to surrender some of the control and desire for control that shapes our current collective ways of dealing with viruses and other pathogens. Although it is obviously controversial to argue against efforts to eliminate contagion when people's lives and livelihoods are at stake, if what we have learnt from the Egyptian experience is right, taking the chance to reflect on the efficacies of current narratives, methods, and practices of living with disease might be one of the most effective biosecurity interventions of all.

NOTES

Acknowledgment: This chapter is indebted to a great many other people and their work, but especially Annemarie Mol and John Law who are continually challenging and inspiring us to think through the multiplicities of disease.

1   United Nations, Food and Agriculture Organization, *Biosecurity Tool Kit* (2007), http://www.fao.org/docrep/010/a1140e/a1140e00.htm.

2   Federation of American Scientists, Case Studies in Dual-Use Biological Research (2007), http://www.fas.org/biosecurity/education/dualuse/.

3   David Fidler and Lawrence Gostin, *Biosecurity in the Global Age* (Stanford, CA: Stanford University Press, 2008).

4   EMRO–WHO, "Avian Influenza," Press Release No. 15 (2005), http://www.emro.who.int/pressreleases/2005/no15.htm.

5   Reported in Stephen Morse, *Emerging Viruses* (New York: Oxford University Press, 1993).

6   Nicholas B. King, "Security, Disease, Commerce: Ideologies of Postcolonial Global Health," *Social Studies of Science* 32, no. 5/6 (2002): 763–89.

7   Joshua Lederberg, Robert Shope, and Stanley Oaks, *Emerging Infections: Microbial Threats to the United States* (Washington, DC: National Academies Press, 1992).

8   Kelley Lee and David Fidler, "Avian and Pandemic Influenza: Progress and Problems with Global Health Governance," *Global Public Health* 2, no. 3 (2007): 215–34.

9   Michel Foucault, *Security, Territory, Population: Lectures at the Collège de France, 1977–78* (London: Palgrave Macmillan, 2007).

10 WHO, Avian Influenza Fact Sheet (February 2006), http://www.who.int/mediacentre/factsheets/avian_influenza/en/print.html.

11 Ibid.

12 Michael Dillon, "Governing Terror: The State

of Emergency of Biopolitical Emergence," *International Political Sociology* 1 (2007): 7–28.

13 Grain, "Fowl Play: The Poultry Industry"s Central Role in the Bird Flu Crisis," *Against the Grain* (February 2006), http://www.grain.org/go/birdflu.

14 Grain, "The Top-Down Global Response to Bird Flu," *Against the Grain* (April 2006), http://www.grain.org/articles/?id=12.

15 For more detail on the history of this sanitation, see Timothy Mitchell, *Rule of Experts: Egypt, Technopolitics, Modernity* (Berkeley: University of California Press, 2002).

16 For more on this notion of interference, see Annemarie Mol, *The Body Multiple: Ontology in Medical Practice* (Durham, NC: Duke University Press, 2002).

17 For more on modes of ordering, see John Law, *Organizing Modernity* (Oxford: Blackwell, 1994).

18 Quoted in Reem Leila, "Poultry Industry Collapses," *Al-Ahram Weekly*, February 3–March 1, 2006, http://weekly.ahram.org.eg/print/2006/783/eg1.htm.

19 J. Gertel and S. Samir, "Cairo: Urban Agriculture and 'Visions' for a Modern City," in *Growing Cities, Growing Food: Urban Agriculture on the Policy Agenda. A Reader on Urban Agriculture,* eds. N. Bakker et al. (Feldafing, Germany: German Foundation for International Development [DSE], 2000).

20 For details, see Mitchell, *Rule of Experts.*

21 Gertel and Samir, "Cairo," 227.

22 For more on the hugely complex relationships in Cairo between the economic practices of marginal groups, NGOs, states, and international organizations such as the World Bank that are too quickly referred to as the "informal" economy, see Julia Elyachar, *Markets of Dispossession: NGOs, Economic Development,*

and the State in Cairo (Durham, NC: Duke University Press, 2005).

23 Sherine El-Madany, "The Cluck Stops Here," Business Today Egypt, May 2006, 2.

24 See Steve Hinchliffe, Geographies of Nature (London: Sage, 2007).

25 M. Gauthier-Clerc, M. C. Lebarbenchon, and F. Thomas, "Recent Expansion of Highly Pathogenic Avian Influenza H5N1: A Critical Review," Ibis 149 (2007): 202–14.

26 BirdLife International, BirdLife Statement on Avian Influenza (updated August 2007), http://www.birdlife.org/action/science/species/avian_flu/index.html.

27 Gauthier-Clerc et al., "Recent Expansion," 207.

28 Juan Lubroth, quoted in Elizabeth Rosenthal, "Smugglers Undercut Fight Against Bird Flu," International Herald Tribune, April 16, 2006.

19 Mike Davis, The Monster at Our Door: The Global Threat of Avian Flu (New York: The New Press, 2005).

30 John Law offers a much more developed version of this argument drawing on the work of Charles Perrow; see "Disaster in Agriculture: Or Foot and Mouth Mobilities," Environment and Planning A 38, no. 2 (2006): 227–39.

CHAPTER EIGHT

From Mad Cow Disease to Bird Flu

TRANSFORMATIONS OF FOOD SAFETY IN FRANCE

Frédéric Keck

In this chapter I argue that the term "biosecurity," which has appeared recently in discussions on the avian influenza pandemic, should be inserted into the scientific controversies between experts, rather than criticized from the outside as an apparatus of hegemonic power, or taken as a self-evident technique of protection. I show that, in France, the avian flu crisis was understood in terms of the bovine spongiform encephalopathy crisis (known as mad cow disease), and raised similar controversies between experts: in particular, it divided the veterinarians, considered as defending the interests of animal husbandry, and the physicians, considered as promoting a public health mission in the service of the consumer. I raise the anthropological hypothesis that these controversies between scientists express a more fundamental contradiction in animal diseases, which can be considered from two points of view: concerning a whole animal spectrum (epizootia) or concerning particularly humans (pandemic). I also try to clarify notions of prevention, precaution, preparedness, conflict of interest, and collective expertise, starting from their use in the controversies between scientists.

"Biosecurity," A Controversial Term

In September 2006, I was a participant-observer among a group of experts called the Groupe d'Expertise Collective en Urgence sur l'Influenza Aviaire (GECUIA) at the Agence Française de Sécurité Sanitaire des Aliments (AFSSA), the French food safety agency. Seated around the table were veterinarians from the Ecole Nationale

Vétérinaire de Maisons Alfort, ornithologists from the Muséum National d'Histoire Naturelle, and a physician from the Institut National de Veille Sanitaire. They were retracing the history of the mutation of the highly pathogenic strain of the H5N1 virus from its first appearance in China to the only case that was found in France, in February 2005. The aim of this collective expertise was to assess the risk of a proliferation of the virus in the country, particularly its interhuman pandemic form. Jokes were made about the turkey farm where the virus appeared in Dombes, a humid area with much traditional poultry breeding and where migratory birds are also numerous. It is still not certain whether this farm was contaminated by the wild duck found dead in a pond a few kilometers from there, or by the journalists and government officials who had come to see the pond and then moved to the farm.[1] The veterinarians felt that everyone should be held responsible for sanitary conditions on poultry farms, not just breeders, but also distributors of animal food, politicians, and journalists.[2] One of them said breeders should have to observe biosecurity precautions, such as wearing plastic caps or washing the wheels of their cars before entering the farm. "I am a biosecurity fanatic," she said. The other veterinarians laughed. "Biosecurity" was just a new word, they said, and it was used unreflectively. In a private interview I had with this veterinarian, she told me she worked as an expert witness in trials where breeders prosecuted those they accused of having contaminated their farms; the veterinarians were often themselves criticized for not observing proper biosecurity measures. Although only recently introduced, she felt that the term "biosecurity" described practices for which there was no better word.

A few weeks later, I had an interview with Muriel Eliaszewicz, a physician who worked with AIDS patients and ran the Direction d'Evaluation des Risques Nutritionnels et Sanitaires (DERNS), which standardized risk assessment in AFSSA. I asked which of the following terms best described what she was doing: urgent decision making, vigilance, preventing catastrophes, biosecurity. "Biosecurity" ranked fourth. She called it a "security delirium," in which every biological being was seen as a threat. As a founding member of AFSSA, she preferred to talk about health safety (*sécurité sanitaire*), which provided a paradigm for thinking about food consumption according to the model of taking drugs. But with the shift in agency priorities, and the new focus on avian influenza (AI), she knew that biosecurity had become more and more prominent. What she disliked about the term was that it stressed food production conditions rather than risks to consumers; it confused risk assessment with risk management (*évaluation* and *gestion*). In her perspective, "bios" was too broad a prefix to qualify the relations of cure and care (*soin*) that needed to be evaluated in their specific contexts. While veterinarians distinguished different animal species that were hosts for a disease, she differentiated consumers by their sanitary conditions, which would expose them to more or less risk. "Biosecurity" was too large to include all the beings that were brought together through the act of eating, although it captured them in an intriguing way.

In this chapter, I want to show how biosecurity has emerged as a problem in the field of discourses and practices that was constituted ten years earlier around food safety. In the two ethnographic examples above, "biosecurity" appeared as a new word that allowed threats to be categorized and blame to be distributed in ways that are still controversial, depending on where the blame is cast and who the victims are considered to be. Before answering the question of how the state should intervene in the face of an uncertain threat and who should accept the blame for the appearance of the threat, one must ask how the problem came to be posed, and why it has been viewed so differently. Since experts disagree on the term "biosecurity," I argue that these disagreements reveal tensions that constitute them as a social group: tensions between physicians and veterinarians, and among veterinarians themselves.[3] The meaning of "biosecurity" depends on the controversies that shape each context, and on how these controversies structure the world of experts.

In the English-speaking world, "biosecurity" actually refers to three domains of intervention: farm-based practices that may allow contamination by animal diseases, border controls that regulate the spread of infectious agents into human populations, and the fight against the intentional use of pathogens for terrorist purposes.[4] In France, the term *biosécurité* was introduced with the controversy over genetically modified organisms, which crystallized a major wave of critiques around food safety.[5] Food safety is then a good ethnographic site from which to investigate how competencies and arguments have been elaborated by experts who have to deal with the problem of biosecurity today. This brings us to the question: How did food safety become a problem, and how did it pit expert professionals such as physicians and veterinarians against one another?

Object: The Meaning of Animal Diseases in Food Safety Crises

I rely here on two years of fieldwork at AFSSA, during which time I observed several expert committees and conducted interviews with scientists both on the committees and in the labs. AFSSA was created in 1998 after the mad cow crisis, to prevent the introduction of infectious agents into the food chain. Following the principle of precaution, it assesses the risks of food products before they are commercialized, and has a mission to ensure public health. As an ethnographer, I was surprised that AI came to be problematized as a food safety issue, since it is clear that cooking the chicken is enough to kill the virus. The official reason is that, after the first case of H5N1 in February 2005, when the media spread the news of a virus that could be transmitted from birds to humans, the consumption of poultry fell by 20 percent; AFSSA, among other institutions such as the Direction d'Information sur les Viandes, had to reassure the public that there was no risk in eating chicken. The bird flu crisis, as it came to be known, was analogous to the mad cow crisis in that it created similar panic among consumers. By talking about "avian influenza" rather than "bird flu," or bovine spongiform encephalopathy (BSE) rather than "mad cow disease," AFSSA responded to sanitary crises with clear and scientifically grounded information on food production. It covered the food chain "from the farm to the fork" (*de la fourche à la fourchette*), since the risks to farmers, who deal with live poultry, are as important as the risks to consumers, who eat dead chicken.

In one way, the entry of AI into the domain of AFSSA was a sign of the organization's success: it had become so legitimate in regard to food safety issues that it could incorporate sanitary problems situated at the outer limits of its field. But there was another reason why AFSSA was mobilized on AI: as an animal disease, it could be addressed either by veterinarians or by physicians, depending on whether the virus was considered from the perspective of its consequences for animals or its impact on humans. In the case of mad cow disease, the collaboration between veterinarians and physicians was necessary, as the BSE agent had already passed from animals to humans. But in the case of AI, this collaboration was more problematic: the H5N1 virus had not (yet?) mutated into an interhuman form, yet plans for a pandemic were already being drawn up by physicians. In another way, AFSSA's success in incorporating bird flu is also a sign of its fragility, revealing an internal tension in its public health mission as to whether it concerns animals or humans. I discovered that the controversy between veterinarians and physicians over animal diseases profoundly structures the field of food safety, and gives a specific meaning to the term "biosecurity" as it emerges in this field. The question I raise is therefore: How has the shift from mad cow disease to bird flu, considered as two major public health crises, transformed the discourses and practices of experts in such a way that biosecurity came to be problematized in terms of the impact of animal diseases on food safety?

This question presupposes another one, which will be addressed only indirectly: Why have animal diseases, among all food safety issues, produced such intense critical activity? My contention is that animal diseases introduce into food safety assessment a tension between two contradictory representations: the animal as good potential food and the animal as a dangerous living being. The English language uses interesting distinctions to express this contradiction: beef and cow, veal and calf, mutton and sheep, chicken and poultry. Experts have to translate this contradiction into their own practices, and they produce intermediary terms to resolve it; "public health" and "risk" take on different meanings when they are considered in animal life or human life. The contradiction between two extreme poles of a human experience (the alimentary act) is what gives food safety crises their significance. The language of risk works ambiguously because it offers provisional compromises to this contradiction.

This contradiction can be expressed in a more historical way: the domestication of animals introduced both a huge stock of food and a new site for viruses. The animals we eat are also those we should be afraid of, as domestication techniques imply new possibilities for mutation and replication of infectious agents. Emerging diseases come from the "livestock revolution" by which we produce and transport animals in an industrial system.[6] Mad cow disease and bird flu have shown that techniques of animal feeding, transportation, and slaughter bring with them new risks of transmission for emerging diseases. As historian William McNeill has observed: "On the time scale of world history, we should view the 'domestication' of epidemic diseases that occurred between 1300 and 1700 as a fundamental breakthrough, directly resulting from the two great transportation revolutions of that age—one by land, initiated by the Mongols, and one by sea, initiated by the Europeans."[7] More recently, physiologist Jared Diamond has talked about the "lethal gift of livestock," and argued that the difference between Amerindians and Europeans was not merely that the latter had military might but that they had become used to the viruses they brought with their domesticated animals, inventing vaccines as a counter gift to the gift of meat and viruses.[8] Far from being natural, animal diseases are related to the way society integrates animals into their milieu; and they tend to make food consumption a problematic act that forces a redrawing of the boundaries between humans and animals in the milieu in which they interact.

It is not enough, however, to content ourselves with broad historical narratives. Rather, it is necessary to observe in each society how the alimentary act problematizes the relations between animals and humans. Philippe Descola recently said that once we abandon the nature/culture divide as a broad anthropological category, it remains an ethnographic task to show how interiorities and physicalities are linked in various contexts, depending on the ontologies that articulate the problems raised by basic attitudes towards things, such as eating animals. Thus, for animist societies that posit animals as sharing with humans the same interiority, food consumption becomes a problem because animals have to be divested of their subjectivity: "A doubt always remains: under the flesh of the animal or the plant that I eat, what subsists of its human subjectivity? What guarantee do I have that I do not (or no longer) eat a subject that is like me?"[9] Starting from very different assumptions, which Descola would call "naturalistic," food safety experts have to answer the same question: If the animals we have domesticated share infectious agents with us, what guarantee do we have that we are not being killed by the living forms we have ourselves produced?

My hypothesis is that animal diseases such as mad cow disease or bird flu reveal anthropological tensions in the alimentary act, which appear as logical contradictions during food safety crises. Relying on the ethnography of AFSSA, I will show how experts deal with these contradictions in a way that is specific to the French context, but that might be analogous to other treatments of the same tensions in other contexts. I assume therefore that the work of expertise is not radically different from the daily cognitive work of those who have to deal with animal diseases (hunters, breeders); it is only more formal, which makes the study of these contradictions easier.

Method: An Anthropology of Contemporary Critique on Human/Animal Relationships

This hypothesis articulates three different theoretical lines. First, it belongs to an anthropology of the contemporary, attentive to the assemblages of discourses, practices, techniques, and institutions that constitute the present through a reconfiguration of older elements.[10] It takes emerging infectious diseases as a site of curiosity and interest in which significant transformations take place in the apparatuses that constitute public health as a stabilized domain. Following Michel Foucault, it raises the question of the biopolitical significance of these diseases, that is, the change they introduce into power relationships between the sovereign power and the power of expertise. In the case of BSE or AI, the dilemma between culling animals and vaccinating them, which has both moral and economic aspects, raises in a specific way the question of the articulation between sovereignty and biopolitics, between the power to "make die and let live" and the power to "let die and make live"—what Foucault called "the acceptability of putting to death in a biopolitical regime."[11]

Second, it relies on an ethnology of human/animal relationships. It presupposes that the separation between humans and animals is not a fixed and given frontier, but needs to be redrawn following certain ideals (such as public health) and depending on specific contexts. It takes this separation as a logical contradiction that constitutes discourses such that they cannot be addressed directly but only through the displacement of binary oppositions. Following Claude Lévi-Strauss, it describes historical change as a transformation of a logical contradiction, showing logical structures that organize the empirical material.[12] It therefore takes the biopolitical as a space of tensions and contradictions, which can be analyzed if they are linked to potentially universal oppositions, such as that between humans and nonhumans.[13] I borrow from Lévi-Strauss the notion of "transformation," which he applies to human/nonhuman relationships in Amerindian mythology, and apply it to the shift from one food safety crisis to another. Food safety crises can be compared because they share a general form, but this form is unstable because it relies on a structural tension in human experience that is oriented in various ways depending on the context in which it appears. Animal diseases are therefore a good site to observe how the term "biosecurity" articulates some constitutive tensions of the *bios* in a new way.

Third, it takes part in a sociology of critique that doesn't consider critique as a denunciatory privilege of the observer, but rather as an activity exercised by the actors themselves.[14] Although it is tempting to denounce biosecurity as a uniform frame of power imposed on life considered as a unified entity, by following the emergence of the word and the differences it reveals in the discourses and practices of experts we can map criticisms of the term to give us a sense of the problems that are at stake. Food safety experts all consider public health as a good to be pursued for its own sake.[15] Since they are asked to evaluate the quality of the food in distribution, they mix forms of assessment that depend on scientific criteria with forms of assessment that draw on other regimes of normativity, relying on much more "familiar" forms of evaluation.[16] They have different views of the good and different expert knowledges (*compétences*) depending on their position in the spectrum that bounds animal health and human health. A sociology of critique is attentive to the ethical dimension of biosecurity in its plurality, and tries to describe the various ethos that enter into a productive tension on biopolitical issues. It therefore raises the problem of the contribution of social sciences to a critical understanding of the present, on which this chapter will conclude.

Tensions between Veterinarians and Physicians: From the Contaminated Blood Affair to Mad Cow Disease

AFSSA was created in 1999 to replace a network of veterinary labs, the Centre National d'Etudes Vétérinaires et Alimentaires (CNEVA). It created the Direction d'Evaluation des Risques Nutritionnels et Sanitaires (DERNS), mostly run by physicians, who oriented risk assessment toward the protection of the consumer and, through collective expertise, added a new form of risk assessment to the older structure of surveillance by laboratories.[17] Veterinary experts who used to work separately under the supervision of the Ministry of Agriculture now came to work collectively for DERNS. The change from *vétérinaire et alimentaire* to *nutritionnel et sanitaire* was significant. Nutrition, a discipline with little prestige in the academic world but much impact on public opinion, was used as a way to reframe the sanitary conditions of food production in terms of its risks to the consumer.

This political decision was significant for the way in which food safety came to be problematized in France as a public health issue. In the context of the formation of the French state, veterinarians were in charge of food safety: they were the representatives of the state all along the food chain, and had to respond to crises that emerged over specific foods, such as milk or meat.[18] The French veterinary surveillance network, developed in the nineteenth century, is organized around four veterinary high schools run by the state (Maisons-Alfort, Lyon, Nantes, and Toulouse). After a century of struggle against the empirical methods of breeders, veterinarians had finally earned the trust of the state, in the context of the rationalization of agriculture as one of the nation's main resources.[19] This relationship was destroyed by mad cow disease. When it was revealed that a new variant of Creutzfeldt–Jakob disease had been transmitted by eating beef, and when the first cases in Great Britain were linked to the reduction in the temperature used to warm meat and bone meal in animal feed, the veterinary network of surveillance came under suspicion. Veterinarians were criticized from both sides: by breeders, because they exposed a disease whose economic consequences were huge and whose health impact was still unknown, and by consumers, who accused them, along with breeders, of having allowed an infectious agent to enter the food chain through an irresponsible use of modern technologies.[20] True, meat and bone meal had been used since the beginning of the twentieth century as a zootechnical measure to increase the amount of protein fed to animals, meanwhile recycling the animal remains and leftovers in slaughterhouses that would have been otherwise useless: it was a constitutive part of the modern agricultural contract. But when the infectious agents responsible for the Creutzfeldt–Jakob disease were discovered to pass through meat and bone meal and cause the degeneration of brain tissue in animals and then in humans, public light was shed on this technical process, which was then denounced as having denatured cows by turning them into cannibals.[21] From the perspective of the veterinarians, mad cow disease was both a professional challenge and a political nightmare. The dissemination of an animal disease was their responsibility, and they were called to the highest levels of the state to try to explain the problem; but the peculiar nature of the infectious agent, and the wave of criticism against the use of meat and bone meal, forced them to open up their field of expertise to other actors with whom they were potentially in competition.

Indeed, the institutionalization of food safety through the creation of AFSSA can be described as a shift in the site of authority over surveillance and control of the food chain from veterinarians to physicians. Physicians had traditionally been in charge of food safety as the hygienic tradition brought food preparation for babies and the elderly under scrutiny,[22] but they left the first stages of the food chain to the veterinarians. From the perspective of physicians, within the patient–doctor relationship, food is one of the basic constituents of a person's health and well being; from the perspective of veterinarians, it is the product of a chain that implies both animals and humans—through breeders and distributors. Mad cow disease shifted the gaze of the physicians from the end of the food chain (the act of consumption) to the possible origin of the disease at the beginning of the chain, the material conditions in which the food was produced. Consequently, the control of food safety was partly transferred from the Ministry of Agriculture, working closely with breeders and veterinarians, to the Ministry of Health, which imported practices from the drug safety industry into food safety.

This transfer had begun in the 1980s after the professional trauma created by the contaminated blood scandal, when it was revealed that HIV had been disseminated through the state-controlled blood transfusion system to hemophilic patients; this called into question one of the core ideals of the medical profession. The French blood transfusion system had shifted from patient-to-patient blood donation to a collective network of distribution that required trust. This trust derived from the model of the World War II Resistance, in which the donation of blood was voluntary, as opposed to the commercial use of blood by collaborators with the Vichy state. The revelation of the presence of HIV in the blood supply had put the moral relationship between the state, physicians, and patients in jeopardy, because it turned out that the precautions to avoid this threat had not been taken for economic reasons.[23] Mad cow disease then appeared as a new battlefield: restoring public health now meant establishing control over the food chain. If an infectious agent such as HIV had been allowed to enter the blood circuit because of a failure of the state, stopping the entrance of the prion into the food chain would reassert the authority of the state.

Thinking about mad cow disease along the lines of the contaminated blood scandal resulted in a redefinition of public health that introduced a potential conflict with animal health. In 1964, Charles Schwabe could write: "The practices of veterinary medicine and public health are based upon identical population concepts. The herd and the flock almost always have assumed a more important place in the veterinarian's thinking than had the individual animal. Similarly, in public health, the individual is not the patient but the community is."[24] In 1998, the object of public health was no longer the population but the individual at risk. Consequently, "viewing man with some objectivity as just another host species in the epidemiological pattern of any particular disease" was no longer sufficient as a public health rationale.[25] The life of a single individual became more important than the economic sustainability of an animal flock. Veterinarians and physicians, who had served the same ideal of public health, now came into conflict, because this ideal had been redefined by the two scandals and had thus become controversial. AFSSA was now a battlefield on which veterinarians and physicians expressed their disagreement in terms of risk assessment. Therefore, expertise in food safety can be described as a conflictual domain between two professions, each blaming the other: physicians accused the veterinarians of allowing mad cow disease to enter the food chain; veterinarians responded that physicians were responsible for the contamination of the blood supply.

Viewing mad cow disease through the lens of the contaminated blood scandal made it a particularly unstable phenomenon, depending on whether it was considered an animal disease or a human disease. An animal disease can be characterized as epizootic, when it concerns only animals, or zoonotic, when it also concerns humans. From the perspective of veterinarians, mad cow disease is the moment when public opinion discovered that animal diseases could spread from animals to humans; incriminating the use of meat and bone meal was just a way to deny this problem by saying that the cows that had gone mad were not really animals. The interpretation of mad cow disease therefore divides two professions serving public health: in one perspective, public health is a prolongation of animal health, but in another, it is not. This makes food safety, rather than a stabilized domain, a field of problematization around a particularly unstable phenomenon. Veterinarians and physicians came into opposition because, in the wake of two scandals, they came to take opposite views of the same phenomenon.[26] Rather than opposing nature (the dissemination of an infectious agent) and culture (the intentional use of biological weapons), I argue that it is better to start from a contradiction in the perception of the living environment—infectious agents pass from humans to animals, yet with radically different consequences—and show how it structures the daily routine of expertise.

Expertise in Daily Life: Transformations of a Contradiction

DEBATE AND THE PRODUCTION OF RECOMMENDATIONS

When I arrived at AFSSA, the tension between physicians and veterinarians had crystallized into a division between the expert committees on which physicians were predominant (e.g., biotechnologies or nutrition), and those on which veterinarians were the majority (e.g., animal health or animal food). Veterinarians and physicians had nonetheless worked together on the expert committee on BSE, but there were now controversies over whether this committee should be absorbed by the animal health committee or remain autonomous. The BSE committee is particularly symbolic as it was the original one—the Comité interministériel sur les ESST et les prions, usually just called the Comité Dormont—on which the others were modeled. Created by the French government in 1996, it gathered around the charismatic figure of a renowned scientist, Dominique Dormont, experts from many areas to identify the BSE infectious agent and issue recommendations (*avis*) to limit its spread. The era of the Comité Dormont is remembered as a period of scientific stimulation, debates, urgent decision making, and a sense of the political importance of the work being done.[27] François Moutou, who took part in the Comité Dormont and now sits on the animal health committee at AFSSA, recalls: "There were a few recommendations in which the majority thought in one direction and some people thought the other way, and the rule was that people should not exercise self-censorship but should dare to express their point of view."[28] Today, many of the experts complain that the work has become routinized, although still led by an imperative of urgency, which becomes a rule in itself. GECUIA is now composed exclusively of veterinarians, as the physicians who were initially contacted gradually declined to serve. Thus the forum of debate tends to become an empty space, as the professions reassert their fundamental doctrines. During the mad cow episode, "collective effervescence" allowed contradictions to be expressed in the pursuit of public health; today, the tensions cannot take the form of a contradiction, and so are expressed in other ways.

One significant event was rewriting the recommendation on Q fever, an animal disease that can be transmitted to humans. Muriel Eliaszewicz recalls: "In December 2004, the expert committee had collectively produced a recommendation that, in the eyes of the director of the agency, underestimated the risk of transmission to humans. Consequently, we at DERNS proposed to add remarks to the published *avis* that were in real contradiction to the opinion of the experts. It became violent: the expert committee on Animal Health worked as a closed microcosm, and we had to break through this fused organization. We then had to give an account to the expert committee on Microbiology: they acted like a tribunal, and asked the secretaries [who write the reports for the head office] to give an account of what had happened. It was a real trauma. Now, when DERNS knows that a recommendation is sensitive—that is, when it concerns agricultural interests—they launch the alert before the recommendation is published."[29] Barbara Dufour, a veterinarian working for AFSSA, who is used to public controversy because of her work with cattlemen's trade unions, teaching at the Ecole Vétérinaire, and interviews with the media, said that the animal health committee, though composed of very different personalities, had suddenly became unanimous: "On one side, there were thirteen experts, some Q fever specialists; on the other, there were the generalists, who wrote something else, in contradiction to the report."[30] This episode is interesting because it is the only moment in the life of the agency when a disagreement was publicly expressed, through the juxtaposition of the opinions of the experts and of DERNS on the same recommendation. Since the contradiction didn't appear between experts, horizontally, it was displaced in a hierarchical way, vertically divided between the expert committees and DERNS. Since this dramatic episode, DERNS has tried to avoid publicizing such disagreement by anticipating the opposition of the animal health committee; contradictions have once again disappeared in the daily routine of expertise.

CONFLICTS OF INTEREST

These tensions can also be observed in the use that is made of the notion of conflict of interest, which guarantees that those who evaluate a project do not have an economic (or political or ideological) interest in the realization of that project. Consumer associations have the right to ask the agency questions, but food industry companies do not, and they are carefully kept outside the process of risk assessment. Experts have to declare their conflicts of interest every three years, when they apply or reapply to the agency, and at the beginning of each expert committee, as a kind of ritual purification that allows them to enter the space of expertise. But this declaration is interpreted differently according to the position of experts in the field. For some physicians, the declaration of conflict of interest is sufficient motive to leave the space of discussion. "If have a conflict of interest, I prefer not to attend the discussion," says Eliaszewicz, referring to the opacity that reigns in certain parts of the hospital where profitability is more important than the protection of human life. When an expert veterinarian says he has previously worked on a project for the Ministry of Agriculture, the president of the animal health committee asks: "Do you feel you have a conflict of interest?" "No," replies the veterinarian, "I have examined this project in terms of collective expertise, and not as an individual expert." This means the expert may speak in two different registers: as a participant in the food chain that he needs to know in order to evaluate the safety of a production technique, and as a participant in the collective expertise organized by its own rules of independence and transparency—causing unique schizophrenia in a scientist who must divide him/herself between the individual and the collective expert.

The division between veterinarians and physicians on this issue should not be overemphasized. Dominique Turck, a physician who runs the nutrition committee, works for milk companies and admits that he cannot evaluate the safety of milk if he is not familiar with the technical and economic aspects of its production. "We all have conflicts of interest," he says, to suggest that talking about the commercial aspects of nutrition issues is what makes the discussion interesting.[31] In a world of experts where economic interests cannot but interfere with pure science, it is better to speak of "interested knowledge" rather than denouncing conflicts of interest.[32] But it is also better to observe how the accusation of having a conflict of interest expresses other tensions between experts: it's the best way to discredit an expert. Declaring a conflict of interest is a delicate task that can affect an expert's legitimacy for a long time: since everyone knows who works for which company, it is considered better not to publicly declare one's conflicts of interest. Because they are suspected of taking the side of breeders on animal diseases, veterinarians are collectively accused of always being in a conflict of interest; but this accusation has no formal value, and only displaces the tension between experts into other arenas of the agency. Therefore, the notion of conflict of interest displaces the opposition between experts from the scene of collective expertise to the halls of the agency, where it takes the form of rumor rather than public judgment.

Having described the shifts of the contradiction between animal health and human health in its more formal aspect (through the different spaces of the agency where it is expressed),[33] I will now turn to its content—that is, to the different visions of the same disease historically produced by this contradiction. Rather than "visions of the disease," which might sound too culturalistic and holistic, I will talk about "rationalities of risk," to show that these different visions are rational because they represent different aspects of the same pathology, the contradiction of which precludes producing a unique and homogeneous conception. My hypothesis is that these different rationalities transform each other, which means they are structural versions of the same contradiction that are transposed to different contents in different contexts.

A Transformation in the Rationality of Risk

FROM *PRÉVENTION* (PREVENTION), TO *PRÉCAUTION* (PRECAUTION), TO *PRÉPARATION* (PREPAREDNESS)

The difference between veterinarians and physicians in risk assessment is clearly expressed by François Moutou, an animal epidemiology specialist and member of AFSSA:

> When we assess risk, from our data, we say the risk should be as high as this and as low as this, with a 95% probability of being between these two levels. The administration that manages risk sees only the highest risk and adapts all the

management measures to this risk. Then the question is: is it worth showing that there is uncertainty; that on the other side they are certain that it should not be at the highest level of risk? If new information leads us to lower the risk level, it is not certain that the administration will modify the prevention plan. Take avian influenza: we are still at the highest risk, even though the epidemiological data do not seem to support the risk of transmission to humans.[34]

This statement illustrates the difference between two rationalities of risk that I will call, according to the French words (which may not be equivalent to their English counterparts), *prévention* and *précaution*. Rather than saying that veterinarians emphasize low risk while physicians emphasize high risk, it is better to analyze the words as indicating two different visions of a disease.

Veterinarians have traditionally practiced prevention; they have established a surveillance network based on epidemiology, in which every single case in farm animals can be detected and analyzed, and they can intervene to minimize the risk of transmission in a population. They view animals as a population among which infectious agents are transmitted before they are passed to humans. The status of animal epidemiology is therefore ambivalent: it is not clear whether the study of the virus aims at reducing the cost of its effects on animals or avoiding its transmission to humans. The infectious agent is the enemy, but the animal livestock is the element through which it propagates. We can read in an epidemiology textbook: "To successfully fight an enemy, one must know the enemy. To do this, we need to classify animals and groups of animals according to their status with respect to diseases."[35] Prevention, in that sense, is an anticipation of the infectious cases in which the animal population is the equivalent of a "milieu" that one must know—in order to be protected against its threats, but also to maximize its economic potentialities. The rationality of animal epidemiology is a rationality of cases and propagation zones: concepts of prevalence and incidence orient the gaze toward the proliferation of cases in order to make them predictable. The fight against diseases implies the accumulation of numbers and the delimitation of zones: it is the knowledge of a certain milieu in which humans and animals are both united and opposed as regards their common exposure to the disease. Animals that are apparently healthy can propagate an infectious agent more rapidly than diseased animals; on the contrary, some animals can be considered as epidemiological dead-ends. Prevention thus opens a spectrum of animal classifications after the incidence of one case: it is based on the confidence of humans in their capacity to cover the animal population with an overarching gaze.

Precaution, on the other hand, implies a space of action based on the limitation of knowledge. Knowledge is not used to clarify the propagation of the infectious agent but to raise doubts about the very possibility of any prediction. François Ewald makes this distinction: "While the attitude of prevention supposes a relation to knowledge that guarantees the veracity of knowledge, the hypothesis of precaution causes us to see a deceitful and malicious demon behind every case."[36] In the principle of precaution, the result of knowledge is itself brought under suspicion: the introduction of meat and bone meal is thus compared to the use of genetically modified organisms as the manipulation of living beings by a science that introduces new risks. But rather than discarding knowledge, precaution implies a new use of knowledge, to protect reflectively a world that science itself has transformed. In a rigorous sense, the principle of precaution can be invoked even when the risk is not known and needs further research before action can be taken. Precaution represents risk as the greatest catastrophe in order to stop commercial action and open a space for scientific reflection. While prevention defines risk in probabilistic terms, precaution implies a public policy in which risks are seen from the perspective of a moral community: a low probability/high consequence epidemiological case becomes a catastrophic event that orients public action.

Mad cow disease opposed prevention and precaution in a schematic way. Veterinarians followed the dissemination of the infectious agents in the food chain, and took into account the interests of all the actors in this chain: if a measure seemed inappropriate for breeders, they would try to minimize the risk. On the contrary, physicians emphasized the worst case scenario (in 2002 the *British Medical Journal* published a study by James Ironside predicting ten thousand human deaths in Great Britain, which was lower than the first estimate of seven hundred thousand in 1996),[37] insisting on the spectacular aspect of the human disease (often young patients suffering from brain degeneration), the difficulty of identifying the pathogenic agent (there is still no consensus on the role of the prion), and the long incubation period. One of the physicians who set up AFSSA admitted to me that there may have been more human deaths from the suicide of cattlemen than from the consumption of contaminated beef, but that the principle of precaution had to be implemented to reorganize the food chain after the disorders revealed by mad cow disease.

Avian influenza has transformed this opposition in an interesting way. After the first hypotheses imputing the spread of the disease to migratory birds, veterinary experts in GECUIA were influential in stressing that the path of the virus was parallel not only to the route of migratory birds but also to the trans-Siberian road, on which there is a lot of commerce in domestic poultry and many industrial farms. This argument is similar to the one that had been proposed for mad cow disease, when the contamination was imputed to the faulty use of animal foodstuff; and yet, the problematization of safety became very different. Avian influenza presented an opportunity for veterinarians to use the logic of prevention in a new way. The question that they asked was not, Is there a risk in the consumption of poultry meat? but, How does the disease propagate, and how can we stop it? The analysis of the risks of AI implied drawing up a spectrum of potential animal carriers: it was said at the start of the epizootia (and then denied) that pigs were carriers, which made it a possible laboratory for mutation to humanly transmissible forms; people even abandoned their cats along the roads when they thought that they could also have the disease. As Marc Savey, one of the veterinarians who founded AFSSA, says: "We expected a huge avian spectrum but the spectrum has not opened itself much. If we say that the spectrum is more or less opened, we cannot come to the same conclusion in terms of risk analysis."[38] Since the nature of the virus was not in question, the point was to classify all animal species with respect to the possibility of its transmission: between sensitive species and receptive species, between carriers and epidemiological dead ends.

But physicians took it in a different direction, and introduced a new rationality of risk. If the H5N1 virus was of the same stock as the one that had killed twenty million people after World War I, it could cause a worldwide pandemic (there was talk of sixty million human deaths), whose effects should be immediately foreseen and mitigated. The question for physicians was not: Is there a risk of mutation of H5N1 to an interhuman form? but: Are we prepared for this catastrophe and what vulnerabilities would it reveal in the public health infrastructure?[39] Physicians thus made the shift from precaution to preparedness (*préparation*). Didier Houssin, in charge of the Direction Générale de la Santé Humaine and Délégué Interministériel de Lutte contre La Grippe Aviaire, characterized this disposition toward preparedness while relying on the language of prevention:

> Contrary to...1918, we are not in a situation that leaves us entirely unarmed. In 1918, our grandparents did not even know it was a virus, they had no capacity for identification, and they had no way to fight or prevent this phenomenon. We are not in the same situation. Today we have a network of surveillance and epidemiology that, even if it is not perfect, has a certain capacity to react. We know it is a virus. We even know it intimately. We know its genome from A to Z. We are able to produce and transmit information rapidly. So we have capacities that give us a certain responsibility.[40]

Because prevention makes it possible to see the dissemination of the virus in its most intimate movements, it places a certain responsibility at the end of the chain of dissemination, even if this end has not yet been attained. To foresee the epidemic means both to prevent its emerging forms and to prepare for its catastrophic effects: buying masks to protect those who work in hospitals, collecting vaccines to cure the population, organizing hospitals so that they can receive patients, schools so that they can teach without students' having to come to school, and businesses so that they can continue to operate with a minimum staff. In this new rationality of risk, precaution is not out of the game, but becomes a necessary step between prevention and preparedness: if the H5N1 virus appears without knowledge of its pathogenicity, precautionary measures can be taken that make it possible to implement the preparedness plan; a cluster of human forms of H5N1 can lead to the launching of the pandemic plan even if no proof exists that there is an interhuman form of the virus. Rather than replacing precaution, preparedness orients it toward a horizon of responsibility that is infinitely opened to the future.

Veterinarians have been surprised by this new rationality of risk. They think that the money spent on preparedness should be dedicated to prevention, arguing that actual problems require more attention than virtual catastrophes. The contradiction between veterinarians and physicians has never been so vast, because it is not just between the two poles of the alimentary act—production and consumption—as was the case with mad cow disease, but between two relations to animal disease—as an actual zoonosis and as a virtual pandemic. Consequently, while physicians talk about avian "flu" to insist on its possible consequences for humans, with symptoms very similar to human flu caused by a broadly spreading virus, veterinarians talk about avian "plague," to suggest that these kinds of symptoms were already present in many animal diseases (such as Newcastle disease). While physicians stress the radical shift that would happen if the H5N1 virus had an interhuman mutation, veterinarians show that low-pathogenic forms of H5N1 are very common among animals and excreted daily without major consequences. Moreover, veterinarians are even more radically dispossessed of the animal disease since the new rationality of risk does not come from food safety but rather from civil defense.[41] Therefore, while the tension between veterinarians and physicians could once be expressed in AFSSA, through the displacements that I have described, they are now expressed outside of the agency, particularly through the opposition between the Ministry of Agriculture and the Ministry of Health. In the discussion on preparedness for AI at the Assemblée Nationale, a veterinarian was thus lambasted by the president of the commission: "The veterinary world should not treat this question in a spirit of competition with the world of public health. Underestimating human pandemic to support the problem of 'avian flu' is the wrong way to communicate. The veterinary world has things to say, including on humanitarian and economic grounds. If you want to help these countries restore their food supply, that's fine, but that doesn't mean you should underestimate the risk of human pandemic to get the message across."[42]

The conflict between the two expert groups should not be drawn too starkly. Veterinarians clearly saw that there was something new with AI: the different occurrences of the disease were not only compared through a surveillance network, but were immediately translated in terms of a genetic sequence, so that it was possible to predict a future mutation of the virus. AI makes prevention necessary not only at a local and symptomatic level (as for its analogous form, Newcastle disease) but also at a global and genetic level (which makes it possible to say that the H5N1 in the Dombes area is from the same lineage as that in Qinghai Lake in China). And since only a few amino acids separate the current H5N1 virus from its interhuman form, prevention is not radically opposed to preparedness. With these three terms (prevention, precaution, preparedness), it is possible to describe the displacement of the tensions between the two professions: each had internal oppositions depending on how experts viewed the relations between these three rationalities of risk. A description of these internal oppositions would be beyond the scope of this chapter. Rather I will focus on how this opposition became problematized when it was confronted by technical measures.

CULLING, CONFINEMENT, VACCINATION

Three technical measures raise similar problems in dealing with mad cow disease or avian influenza. They aim at stopping the disease, yet with different rationalities of risk assessment.

Culling (massive slaughter, and usually destruction, of animals) is the most impressive act in the fight against the spread of animal diseases. It can be described as a sacrifice of innocent animals in order to assert the public health ideal, which would account for both its emotional impact and the difficulty of its being represented (representing culling is often forbidden by the states that practice it as a public health measure). But it can also be described as the opposition between two rationalities of risk: prevention and precaution. In June 2001, when AFSSA had to recommend culling after the discovery of a BSE case in a cattle herd, the veterinarians were in favor of selective culling whereas the physicians were for total destruction of the herd. As the modes of contamination by the prion were not known, it was a precautionary measure to kill all the cows that were in contact with the contaminated case; but from an epidemiological point of view, it is a fact that only rarely have two cases been found in the same herd. The recommendation was therefore a compromise between the logics of prevention and precaution, which was considered unclear by the major actors: it proposed adapting culling measures to the results of expert studies, while maintaining the same level of safety for the consumer. As the director of the agency explained, the logic of precaution was necessary because it restored the public trust: it protected the government from all critics that might accuse it of endangering consumers, and the responsibility was delegated to the experts. The director of AFSSA, physician Martin Hirsch, writes: "The government could say it was a preoccupation with precaution, and that it was due to scientists. And total culling could reassure both the consumer, to whom it was explained that a radical measure was taken, and the countries to which exports were made."[43] Marc Savey, who publicly disagreed with this policy, says: "You control an animal disease mechanically; but with mad cow disease there was massive culling, which became morally unacceptable for our contemporaries."[44] For veterinarians, the massive culling showed that precaution was a moral, not a scientific, principle; it reassured consumers even though it shocked their sensibilities: it was not a technical measure, that is, a way to limit the propagation of the infectious agent.

The first cases of H5N1 in France triggered a similar disagreement on confinement, that is, on the necessity to close off the farms situated along the route of migratory birds suspected of carrying the H5N1 virus. If the transmission of the virus is airborne (and not, as with mad cow disease, through consumption), domestic birds have to be confined so that they don't get the virus from migratory birds, or spread it to humans. But this disagreement took place not within the agency but between the agency and the government. On October 19, 2005, AFSSA published a recommendation in which veterinarians claimed that the risk of transmission was not high enough to justify the confinement (*claustration*) of poultry farms outside of the zone where the first H5N1 virus had appeared; they said they would reconsider the measure in light of epidemiological data. On October 15, 2006, the Minister of Agriculture, Dominique Bussereau, decided to impose confinement on farms in twenty-one departments, arguing: "As far as confinement is concerned, we lean heavily toward the application of the principle of precaution. If we have extended confinement, it is not only because of the events in Turkey [ninety-seven infectious cases], but also to prepare our farmers for a return of migratory birds in February and encourage them to think about the way they work."[45] The government argument mixed the rationalities of precaution and preparedness: the limits of precaution were pushed so far that it became preparedness. Precaution would imply building a space of transparency in which the conditions of dissemination of the virus could be studied. Confinement is a technical measure that establishes frontiers so as to institute a space of mobilization in the expectation of catastrophe. But confining farms in places where the virus was not supposed to be able to spread created obscurity and caused confusion; the aim was to prepare breeders for higher biosecurity measures when the virus really appeared, through an "imaginative enactment" of the event.[46]

The alternative to culling, and the complementary measure to confinement, is vaccination. In the epidemiological rationality of veterinarians, vaccination is used as a preventative measure around the zone where culling has been practiced. Culling and vaccination delimit two concentric zones around the point of appearance of the infectious agent. This is what made the culling of mad cows so scandalous: there was no vaccination possible. Vaccination is possible for AI, since the virus is perfectly known, but it is costly: animals who have been vaccinated cannot be transported for a certain period, and distributors fear that consumers might not want to buy meat that has been vaccinated. Vaccination of animals requires identification and a form of surveillance and tracking. It implies an economic rationality: What is the benefit of the vaccination in relation to its cost? When China announced that it would vaccinate thirteen billion chickens, an announcement criticized by all other countries as unrealistic, it pushed the logic of prevention to its limit. But the question of vaccination is totally different if seen from the vantage point of pandemic preparedness, since it becomes a question of human vaccination. As the interhuman form of the virus has not (yet) appeared, laboratories that work on the vaccines would have to produce forms that evolve as the virus mutates. People would be asked to stay at home until an adequate vaccine could be produced, and once this vaccine was available, it would first be administered to physicians and nurses. The question of vaccination becomes an ethical one: Who will receive the vaccines first, and how can the population be convinced to wait until the adequate vaccines are produced?

FROM HEALTH SAFETY TO BIOSECURITY

With this set of distinctions between different rationalities of risk we can now look at how biosecurity has transformed food safety. My hypothesis is that biosecurity introduces the rationality of preparedness into a field that was formerly structured by the opposition between prevention and precaution. It is necessary, therefore, to move beyond the conflict between two groups of experts to see how each of them understood the term "biosecurity." Starting with a contradiction that appeared with the founding of AFSSA and its displacements in the daily life of expertise, we have seen that this contradiction does not pass formally between two professions, but more profoundly structures different visions of disease that give different meanings to biosecurity measures and to the notion of "security" itself.

The term *sécurité sanitaire* (health safety) was coined as an answer to mad cow disease, and defines security as the restoration of trust and transparency in a domain where relations have become opaque and indeterminate. Health safety, in terms of the law that created AFSSA in 1998, is a relationship between those who commercialize substances, be they food or drugs, and those who consume them, guaranteed in such a way that the risks of consumption are not greater than the benefits.[47] Biosecurity refers to production rather than consumption: it points to technical measures aiming at the control of beings situated at the limit of production. Migratory birds, in the case of poultry farms affected by AI, are a paradigmatic example, as they are considered to be either food machines or virus carriers. These are two different conceptions of the social space: while health safety aims at restoring solidarity in a community that has become opaque to itself, biosecurity produces solidarity with living beings at the limits of the social space.

The biological characteristics of the pathogen itself structure the types of security practices that emerge in response. The mad cow infectious agent was a protein whose mechanism was not known but whose presence was certain: health safety aimed at making visible what had been invisible, and thus avoiding the long-term effects of the disease. The structure of the H5N1 virus is perfectly known, as it has been analyzed since the 1997 Hong Kong outbreak, but what is not known is when it will mutate into an interhuman form; therefore, the security measures aim at delaying the moment of the catastrophe. Marc Savey says:

> Being an expert on mad cow disease is like watching a movie in slow motion: when we know the beginning, we know the end. If there was a risk, in terms of public health, it has already been taken. For avian influenza, it is a classic science fiction film scenario: we know all the amino acids, we just don't know how they will combine. Hence the role of wild fauna, where combination can occur; we can assess the risk when we know what animals have been involved. Avian influenza moves very quickly and we have to be very calm when people talk about virus-bombs; mad cow disease moves very slowly, it has great inertia, and we need to think quickly to stay ahead of the disease.[48]

Here a paradox appears. While BSE is a slow-developing disease (due to a long incubation period), the experts had to identify it very quickly because of the many economic interests at stake, not to mention some human casualties. AI, on the other hand, strikes quickly, raising panic among consumers as well as opportunism among breeders, who could take advantage of the panic to sell their products immediately; in this scenario experts have to be very cautious. In other words, the speed with which each disease appears (and public reaction occurs) is inversely proportional to the speed with which experts must react.

Biosecurity and health safety, in the realm of animal disease, cast the questions of causality and responsibility in different lights. From the perspective of health safety, the institution is responsible for the quality of the substances in circulation: if a problem has occurred in the production of a food or drug, the role of the agency is to bring it to light, and to assess its risk. Causality is transformed into responsibility by the collective framework of public health. Through the use of the term "biosecurity," in contrast, responsibility is borne by those who stand at the outskirts of the human community, where viruses appear. When there are controversies about who should pay for the contamination of a poultry flock, responsibility is most often imputed to the breeder who has not taken sufficient biosecurity measures. The role of the agency is then to retrace the chain of contamination so that the first actor in the chain appears as a causal agent. In a similar way, when veterinarians redraw the itinerary of the H5N1 virus, they point to China as a "rogue state," where information is concealed and sanitary practices are considered dubious. Biosecurity for animal diseases implies a politics of declaration and suspicion: if the H5N1 virus concerns the world community, all countries have to declare both their animal cases and their human cases to the World Organization for Animal Health (OIE, based in Paris), and countries that declare only human cases, such as Indonesia, are considered untrustworthy.

As for the moral issues, health safety and biosecurity are also two different conceptions of nature. Health safety, as it was problematized by physicians referring to the contaminated blood affair and mad cow disease, points to a nature that has been altered, in which regular lines of production and exchange have been "denatured" for economic reasons. The role of the institution, in that perspective, is to restore a "second nature" by qualifying substances—even if most actors agree that there is no such thing as "pure nature." With biosecurity, as it is problematized by veterinarians for AI, nature is seen as proliferating diseases: migratory birds are suspected of propagating the virus, and those who live closer to animals are considered most exposed to the disease. Therefore, biosecurity measures, such as confinement and sanitary cleansing, are aimed at limiting this proliferation. We can speak of a "supernature" in the sense that the transformation of the environment has put natural phenomena out of control, in such a way that nature seems to take revenge against those who have transformed it. The demand for biosecurity is infinite since living beings appear as proliferating when the divide between nature and culture is no longer available to contain it.

Finally, biosecurity and health safety address the issue of sovereignty differently. Health safety clearly points to the horizon of the sovereign state: even if AFSSA only has consultative power, it addresses its recommendations to the state which can, through its organizations such as the Direction Generale du Commerce, de la Consommation et de la Repression des Fraudes (DGCCRF), halt the commercialization of a dubious substance. Mad cow disease can be seen as the reaffirmation of sovereignty in an economy of global circulation, particularly through the use of the embargo. In the case of AI, it is less clear who has the power to stop the global transportation of poultry. The World Health Organization has published an international sanitary rule that describes safety measures proportionate to the levels of risk. But if an interhuman case appears in a state, will it have the power to cut off its relationships with other states? There remains the question of the level of responsibility at which biosecurity is exercised—which raises, in turn, the question of the critiques that can be made of it.

A Critique of Biosecurity?

How can the social sciences produce a critical discourse on biosecurity, that is, a discourse that renders its stakes intelligible and raises the question of justice? One possible answer is that biosecurity is an encompassing form of power, a waste of time and money in the name of an imaginary catastrophe, and that the social sciences have to give voice to those who suffer under biosecurity measures. This chapter contends that biosecurity should rather be situated in a conflictual field of discourses and practices, in which the question of its social and human cost is raised by the actors themselves, and which it transforms in light of a future catastrophe. Biosecurity does not have the same meaning when it is used by veterinarians, who refer to the responsibility of breeders, or by physicians, who organize a pandemic plan for hospitals: they both refer to the same virtual event—the mutation of the H5N1 virus to an interhuman form—but they see it from opposite points of view in the chain of production of living beings. Food safety crises offer a window on these varying perspectives by revealing the potential tensions in the alimentary act: the two poles, production and consumption, are both united and separated by health crises.

The task of the social sciences regarding biosecurity is, therefore, threefold: first, to offer a genealogy of its emergence on a preexisting field of social relationships, so as to bring to light the potential tensions and actual contradictions that account for both its fragility and dynamism; second, to clarify its conceptual meaning in a given domain of public health, where it captures practices and distributes responsibilities in ways that are not yet established; and third, to found it on some universal anthropological tension, so that its similarities to and differences from other discourses and practices in the world can be made meaningful. Social sciences can give historical and anthropological resonance to the notion of biosecurity, which does not mean that they legitimate it: they can show how it takes hold of previous experiences, while playing on the margins of indeterminacy.

To clarify this last point, let us return to the discussion of the veterinarians who laughed when one of their colleagues talked about biosecurity. My fieldwork showed that the different rationalities of risk were anchored in specific experiences that were formative of professional groups: for veterinarians, helping a breeder give birth to a calf; for physicians, refusing to be bribed by pharmaceutical companies. Biosecurity lacks this form of experience since it puts all the blame on the breeders (whereas health safety introduced the expert as intermediary between the breeder and the consumer), and prepares for a catastrophe that is still virtual (whereas health safety started with a real contamination). It is a rationality of risk that has not been tested in reality.[49] Through their controversies experts integrate biosecurity into an already-established field of experience with animal diseases. Starting with different assumptions, they view this all-encompassing word as reflecting in strange

Figure 8.1: The AFSSA: An Institution and Its Internal Tensions

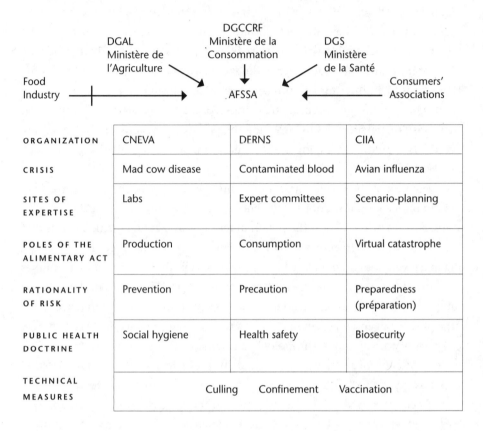

ORGANIZATION	CNEVA	DFRNS	CIIA
CRISIS	Mad cow disease	Contaminated blood	Avian influenza
SITES OF EXPERTISE	Labs	Expert committees	Scenario-planning
POLES OF THE ALIMENTARY ACT	Production	Consumption	Virtual catastrophe
RATIONALITY OF RISK	Prevention	Precaution	Preparedness (préparation)
PUBLIC HEALTH DOCTRINE	Social hygiene	Health safety	Biosecurity
TECHNICAL MEASURES	Culling Confinement Vaccination		

ways their own practices and rationality, and use their critical sense to give it some meaning. The role of the social sciences, from that perspective, is to illuminate this field of experience in which expert knowledges are formed, with the hope of transforming "biosecurity fans" into critical actors of the contemporary.

NOTES

Acknowledgment: I thank Steve Collier and Andrew Lakoff for their invitation to attend the workshop at the Social Science Research Council in New York on April 6–7, 2007, and for their reading and helpful suggestions for improvement of the text. I also wish to thank Paul Rabinow and Janet Roitman for their helpful remarks, and François Moutou for his native's feedback.

1   See V. Manceron, "Les oiseaux de l'infortune et les conflits réparateurs: chronique d'une crise aviaire en Dombes," *Ethnologie française* (forthcoming).

2   The H5N1 virus had appeared in France just a few weeks before the outbreak of riots in the Parisian suburbs, when the media were criticized for having themselves helped to spread the phenomenon they were supposed to be observing and reporting on.

3   Andrew Abbott has shown that the structure of the relations between professional groups determines the content of their work and leads them to see different aspects of the same object; see *The System of Professions: An Essay on the Division of Expert Labor* (Chicago and London: University of Chicago Press, 1988).

4   See the chapter by Nick Bingham and Steve Hinchliffe in this volume.

5   Hervé Kempf, *La guerre secrète des OGM* (Paris: Flammarion, 2003).

6   Michael Greger, *Bird Flu: A Virus of Our Own Hatching* (New York: Lantern Books, 2006).

7   William McNeill, *Plagues and People* (New York: Anchor, 1976), 198.

8   Jared Diamond, *Guns, Germs and Steel: The Fate of Human Societies* (New York: Norton, 1997).

9   Philippe Descola, *Par-delà nature et culture* (Paris: Gallimard, 2005), 391.

10   Paul Rabinow, *French Modern: Trouble in Purgatory* (Chicago: University of Chicago Press, 1999), and *Anthropos Today: Reflections on Modern Equipment* (Princeton, NJ: Princeton University Press, 2003).

11   Michel Foucault, *"Il faut défendre la société": Cours au Collège de France, 1976* (Paris: Seuil/ Gallimard, 1997).

12   Frédéric Keck, *Lévi-Strauss et la pensée sauvage* (Paris: Presses Universitaires de France, 2004).

13   Frédéric Keck, "Comment les foetus sont devenus visibles: Approches phénoménologiques et structuralistes des contradictions biopolitiques; à propos de *La condition fœtale* de Luc Boltanski," *Annales HSS* 61, no. 2 (2006): 505–20.

14   Luc Boltanski and Laurent Thévenot, *De la justification: Les économies de la grandeur* (Paris: Gallimard, 1990); Luc Boltanski, "La dénonciation," in *L'amour et la justice comme compétences* (Paris: Métailié, 1992).

15   Nicolas Dodier, *Leçons politiques de l'épidémie de sida* (Paris: EHESS, 2003).

16   Laurent Thévenot, "Un gouvernement par les normes: Pratiques et politiques des formats d'information," in *Cognition et information en société, Raisons Pratiques No.8*, ed. Bernard Conein and Laurent Thévenot (Paris: EHESS, 1997), 205–41.

17   When I arrived at AFSSA, its director, Martin Hirsch, told me there was nothing interesting to see in the labs. That is highly provocative to an anthropologist of science who looks at labs as the places where science is "in the making." It showed me that the type of scientific truths produced by expert comittees was very different from that produced in the labs; I consequently did not observe labs but expert committees. However, I found within the different expert committees an opposition

(between veterinarians and physicians) that in many respects displaces that between labs and expert committees (veterinarians defending the labs when their money is cut or their data overlooked). This chapter is about this opposition, which I consider as structural for the field of animal diseases.

18 See Alessandro Stanziani, *Histoire de la qualité alimentaire, XIXe–XXe siècle* (Paris: Seuil, 2005).

19 Ronald Hubscher, *Les maîtres des bêtes: Les vétérinaires dans la société française, XVIIe–XXe siècle* (Paris: Odile Jacob, 1998).

20 See Francis Chateauraynaud and Didier Torny, *Les sombres précurseurs: Une sociologie pragmatique de l'alerte et du risque* (Paris: EHESS, 1999), 316ff.

21 Maxime Schwartz, *How the Cows Turned Mad: Unlocking the Mysteries of Mad Cow Disease* (Berkeley and Los Angeles: University of California Press, 2003).

22 Lion Murard and Patrick Zylberman, *L'hygiène de la République: La santé publique en France ou l'utopie contrariée* (Paris: Fayard, 1996); Madeleine Ferrière, *Histoire des peurs alimentaires du Moyen-Âge à nos jours* (Paris: Seuil, 2003).

23 Aquilino Morelle, *La défaite de la santé publique* (Paris: Flammarion, 1996); Dodier, *Leçons politiques*.

24 Calvin W. Schwabe, *Veterinary Medicine and Human Health* (Baltimore, MD: Williams and Wilkins, 1964), 4.

25 Ibid.

26 Annemarie Mol talks about "various enactments of a particular disease"; see Annemarie Mol, *The Body Multiple: Ontology in Medical Practice* (Durham, NC: Duke University Press, 2002). I rely on her perspectivist method, which allows for the translation of scientific debates into ontological premises. I add to her work the notion of contradiction, that she would probably refuse for philosophical reasons.

27 Jacqueline Estades and Elizabeth Rémy, *L'expertise en pratique* (Paris: L'Harmattan, 2003).

28 Personal interview, AFSSA, January 29, 2007.

29 Personal interview, AFSSA, March 28, 2007.

30 Personal interview, AFSSA, May 22, 2006.

31 Personal interview, AFSSA, May 24, 2005.

32 Andrew Lakoff, *Pharmaceutical Reason: Knowledge and Value in Global Psychiatry* (New York: Cambridge University Press, 2005), 141.

33 To be complete, this description of the tensions at the agency should look at the contradiction beween the data produced in the labs and that used in the expert committees. Unfortunately, I could not pursue this extensively, although I have interviews showing that these contradictions exist.

34 Personal interview, AFSSA, January 29, 2005.

35 Bernard Toma et al., *Épidémiologie appliquée à la lutte contre les maladies animales transmissibles majeures* (Paris: AEEMA, 2001), xxvii.

36 François Ewald, "Philosophie de la précaution," *L'Année sociologique* 46, no. 2 (1996): 402.

37 James Ironside et al., "Accumulation of Prion Protein in Tonsil and Appendix: Review of Tissue Samples," *British Medical Journal* 365 (2002): 633–34.

38 Personal interview, AFSSA, November 6, 2006.

39 See Stephen J. Collier and Andrew Lakoff, "Vital Systems Security," Laboratory for the Anthropology of the Contemporary, Discussion Paper (2006), http://anthropos-lab.net/wp/publications/2007/01/collier_vital-systems.pdf.

40 Didier Houssin, "Les risques potentiels pour la santé humaine: Politiques de prévention," in *Réunion d'information sur la grippe aviaire*, Région de Pays de la Loire, 2006, 36.

41 A. Lakoff, "Preparing for the Next Emergency," *Public Culture* 19, no. 2 (2007): 247–71.

42 Jean-Marie Le Guen and Jean-Pierre Door, *Le H5N1: une menace durable pour la santé animale,*

Rapport de l'Assemblée Nationale II, no. 2833 (2006), 252.

43 Martin Hirsch, *Ces peurs qui nous gouvernent: Sécurité sanitaire, faut-il craindre la transparence?* (Paris: Albin Michel, 2002), 223.

44 Personal interview, November 6, 2006.

45 Le Guen and Door, *Le H5N1*, 127.

46 Collier and Lakoff, "Vital Systems Security."

47 Didier Tabuteau, *La sécurité sanitaire* (Paris: Berger-Levrault 2002).

48 Personal interview, AFSSA, November 6, 2006.

49 I raise this hypothesis following Luc Boltanski and Eve Chiapello's analysis of the new forms of capitalism as lacking "tests" (*épreuves*); see Luc Boltanski and Eve Chiapello, *Le nouvel esprit du capitalisme* (Paris: Gallimard, 1999).

CHAPTER NINE

Biodefense

CONSIDERING THE SOCIOTECHNICAL DIMENSION

Kathleen M. Vogel

In U.S. biosecurity policymaking, biodefense activities and government transparency have had a long and contentious relationship dating back several decades.[1] In 2001 (exactly one week prior to the U.S. anthrax attacks), these tensions were reignited when the *New York Times* published a story alleging that the U.S. Department of Defense (DoD) and Central Intelligence Agency (CIA) funded and carried out several secret biodefense projects that could be considered as offensive projects, and therefore, in contravention to U.S. treaty commitments under the Biological and Toxins Weapons Convention (BTWC).[2] The controversial projects, referred to as Project Jefferson, Project Bacchus, and Project Clear Vision, involved the creation of a genetically engineered strain of anthrax bacteria, the development of a mock bioweapons facility, and the reverse engineering of a Soviet biological munition. The Clinton administration initiated these projects in response to growing post–Cold War concerns about the use of biological weapons by "rogue" states and nonstate actors.[3] Critics argued that such projects should have been declared per requirements of biodefense disclosure under the BTWC; additional concerns were voiced about the lack of U.S. government oversight and review on these classified projects. At the time, government officials countered that the projects had been internally reviewed and deemed as legitimate biodefense activities under the BTWC.[4] Officials stated that information about the biodefense projects was not released to the public to avoid the revelation of potential U.S. vulnerabilities to adversaries.

Although these controversial projects were initially funded and completed under the Clinton administration, the Bush administration has continued to support next-generation biodefense research and threat assessments in order to develop bet-ter countermeasures for protecting the American public against a bioweapons (BW) attack and to provide early warning against technological surprise in BW develop-ment.[5] Since September 11 and the 2001 U.S. anthrax attacks, over $40 billion of new government funding has been allocated to the U.S. biodefense program.[6] This funding supports four main categories of biodefense activities: (1) research, devel-opment, and acquisition of medical countermeasures and related protective equip-ment; (2) enhancing medical surveillance and detection of bioweapons agents in the environment; (3) conduct of bioweapons threat assessments; and (4) improving state, local, and hospital preparedness to deal with bioterrorism attacks. Arguments continue over the appropriate level of transparency in these activities.[7]

One recent catalyst to these debates has involved efforts by the U.S. Depart-ment of Homeland Security (DHS) to establish a new multimillion dollar, high containment biodefense research initiative under the National Biodefense Analysis and Countermeasures Center (NBACC).[8] The NBACC will use simulations, com-putational modeling, laboratory experimentation, and forward-looking techni-cal analyses of emerging biotechnologies to anticipate future bioterrorist threats. Although the facility will have unclassified work areas, NBACC has the potential to operate in a highly classified environment that may not be subject to public dis-closure. Additional highly classified biological experiments and threat assessments are being carried out by the U.S. DoD, defense contractors, and the intelligence community.[9]

Critics of these programs argue that invoking high levels of secrecy for such biodefense research could create new security risks, especially if rigorous oversight mechanisms are not in place. These debates over appropriate levels of transparency are indicative of sustained tensions between the security policy community, life science researchers, and the public regarding appropriate levels of open commu-nication and public input on U.S. biodefense activities. Capturing one essence of this conflict, John Steinbruner states,

> there's a battle going on here as yet unresolved between the basic principle of
> protection and out of the public health tradition, the basic principle is transpar-
> ency.... The basic principle in the security community is quite the opposite. It

has sequestered the information for national advantage. I personally believe very strongly that ultimately the only protection is in public health transparency and that we've got to avoid the attempt to utilize this or sequester it within the security community. But to put it mildly, this is an ongoing battle. It has not yet been won by either side.[10]

Alan Pearson has described how these tensions reflect a broader, government-wide philosophical debate on how to approach biosecurity issues, in which questions of openness, transparency, and sharing of vital information remain under dispute.[11]

Current Policy Perspectives on Biodefense Transparency

As Steinbruner and Pearson's comments highlight, within the security community there exist different norms with respect to the secrecy/transparency divide in biodefense activities.[12] Below, I will describe two polarized perspectives that reflect some of the key issues structuring current biodefense debates. In examining these two perspectives, I will describe the different norms and logics that structure their thinking and shape their particular policy positions on biodefense. One key difference between these two positions turns on questions of access: How much information about U.S. biodefense activities should be open to public scrutiny?

One end of the debate is reflected in current U.S. government biodefense policy formulation and planning. In 2004, President Bush issued Homeland Security Presidential Directive (HSPD) 10, *Biodefense for the 21st Century*. In calling for a new U.S. biodefense agenda, President Bush describes the need for this new initiative:

> Armed with a single vial of a biological agent...small groups of fanatics, or failing states, could gain the power to threaten great nations, threaten the world peace. America, and the entire civilized world, will face this threat for decades to come. We must confront the danger with open eyes, and unbending purpose.[13]

Government and nongovernmental experts have often emphasized three key problems that have stimulated this biosecurity concern: (1) poor intelligence on adversary intentions and motivations for biological weapons; (2) recent advances in biotechnology and the life sciences; and (3) lags in the development of effective defensive countermeasures behind offensive innovations.[14] To address some of these problems, HSPD 10 calls for "more forward-looking analyses...to understand new scientific trends that may be exploited by our adversaries to develop biological weapons."[15] Before and after coming to hold high-level biodefense policy positions in the Bush White House, Drs. James B. Petro and W. Seth Carus have advanced the need for these forward-looking research projects by arguing for what they describe as a "capabilities"- or "science"-based approach to biodefense.[16]

Under this model, justification for U.S. biodefense activities moves away from a tight coupling to intelligence assessments on specific adversaries. Instead, biodefense priorities would be based on exploring the technical feasibility of plausible current and future bioweapons (BW) threats.[17] As Petro describes it, "much of this work would involve the study of organisms, materials, methodologies, and technologies to characterize the hazard presented by their use in BW."[18] In light of poor intelligence information and the unpredictability of advances in life science, this science-based approach is seen as providing a more robust and rapid mechanism for developing countermeasures against a broad range of potential BW attacks.

Under this program, Petro and Carus state that the most contentious types of biodefense research would necessitate a centralized, coordinated federal oversight mechanism, which could include arrangements involving new partnerships between the security, life science, and other relevant communities. Yet even with their calls for greater oversight, Petro and Carus maintain that high levels of secrecy are necessary in some biodefense work. They argue that complete transparency is impossible (and risky) to achieve in the biodefense area in order to prevent the revelation of U.S. vulnerabilities, the compromise of intelligence sources and methods, or the proliferation of bioweapons-related knowledge that could be readily picked up and used by adversaries. Defending this need for high levels of secrecy on certain kinds of biodefense research, Bernard Courtney, NBACC's scientific director, states: "Where the research exposes vulnerability, I've got to protect that, for the public's interest. We don't need to be showing perpetrators the holes in our defense."[19] This focus on potential acquisition of information about American vulnerabilities has pushed the U.S. biodefense program into greater levels of classification and compartmentalization. Thus, despite Petro and Carus's calls for some levels of transparency, in practice, many details of the most controversial aspects of the U.S. biodefense program remain shrouded in secrecy.[20]

At the other end of the debate, others call for a much greater level of oversight and transparency in biodefense activities. Proponents of this perspective argue that capabilities-based biodefense activities, as described by HSPD-10 and Petro and Carus, have proliferated across the health, agriculture, defense, intelligence, and contractor communities, without rigorous oversight mechanisms to make sure that the activities do not cross over into offensive work.[21] Some have argued that this could fuel suspicions about a resurgent U.S. offensive program, potentially leading to a biological arms race with other countries (or with ourselves).[22] Also, Mark Wheelis has expressed concern that ongoing and proposed biodefense activities would allow the United States to develop a short-notice offensive capability involving "a range of new genetically engineered pathogens, new production capabilities suitable for covert production of biological weapons agents, new methods of dissemination, and new ways of extending the longevity of pathogens in the environment."[23] Other critics of the biodefense buildup charge that a lack of oversight on a growing number of activities can also obscure problems in the design, operation, maintenance, and safety of high containment facilities involved in such work.[24] The June 2007 shutdown of research in five biodefense labs at Texas A&M University due to staff worker infections with biodefense agents and problems with their institutional review board (IRB) have been cited as a worrisome harbinger of the problems in expanding biodefense activities without adequate transparency and oversight mechanisms in place.[25]

Due to these concerns, some critics argue that transparency into biodefense activities needs to be increased. These advocates argue that, without revealing critical U.S. vulnerabilities, information should be released on what studies are being conducted and why they are being done in order to reassure the public and foreign governments that the United States does not have an offensive program. Many holding this perspective question the proliferation of U.S. biodefense activities, emphasizing the national and international security benefits from increasing the amount and quality of information released publicly about the U.S. biodefense program. Debates remain, however, as to exactly what quality and quantity of information should be released and who should have access to this information.

To move the transparency discussion forward, biosecurity scholars in nongovernmental organizations (NGOs) and academia have proposed specific mechanisms for increasing the levels of biodefense transparency. These proposals outline new oversight mechanisms for the review, conduct, and publication of biodefense research. Perhaps the most stringent oversight proposal comes from John Steinbruner and others at the University of Maryland, who argue for the need for a global biosecurity oversight system. This new system, which they call "enforced transparency," would require the establishment of a coordinated local, national, and international system to review and approve the most contentious biodefense and dual-use research.[26] This system would involve two key components: (1) a requirement for the licensing of researchers and facilities engaged in dual-use or biodefense research, including security background checks of scientific personnel; and (2) procedures for a tiered peer review and approval system (local, national, international—depending on risks posed by a given experiment) prior to funding, taking into account both the pathogen to be studied and the techniques to be employed to assess the level of danger and oversight needed. The system would be comprehensive (covering government, academia, and industry), mandatory (with legally binding obligations), and universal (with internationally harmonized procedures and rules).

Other prominent proposals examining governance for biodefense activities focus more on different types of national and international oversight and information-sharing mechanisms. Some examples include: (1) Jonathan Tucker's analysis of the World Health Organization's oversight of smallpox research as a template for biodefense review;[27] and (2) Brian Gorman's proposal for the establishment of a "Due Process Vetting System."[28] Tucker's proposal discusses how institutional arrangements and mechanisms (e.g., funding, scientific expertise, guidelines) could be designed to create an international oversight committee to evaluate dual-use biological research. In contrast, Gorman's proposal would establish a new federal agency called the Biologic Regulatory Commission. This commission would be responsible for reviewing biodefense research activities of concern and would establish a mechanism that would enable rapid communication and dialogue between the scientific and national security communities on new and potentially sensitive life science research prior to publication and public release.

In spite of these proposals, however, little progress has been made in resolving the existing tensions over questions about the quality and quantity of information to be released and who should have access to this information. For example, much of the transparency debate remains fixated on (1) how much specific information (e.g., experimental protocols, descriptions, results) should be publicly declared or kept classified; (2) who should have access to such information; (3) what kinds of access should be granted for this information and who should provide oversight to this process. Thus, because many of the disputes revolve around questions of access, little progress has been made in government circles on the more fundamental and complex issues underlying the issue of transparency in biodefense activities.

Biodefense Transparency Debates: A Flawed Biotechnological Frame?

Although often at odds over secrecy norms and appropriate policy prescriptions, both ends of the transparency debate share the same framework for understanding biotechnology—largely predicated on the conceptual framework of a "biotechnology revolution." This framework incorporates particular assumptions and conceptualizations of biotechnology, consisting of specific foci of attention, temporal and spatial orientations, and certain beliefs about technological trajectories.[29] Because I have described this dominant frame in more detail elsewhere,[30] I will summarize here only two elements that I see as being particularly relevant to the current biodefense transparency debate: materiality and globalization (described in more detail below). Due to the dominant reliance on this framework, policy attention remains on classification/oversight and technological solutions to biodefense or the perceived BW threat. Yet, the current focus on a narrow conceptualization of biotechnology leaves out important factors that remain critical to understanding biosecurity threats and designing appropriate biodefense policy responses to those threats.

One element of the common biotechnology frame is a focus on various material aspects constituting biotechnology. For example, codified biological knowledge, such as information found in journal articles, scientific textbooks, websites, databases (e.g., genome sequences), or other written sources, has been a central theme in these discussions.[31] In describing the perils of transparency in the current "information society" Brian Gorman states, "recent advances in communication technologies can aid in the acquisition and instantaneous delivery of entire volumes of the world's most sophisticated science and technology journals to any interested party the world over. Today...an adversary would be walking off with more dual-use articles having WMD proliferation than ten years ago."[32] In addition, a report issued by the Center for Strategic and International Studies plainly states, "know-how that is generated in the course of scientific research is available to anyone participating in that research. If the results of that research are published openly, they become available to all—including those who may seek to use those results maliciously."[33] These discussions, however, rarely differentiate between the tacit and explicit knowledge comprising scientific and technological developments.[34]

In addition to codified knowledge, another focus is on biological materials (e.g., pathogens, oligonucleotides), biological supplies (e.g., reagents, prep kits), infrastructure (e.g., DNA synthesizers, laboratory benches), and other tangible items (e.g., monetary resources, computers). With respect to biological materials, a 2005 U.S. National Academies of Science (NAS) report notes:

> the number of agents created by the life sciences revolution (e.g., via recombinant and transgenic technology and even synthetic biology) is increasing practically exponentially. So while there are only half a dozen fissile nuclear materials and dozens of "dual-use" chemicals that could be diverted for malevolent purposes, the number of potentially harmful biological agents is virtually limitless.[35]

Even biodefense critics, such as the ETC Group, have focused on material aspects in their critiques: "Using a laptop computer, published gene sequence information, and mail-order synthetic DNA, just about anyone has the potential to construct genes or entire genomes from scratch including those of lethal pathogens."[36]

Moreover, biotechnology is often given a globalized and diffused character in these policy discussions. A 2004 NAS report argued that given the global character of biotechnology, "it is unrealistic to think that biological technologies and the knowledge base upon which they rest can somehow be isolated within the borders of a few countries."[37] Swedish biodefense expert Roger Roffey adds, "The combination of the increased movement of people, knowledge, and products across borders as well as the greater availability of expertise and information via the Internet has made it easier to acquire BW materials and know-how."[38] An implicit corollary of the globalization argument is that emerging biotechnologies are becoming standardized, routinized, and even automated, removing the need for expert, local, or other kinds of specialized know-how.

Thus, in looking at the biodefense debates, one sees a predominant focus on the material aspects of biotechnology and their inevitable diffusion. For example, there remains a preoccupation with controlling the release of biodefense information and other material aspects that might aid terrorists or proliferant states. This is reflected in the considerable resources and programs within U.S. biodefense that focus on science-based threat assessments, R&D for countermeasures, and surveillance and detection systems. These programs, which account for 98 percent of the U.S. biodefense budget, remain largely focused on finding technological solutions to counter potential bioweapons threats. Analogously, those at the other end of the debate see the ubiquitous and global diffusion of biotechnology as demanding (some would argue, urgently mandating) an entirely new oversight and accounting system and infrastructure that tracks various material factors in biodefense and dual-use research programs, such as people (e.g, licensing), biological materials, experimental protocols, countermeasures, manuscripts, publications, and funding proposals.

These foci have some merit, but their predominant concern on material aspects and their inherent assumptions about biotechnology miss other critical aspects of biotechnology that are pertinent to understanding the true nature of bioweapons threats and, consequently, how to consider and evaluate biodefense activities and their transparency. To illustrate this point, I will briefly discuss three relevant case studies: (1) the development of the Soviet anthrax biological weapon (Anthrax 836); (2) the 2002 poliovirus synthesis experiment; and (3) the 2003 phiX synthesis experiments.[39] An in-depth analysis of these cases questions some of the predominant assumptions and logics about biotechnology underpinning both the security and public health perspectives on biodefense. Moreover, examining how these cases are discussed within the transparency debates provides a lens to see the limitations of the current way of thinking and structuring biodefense and biosecurity policy issues and suggests alternative avenues for policy attention.

Opening Up the Black Box of Biotechnology:
Anthrax 836, Poliovirus, phiX

CASE 1: ANTHRAX 836

The Soviet's premier anthrax biological weapon, Anthrax 836,[40] was developed by the Scientific and Experimental Production Base (SNOPB) in Stepnogorsk, Kazakhstan. When SNOPB bioweaponeers were tasked by the Soviet Ministry of Defense (MOD) to develop this new weapon, they were given orders to add modifications to an older Soviet anthrax recipe. As a starting point, the MOD provided SNOPB with extensive classified technical papers (over 400 pages) that summarized previous MOD work in developing their older anthrax weapon. These papers described different parameters, equipment, and biosafety conditions for the cultivation and production of the anthrax strain. Other documents detailed how to fill and assemble bombs and warheads with the agent, and listed the various suppliers for all the necessary raw materials.

In spite of the extensive classified documents provided by the MOD, however, the original SNOPB staff experienced problems in applying this information at their facility. For example, they found that the Anthrax 836 documentation was specific to growth in MOD fermenters and equipment. As a result, SNOPB technical staff experienced difficulties in trying to replicate previous MOD anthrax work in SNOPB's fermenters and had to go through painstaking efforts to adapt the MOD classified production protocols to the existing SNOPB system. Because of these early technical difficulties (even with the extensive classified information sent to the facility), the MOD ultimately decided to transfer sixty-five biological weapons specialists from MOD facilities in Sverdlovsk and Kirov to SNOPB. As developers of the older Soviet anthrax weapon, these individuals had specialized know-how in research and manufacturing techniques for weaponizing anthrax bacteria. Upon being transferred to SNOPB, these individuals were placed in key managerial, technological, manufacturing, and biosafety positions, and also served as "master trainers" to all new biological weapons employees. At its peak of 300 employees, SNOPB bioweaponeers were organized in interdisciplinary teams across the various technological processes involved in R&D, production, and weaponization of the anthrax weapon. And, despite the transfer of experienced MOD staff to SNOPB, creating the new Anthrax 836 weapon was not trivial and ultimately took five years of dedicated effort, even though it was based on an already developed weapons technology outlined in great detail in available classified documents.

CASE 2: 2002 POLIOVIRUS EXPERIMENT

In 2002 virologist Eckard Wimmer and members of his research group published their artificial synthesis of the poliovirus in *Science*.[41] When the poliovirus experiment is discussed in policy circles, the focus tends to be on how the Wimmer group obtained information about the poliovirus genome sequence off the Internet and ordered commercially available oligonucleotides to make the virus. Not widely known, however, is that the most difficult part of the poliovirus synthesis involved making good HeLa cell-free cytoplasmic extracts to yield a fully intact, infectious poliovirus.[42] Although the extract procedure has been around for more than twenty years and various methods papers give detailed step-by-step instructions for it, there remains considerable contingency in using these written experimental protocols to make the synthetic poliovirus.

In my interviews with the small sub-community of polio virologists who use this extract for studying viral synthesis, I have learned that specific kinds of localized know-how underpin extract preparation and other steps in the synthesis. These virologists claim that this know-how is critical to making the virus synthetically using the published method. This know-how is not written down, but resides in the heads and hands of laboratory members within this specialized polio virology community; individuals who have not been able to master this hands-on know-how have not been able to synthesize the virus. For example, these polio virologists describe the importance of specialized and localized training, practices, and attention to detail across steps of the synthesis experiment, from growing the HeLa cells, to various processes involved in making the extract, and working with the RNA of the virus. The virologists maintain that retaining experienced technicians in the laboratory (who have developed the critical know-how through years of trial-and-error work) is a key part of inculcating and sustaining the institutional memory of this know-how as students and postdoctoral researchers rotate through the laboratory. Yet, these polio virologists maintain that making good extract and viable synthetic poliovirus is a difficult process, fraught with failures, even for experienced researchers who have been using these techniques and practices for decades.

CASE 3: 2003 PHIX BACTERIOPHAGE SYNTHESIS

In December 2003, a mere eighteen months after the synthetic poliovirus experiment was published, researchers from the J. Craig Venter Institute published an alternative method for artificially synthesizing the ϕX174 bacteriophage (hereafter referred to as phiX) in a mere two weeks; their method was reported to be a substantial improvement over the poliovirus synthetic method.[43] Public discussions of the phiX synthesis focused on the security risks of its open scientific publication—perhaps creating a widely available blueprint for terrorists to make a larger and more lethal virus from this published method. In interviews with Venter Institute researchers, however, what I found again is more experimental contingency than is represented in public or policy accounts.

Although the synthesis was ultimately carried out over a two-week period, work on the project began nearly seven years earlier (1996) when one of the researchers, Clyde Hutchinson, on sabbatical at the J. Craig Venter Institute, began working on the phiX bacteriophage as a model for synthesizing a larger bacterial genome. Initially, Hutchinson tried a "quick and dirty" method by merely copying a published protocol that described using a modified technique of polymerase chain reaction (PCR) and commercially available oligonucleotides to build a synthetic plasmid.[44] In applying this published protocol to phiX, Hutchinson was able to produce DNA that was the right length of the phage. But, when he put the DNA into *E. coli* to check for the infectivity of the phage, Hutchinson did not obtain any plaques, signifying that the bacteriophage had deleterious mutations and was therefore not viable (infectious).[45] Due to other work priorities, Hutchinson did not have time to troubleshoot the experiment and so he set the failed project aside.[46] Although ultimately the experiment was completed in 2003, success involved bringing in two additional researchers who each brought unique sets of experience and expertise to the project that generated new intellectual insights for how the synthesis could be developed. The success of the project resided not in merely copying a published protocol, but in developing new laboratory methods and significant trial-and-error problem solving by all three researchers working on the project.

Moreover, the straightforward applicability of the published phiX protocol to build larger genomes is questionable. In order to identify the formation of an intact, infectious bacteriophage with this method, an important part of the experiment involved the use of a plaque assay. Since the phiX experiment produced only one plaque-forming genome per ten thousand colonies, the plaque assay allowed rapid visual identification of fully infectious genomes generated from the synthesis reaction without having to go through laborious and lengthy sequencing. Such a plaque assay, however, is problematic in building larger viral genomes and has been cited as a limitation of this synthetic method in subsequent scientific publications.[47] The inherent limitations of this published protocol for creating larger genomes have not, however, been included in public biosecurity policy discussions; instead, policy attention focuses on the "rapid" two-week synthesis of the phage.

Biotechnology as a Sociotechnical Assemblage

As illustrated by a closer look the Anthrax 836, poliovirus, and phiX cases, there are a number of contingencies and factors at play in these experiments that challenge the "biotechnology revolution" framework currently dominating biodefense policy discussions. In each of these experiments, the material components (e.g., classified documents, published protocols, oligos) played a limited role in their ultimate success. Rather, success in getting these experiments to work lay in the development of particular kinds of know-how and expertise, assembled and configured in particular ways, with extensive troubleshooting efforts. Moreover, these studies also reveal that the applicability of the experimental results to new and different contexts does not appear to be facile or straightforward. For example, in the Anthrax 836 case, many SNOPB problems were not remedied by the availability of detailed classified technical information, but were more fundamentally related to solving different types of novel sociotechnical problems that were unique to SNOPB and contingent on local conditions. Turning the MOD paper-based concept of Anthrax 836 into a working technology required the endogenous development of new materials, protocols, equipment, and infrastructure, as well as the transfer of experienced personnel with particular kinds of weapons know-how and the hiring of several hundred additional personnel. All of these personnel then had to be organized into new interdisciplinary knowledge teams, and appropriately configured into the existing infrastructure in order to translate existing scientific knowledge, as well as create new types of local, site-specific knowledge, to produce large quantities of bioweapons agents at SNOPB. The difficulties of establishing such a stable and functional system are reflected in the myriad problems that bioweaponeers at SNOPB faced in developing the new 836 anthrax weapon. Even with generous funds, government pressure, extensive classified technical information, resources, critical infrastructure, and experienced personnel at SNOPB's disposal, the Soviet's 836 anthrax weapon still took several years to produce.

In the poliovirus and phiX experiments, the success of both synthetic approaches was limited with respect to the availability of written protocols and other types of published scientific information. With phiX, one of the researchers tried to simply take a published protocol and apply it directly to synthesize his bacteriophage, with no success. Other scientists have commented on the problems of applying the published phiX synthetic method to create a larger virus. In the synthetic poliovirus case, the success and replication of that experimental method has depended on the specialized laboratory know-how developed within a very small and localized subset of the poliovirus community. Also, as the SNOPB case illustrates (and other historical state offensive programs suggest), in order to turn either of these viruses (or others) into mass casualty biological weapons, additional experimentation and troubleshooting with particular kinds of expertise and infrastructure would be required to produce, stabilize, weaponize, and disseminate these agents to kill large numbers of people.

The case studies described here add to a growing set of qualitative and quantitative empirical studies that have argued against the dominant frame of a "biotechnology revolution" to describe biotechnology.[48] Instead, these studies suggest that we need to consider biotechnology more as a *sociotechnical* assemblage, which takes into equal account *both* the social and the technical character of biotechnology. In this way, one would examine how the social component of biotechnology is co-constructed with the technical, how this assemblage infuses and shapes how materials and infrastructure are used, and how experiments and technological developments are structured and carried out for particular purposes. Thus, this approach would examine qualitative aspects of biotechnology as a way to ground and refine purely technical analyses.

Conceptualizing biotechnology as an assemblage helps to explain the problems that have been encountered in moving biotechnology from the research bench to more applied uses. For example, a number of recent qualitative studies find that significant bottlenecks have been found to emerge across various biotechnology development pathways, bottlenecks that involve both technical (e.g., contingency and complexity of biological systems, problems in engineering or industrial processes) and socio-organizational components (e.g., know-how, communities of practice, teamwork, organizational schemes). These bottlenecks can constrain and structure the adoption of new biotechnologies, in many cases taking several decades to resolve. The studies emphasize the importance of understanding the particular sociotechnical assemblages that are co-constructed with, and are an intimate part of, biotechnology developments to more fully understanding the dynamic and contingent character of biotechnology.[49] Thus, instead of having an established globalized and materialistic character, biotechnology can be expected to have some unique localized and social components that should be explored and taken into account.

Thinking about Biodefense as a Sociotechnical Assemblage

If one were to reconsider biotechnology as a sociotechnical assemblage, what would this have to offer for thinking about biodefense activities and transparency? To begin, it would move the existing policy focus away from material elements in biodefense with its focus on questions of access, to a more *contextual* consideration of how a sociotechnical assemblage constitutes specific biodefense activities and the overall biodefense program. This alternative approach offers new perspectives for how to conceptualize biodefense policy responses. Below, I discuss how a sociotechnical understanding of biodefense can offer different micro- and macro-level policy-relevant insights in current policy debates on biodefense.

MACRO-LEVEL POLICY IMPLICATIONS FOR BIODEFENSE

To date, much public focus on biodefense transparency has involved requests for declarations or detailed review of particular experiments, quantities of agent, and infrastructure constituting U.S. biodefense activities. Although such data provide useful baseline information, they do little to shed light on how all U.S. biodefense activities fit into a larger context—and to what extent that context is suggestive of an intentional or unintentional buildup of an offensive program or offensive capabilities. Gerald Epstein points out the inherent problem in evaluating specific biodefense projects: "The problem is the treaty [BTWC] doesn't have clear, objective criteria of what types of activities are or are not in compliance, and so people may disagree on the compliance of any specific activity. The treaty doesn't mention research, only development. So, when does research slip into development and over the line?"[50] Epstein's comment reflects the difficulties in trying to discern the offensive character of a project from a purely technical analysis or by looking solely at very specific projects or activities.

Historian of science Michael Dennis explains that such a focus on data (e.g., specific materials, information, research) reflects an "access" view of secrecy, which operates under the belief that if such restricted data is declassified, then one will automatically be able to assess what is going on.[51] As Dennis explains, however, this assumes that classified and unclassified information are linked in some directly observable and unmediated fashion. Instead, Dennis points out that knowing reams of restricted data might not go far in understanding and reconstructing the larger picture because the contextual basis for the activities is absent. This suggests that evaluations that focus on examining specific research projects to assess the offensive character of the U.S. biodefense program may give a meaningless or incorrect picture.[52]

To date, there is no government-wide review process for evaluating treaty compliance for U.S. biodefense activities.[53] Yet, as the three case studies above illustrate, a more insightful picture of evaluating the character of the U.S. biodefense program would involve understanding the various sociotechnical assemblages that constitute particular experiments and programs occurring in particular government agencies, as well as how all of these activities fit into a larger sociotechnical system across the U.S. government (and defense contractors). With this in mind, criteria for evaluating and enhancing transparency would necessitate a more contextual elucidation of the technical work occurring within the U.S. biodefense program, one that moves beyond specific projects

Figure 9.1: Defensive or Offensive Research?
Common Laboratory Techniques at Outset,
BUT Different Experimental Hypotheses[55]

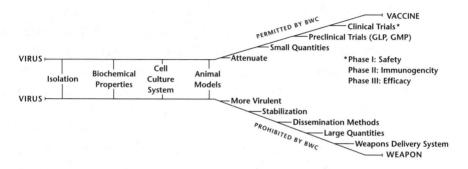

and data and looks more at the unique knowledge networks and structures being developed and maintained.

Some historical examples offer up insights for how one could initially approach this type of contextual analysis. For example, David Huxsoll, former commander at the U.S. Army Medical Research Institute of Infectious Diseases (USAMRIID), has provided a useful schematic for how to differentiate between defensive and offensive activities (see figure 9.1). In a 1989 congressional testimony, Huxsoll stated,

> From the outset, defensive research is based on different postulates and hypotheses than is research directed toward offensive ends, and the rationales for data collection and analysis are different. At the basic research level, the laboratory techniques used would be very similar, but the objectives are markedly different. Beyond the basic research level, there is a marked divergence in the type of work that would be done. If a vaccine were to be produced, one would pursue ways of crippling, weakening, or lessening the virulence of the agent in question so that it could be used in humans without fear of inducing disease…. This type of work is permitted by the Biological Weapons Convention. If, however, the goal were to create a weapon, the opposite objectives would be pursued. Efforts to enhance virulence or toxicity and to produce enormous quantities of agent far larger than those required for vaccine production would be undertaken. In addition, the issues of stability, dissemination, and weapons delivery systems would

have to be addressed. These activities are clearly prohibited by the Biological Weapons Convention.[54]

According to Huxsoll, one should be able to differentiate between offensive and defensive work as one moves down the development chain.[55] Huxsoll's model, however, primarily focuses on purely technical characteristics to guide an analysis. Additional complementary evaluation criteria have been put forward in a report by the Armed Forces Medical Intelligence Center (AFMIC).[56] In 1993, AFMIC created a set of categories and indicators for biological weapons activities, which included: (1) funding and personnel; (2) facility design, equipment, and security; (3) technical considerations; (4) safety; and (5) process flow. Although the AFMIC criteria are an improvement to augment Huxsoll's analysis, the predominant focus here remains on counting or documenting specific items (e.g., refrigerated bunkers, air filters, number of scientists, aerosol chambers, pathogens, waste treatment). In contrast, a sociotechnical analysis would build on Huxsoll and AFMIC's proposals by looking at the socio-organizational components and dynamics of biodefense programs and how they are structured across the U.S. government. This would involve asking questions such as:

- How are biodefense activities, institutions, people, and practices being organized and connected?
- What kind of knowledge or know-how is being generated through these activities? How is it being accumulated, integrated? For what purposes?
- How could these existing or new sociotechnical assemblages contribute/not contribute to a weapons development chain or offensive capability (either within a particular agency or across agencies)?

Using these markers as a guide, a more holistic, strategic-level assessment could be carried out to focus specifically on an internal evaluation of the U.S. biodefense program and BTWC compliance.[57] This assessment should involve governmental and nongovernmental experts with backgrounds in the life sciences and social sciences (including some who understand technology as a sociotechnical assemblage). The analysis could be conducted with oversight by the White House, Congress, or a special interagency group.[58] Such large-scale assessments have been previously carried out to inform U.S. biodefense programmatic and budgetary priorities for the future and so could be adapted to examine treaty compliance. Once this assessment is completed, one would have a better sense of the nature of biodefense activities occurring within particular agencies and across the U.S. government. Given the current political climate, this type of exercise would most likely only be feasible in a new administration.

Although one could debate the utility and prudence of biodefense activities like Project Jefferson, Bacchus, and Clear Vision, a more worrisome finding would be if an comprehensive assessment revealed that a concerted government effort existed to construct these three projects together in a way that would build specific sociotechnical assemblages (e.g., people, knowledge, practices, institutions) leading to a dedicated offensive bioweapons capability. Thus, my proposed sociotechnical assessment, which would move beyond focusing on specific experiments to look at the larger picture, would provide a more holistic understanding and evaluation of such activities occurring within the U.S. biodefense program. Although some critics of the U.S. biodefense program have expressed concern over specific experiments because they might allow a short-term offensive break-out capability, a sociotechnical assemblage perspective of biotechnology (as the Anthrax 836 case has illustrated), would appreciate the complexity of constituting and maintaining a sociotechnical system for a large, robust offensive bioweapons program or break-out capability that would pose a significant security threat. My current research on the former Iraq bioweapons program suggests that even when people, infrastructure, and materials were available, the larger sociotechnical context comprising this program (post–1st Gulf War) led to significant problems for Iraq to reconstitute, maintain, and advance an offensive program.[59] These findings would recommend that more attention needs to be given to better understanding the unique sociotechnical assemblages constituting state and nonstate bioweapons programs to more accurately assess bioweapons threats and policy responses.

MICRO-LEVEL POLICY IMPLICATIONS FOR BIODEFENSE

One of the main concerns about increasing transparency on biodefense activities involves the risks of revealing U.S. vulnerabilities to adversaries by relaxing classification and/or promoting public release of information on specific projects. If one considers biodefense as a sociotechnical assemblage, however, then information about an experiment would only be one component among several in understanding U.S. biodefense capabilities and vulnerabilities. This would open up the possibility that more transparency on certain details could be allowable within specific biodefense activities.

For example, in the review of particular biodefense experiments, one could examine to what extent certain specialized or localized communities of practice, know-how, institutional structures, or other components are critical to replicating a particular experiment. Taking into account these sociotechnical factors, a useful spectrum of laboratory know-how across a range of biodefense projects could be constructed to inform transparency evaluations. In addition, one could examine the role of "transactional knowledge," or how different kinds of interdisciplinary scientific knowledge (e.g., knowledge networks, organizational structures) are involved in biodefense work.[60] For example, there appears to be very specialized and localized know-how that was involved in replicating the poliovirus experiment; for other biodefense projects the know-how threshold may be lower or organized differently.

Using this type of sociotechnical analysis would help more accurately assess the level of classification needed for a particular biodefense project; a contextual analysis would likely narrow the range of cases considered contentious or subject to more rigorous oversight. My poliovirus and phiX case studies suggest that much of this analysis could take place at the unclassified level. For a small number of biodefense projects that pose special risks due to the lack of specialized know-how, some of this analysis could be done at a classified level, with certain key pieces of data kept classified. Huxsoll, who was at USAMRIID during the height of U.S. suspicions of a Soviet BW program during the Cold War, has pointed out the importance of keeping a fair amount of biodefense research unclassified: "It's a whole lot easier to do the work if it's unclassified. You do not have that barrier to acquisition of good research—whether it's in house or a contract...you have a personal responsibility to see that [the openness of the research program] continues."[61] Adding to Huxsoll's remarks, another former commander of USAMRIID explains that keeping biodefense research unclassified facilitates the sharing of know-how and other types of knowledge among biodefense researchers to aid in the development of new countermeasures.[62]

Having more contextual knowledge about activities within the U.S. biodefense program can help the public and government better assess the potential bioweapons threat. To illustrate, let us revisit the controversial Project Bacchus experiment, which involved the construction of a mock BW production facility in Nevada. The project was carried out in order to ascertain the ease by which a rogue state or terrorist group could assemble a BW facility without detection. The facility was constructed largely through the purchase of commercially available components and resulted in the production of approximately two pounds of anthrax simulant. After the completion of the project and its public disclosure, many inside and outside the government pointed to its success as a clear indicator that rogue states and terrorists could easily acquire the necessary components and build such a facility, without weapons expertise. What is not widely reported or discussed is that the establishment of this mock BW facility was guided by individuals with specific bioweapons expertise and know-how.[63] This piece of information would suggest that specific BW know-how is still critical for developing a mass casualty BW capability, further indicating the need to take into account the sociotechnical character in accurately assessing bioweapons threats to inform biodefense planning.

Judith Reppy has described a curious paradox between transparency and secrecy: "Transparency is important for building trust and providing accountability in a democratic society; so is secrecy."[64] Within this paradox, however, how biotechnology and biodefense are framed shapes how certain types of problems and approaches become the focus and attention of policymaking. In this chapter, examining existing biodefense transparency debates and specific case studies provides a lens through which to see the limitations and problems with the current policy framing of the issue, which focuses on an assumed materialistic and globalized character of biotechnology.

My call for an alternative yet complementary frame, one that takes into account the sociotechnical dimensions of biotechnology, suggests a different focus of attention and resources in overall U.S. biodefense programmatic priorities. For example, the current policy focus on detection, surveillance, and preparedness activities has garnered 98 percent of the U.S. biodefense budget since 2001; only 2 percent of the budget during this same period has been directed at prevention activities that aim to more rigorously understand adversary capabilities (e.g., in a larger sociotechnical context) for developing mass casualty biological weapons.[65] My research suggests that the current capabilities- or science-based approach to biodefense, which is based on a limited conceptualization of biotechnology, needs to be broadened to include more attention to contextual factors in BW threats and responses. This approach would recognize that biotechnology knowledge is embedded within a larger sociotechnical assemblage that can modulate the extent to which biotechnology can be readily adopted by terrorists or proliferators.

Current policy attention that is focused primarily on technical solutions to the bioweapons problem, however, has tended to marginalize the analysis of social components of the BW threat. Seeing biodefense as a sociotechnical assemblage, however, would suggest that greater effort should be given to reform intelligence collection and analysis to consider the sociotechnical dimensions in evaluating state and nonstate bioweapons means and aspirations.[66] For example, CIA analysts focused on BW assessments could be reorganized to work much more closely with other intelligence analysts who consider the political, economic, social, and cultural dimensions of terrorist and state-level programs.[67] As a model, efforts are already underway to place more technical intelligence analysts within the CIA's Directorate for Operations in order to help members of the clandestine services improve their collection efforts on technical information related to weapons of mass destruction. Similarly, new collaborative linkages could also be forged between technical and social science analysts to guide collection and analysis on bioweapons-related intelligence. My preliminary analysis of the U.S. intelligence failures regarding Iraq's bioweapons program indicates this type of collaboration is lacking within the intelligence community and provides a partial explanation for how U.S. intelligence analysts misjudged the nature of the Iraqi BW program. Although technical analyses of weapons programs are important, a more careful reading of history suggests that technical issues are only one component of the more complex character constituting bioweapons threats.

Furthermore, a focus on particular experiments also tends to obscure the larger context in which the U.S. biodefense program is being conducted and the extent to which all of these activities are creating a sociotechnical assemblage conducive to an offensive capability. Although many charges have been made against the U.S. government regarding this purported capability, my contention is that one needs to move beyond looking at specific activities or material aspects to adequately assess whether an offensive program/activity truly exists. Finally, because the predominant focus has remained on the material aspects of biodefense (e.g., protocols, pathogens, publications), the focus of U.S. policy attention remains on information control, new oversight mechanisms, or technological responses to the material threat (e.g., detection, surveillance, countermeasures). These calls for change are often voiced with a need for a rush to action (e.g., more technology, oversight, or classification) to deal with an increasing and presumed BW threat. Thus, currently, a flawed assumption of the materiality and globalization of biotechnology has led both sides in the biodefense debate to put forth policy proposals and responses that do not reflect the more complex sociotechnical character of biotechnology underpinning biodefense. In talking about biosecurity threats President Bush is correct in stating: "We must confront danger with open eyes and unending purpose."[68] This chapter argues, however, that a more cautious and studied approach to assessing bioweapons threats and biodefense, which incorporates more contextualized elements, is critical to good and democratic governance on these policy issues.

NOTES

Acknowledgment: Thanks to Andrew Lakoff, Stephen Collier, and participants in the SSRC workshop on biosecurity for lively discussion and insightful comments on earlier versions of this chapter. I also thank Alan Pearson for his comments on an earlier version of this manuscript, as well as the Center for Arms Control and Nonproliferation for the opportunity to give a version of this paper at their October 19, 2007, conference on "Transparency in Current and Emerging Approaches to Biosecurity," held in Washington, DC.

1 Julian Perry Robinson and Milton Leitenberg, *The Rise of CB Weapons* (Stockholm: Almqvist & Wiksell, 1971); Milton Leitenberg, *Biological Weapons Arms Control* (College Park, MD: CISSM Project on Rethinking Arms Control, May 1996); Erhard Geissler and John Ellis van Courtland Moon, eds., *Biological and Toxin Weapons: Research, Development and Use from the Middle Ages to 1945* (Oxford: Oxford University Press, 1999); Charles Piller and Keith Yamamoto, "The U.S. Biological Defense Research Program in the 1980s: A Critique," in *Preventing a Biological Arms Race,* ed. Susan Wright (Cambridge, MA: The MIT Press, 1990), 133–68; U.S. Senate, Committee on Governmental Affairs, *Hearings on Global Spread of Chemical and Biological Weapons,* 101st Cong., 1st sess. (May 1989).

2 Judith Miller, Stephen Engelberg, and William J. Broad, "U.S. Germ Warfare Research Pushes Treaty Limits," *New York Times,* September 4, 2001; for more details, see Judith Miller, Stephen Engelberg and William J. Broad, *Germs: The Ultimate Weapon* (New York: Simon & Schuster, 2001): 290–96. The United States has been a member of the BTWC since the treaty entered into force in 1975. Under Article I of the BTWC, no part of an offensive biological weapons program (pathogens/toxins, equipment, weapons, delivery systems, or facilities), such as development, production, stockpiling, acquisition, or retention, is allowed by state parties under the BTWC. Research, however, is allowed for defensive and prophylactic purposes; see *Convention on the Prohibition of the Development, Production and Stockpiling of Bacteriological (Biological) and Toxin Weapons and on Their Destruction,* http://www.state.gov/t/ac/trt/4718.htm#treaty (accessed August 3, 2007).

3 For background on these policy concerns, see Susan Wright, "Terrorists and Biological Weapons: Forging the Link in the Clinton Administration," *Politics and the Life Sciences* 25, no. 1–2 (February 15, 2007): 57–115; Brad Roberts, ed., *Hype or Reality: The New Terrorism and Mass Casualty Attacks* (Alexandria, VA: CBACI, 2000); Milton Leitenberg, *Assessing the Biological Weapons and Bioterrorism Threat* (Carlisle Barracks, PA: U.S. Army War College, December 2005).

4 Victoria Clarke, DoD news briefing, September 4, 2001, http://www.defenselink.mil/transcripts/transcript.aspx?transcriptid=1605 (accessed July 27, 2007). There were internal disagreements, however, between DoD, CIA, and State Department lawyers on the treaty permissibility of these projects. For a discussion of these disagreements, see Miller, Engelberg, and Broad, *Germs.*

5 The White House, *Biodefense for the 21st Century,* April 28, 2004, http://www.whitehouse.gov/homeland/20040430.html (accessed August 3, 2007).

6 Alan Pearson, "Federal Funding for Biological Weapons Prevention and Defense,

Fiscal Years 2001 to 2008," http://www. armscontrolcenter.org/resources/fy2008_bw_ budget.pdf (accessed July 25, 2007).

7   Laura H. Kahn, "A Dangerous Biodefense Path," *The Bulletin of Atomic Scientists*, March 5, 2007, http://www.thebulletin.org/columns/ laura-kahn/20070305.html (accessed August 3, 2007); Joby Warrick, "The Secretive Fight Against Bioterror," *Washington Post*, July 30, 2006, A01; Lois R. Ember, "Testing the Limits: Biodefense Research to Characterize Threats May Violate the Biological Weapons Treaty, Experts Say," *Chemical & Engineering News* 83, no. 33 (August 15, 2005): 26–32, http://pubs. acs.org/cen/government/83/8333gov1.html (accessed March 25, 2008); Milton Leitenberg, James Leonard, and Richard Spertzel, "Biodefense Crossing the Line," *Politics & The Life Sciences* 22, no. 2 (May 17, 2004): 1–3.

8   Dana A. Shea, "The National Biodefense Analysis and Countermeasures Center: Issues for Congress," *CRS Report for Congress*, RL32891, February 15, 2007, http://fpc.state.gov/ documents/organization/77714.pdf (accessed March 25, 2008).

9   For example, see: Yudhijit Bhattacharjee, "Bioterrorism: Panel Provides Peer Review of Intelligence Research," *Science* 318 (December 7, 2007): 1538.

10   John Steinbruner, remarks made at 2007 Carnegie Nonproliferation Conference, "Biotechnology Proliferation: Benefits, Dangers, and Management," http://www.carnegie endowment.org/static/npp/2007conference/ transcripts/biotechnology_proliferation.pdf (accessed July 25, 2007).

11   Ember, "Testing the Limits," 28.

12   Andrew Lakoff describes current U.S. security policy responses as maintaining a "preparedness" perspective; for more background on how this perspective came to influence U.S.

policymaking, see Andrew Lakoff, "Preparing for the Next Emergency," *Public Culture* 19, no. 2 (2007): 247–71.

13   The White House, *Biodefense*, 1.

14   For a few examples, see U.S. National Academies of Science, *Globalization, Biosecurity, and the Future of the Life Sciences* (Washington, DC: The National Academies Press, 2006); Christopher F. Chyba, "Biotechnology and the Challenge to Arms Control," *Arms Control Today* 36, no. 8 (October 2006): 11–17; Eileen R. Choffnes, Stanley M. Lemon, and David A. Relman, "A Brave New World in the Life Sciences," *Bulletin of the Atomic Scientists* (September/October 2006): 26–33; U.S. Central Intelligence Agency, *The Darker Bioweapons Future* (November 3, 2003), http://www.fas.org/irp/cia/product/ bwi103.pdf (accessed March 7, 2007).

15   The White House, *Biodefense*, 4.

16   James B. Petro and W. Seth Carus, "Biological Threat Characterization Research: A Critical Component of National Biodefense," *Biosecurity and Bioterrorism: Biodefense, Strategy, Practice, and Science* 3, no. 4 (2005): 295–308. James B. Petro is currently Director for Biological and Chemical Defense Policy, White House Homeland Security Council; W. Seth Carus was the lead bio-official in the Office of the Vice President in the early years of the George W. Bush administration and is currently a professor at National Defense University. As Petro and Carus state in their article, this capabilities-based approach to biodefense is consistent with former Secretary of Defense Donald Rumsfeld's interest in a capabilities-based approach to military transformation, where technology has been envisioned as a critical centerpiece and force multiplier. For analyses that describe the limitations of this approach to broader defense policy issues, see Stephen D. Biddle, "Allies, Air Power, and Modern Warfare,"

International Security (Winter 2005–2006): 161–76; John Mearsheimer, "Hans Morgenthau and the Iraq War: Realism versus Neo-conservatism," http://mearsheimer.uchicago.edu/pdfs/A0037.pdf (accessed on July 26, 2007).

17 In choosing to focus on a science-based approach to biodefense, Petro and Carus describe the problem of assessing adversary intentions because this information is seen as scarce, dated, incomplete, contradictory, or insufficient for prioritizing biodefense resources and activities.

18 Petro and Carus, "Biological Threat Characterization Research," 297.

19 Warrick, "Secretive Fight Against Bioterror."

20 However, Gerald Epstein argues that classified research constitutes a very small portion of the U.S. biodefense program (although he acknowledges that this small subset of projects is likely to raise public concerns). See Gerald L. Epstein, "Biodefense in the Department of Homeland Security, FY08 Science and Technology Budget," Testimony to the Subcommittee on Technology and Innovation, Committee on Science and Technology, U.S. House of Representatives, March 8, 2007.

21 Jonathan B. Tucker, "Biological Threat Assessment: Is the Cure Worse Than the Disease," *Arms Control Today* (October 2004); Leitenberg et al., "Biodefense Crossing the Line"; and "Avoiding the Biological Security Dilemma: A Response to Petro and Carus," *Biosecurity and Bioterrorism: Biodefense Strategy, Practice, and Science* 4, no. 2 (2006): 195–99.

22 Tucker, "Biological Threat Assessment."

23 Ember, "Testing the Limits," 28.

24 The Sunshine Project, *Mandate for Failure: The State of Institutional Biosafety Committees in an Age of Biological Weapons Research* (October 2004), http://www.sunshineproject.org/ (accessed July 27, 2007).

25 Editorial, "Safety Clause," *Nature,* July 12, 2007.

26 John Steinbruner et al., *Controlling Dangerous Pathogens: A Prototype Protective Oversight System* (College Park, MD: CISSM, March 2007). Dual-use research is defined here as biological research that has peaceful scientific applications, but could also be misused to create biological weapons.

27 Jonathan B. Tucker, "Preventing Misuse of Biology: Lessons from the Oversight of Smallpox Virus Research," *International Security* 31, no. 2 (Fall 2006): 116–50.

28 Brian J. Gorman, "Balancing National Security and Open Science: A Proposal for Due Process Vetting," *Yale Journal of Law & Technology* (2004–2005): 1–43.

29 For a general description of the "biotechnology revolution" framework, see Choffnes, Lemon, and Relman, "A Brave New World"; Robert Carlson, "The Pace and Proliferation of Biological Technologies," *Biosecurity and Bioterrorism: Biodefense Strategy, Practice, and Science* 1, no. 3 (August 2003): 203–14.

30 Kathleen M. Vogel, "Framing Biosecurity: An Alternative to the Biotech Revolution Model?," *Science and Public Policy* 35, no. 1 (February 2008): 45–54.

31 For some examples, see Dana A. Shea, "Balancing Scientific Publication and National Security Concerns: Issues for Congress," *CRS Report for Congress* (2006), http://www.fas.org/sgp/crs/secrecy/RL31695.pdf (accessed August 3, 2007); U.S. National Research Council, "Scientific Openness and National Security Workshop" (January 2003), http://www7.nationalacademies.org/DSC/Scientific_Openness_Agenda.html (accessed August 3, 2007); Editorial, "Uncensored Exchange of Scientific Results," *PNAS* 100, no. 4 (2003): 1464; U.S. National Academies of Science, *Seeking Security: Pathogens, Open Access, and Genome*

Databases (Washington, DC: U.S. National Academies Press, 2004); Defense Threat Reduction Agency, *Quantification of Open Source Research Publications in Biological Sciences for Biological Weapons Development Utility* (2003), http://www.dtra.mil/documents/asco/ publications/BioliteratureReviewFinalReport TR03557.pdf (accessed August 3, 2007).

32 Brian J. Gorman, "Biosecurity and Secrecy Policy: Problems, Theory, and a Call for Executive Action," *I/S, A Journal of Law and Policy* 2, no. 1 (2006): 79.

33 Center for Strategic and International Studies, *Security Controls on Scientific Information* (June 2005), http://thefdp.org/CSIS_0506_cscans.pdf (accessed July 25, 2007).

34 Tacit knowledge is the unarticulated personally held laboratory knowledge that one acquires through a practical hands-on process, either through "learning by doing" or "learning by example." In contrast, explicit knowledge is codified knowledge that can be communicated through print media (e.g., information found in laboratory notebooks, scientific publications, textbooks). For an excellent overview of the different types of tacit knowledge in scientific work, see H. M. Collins, "Tacit Knowledge, Trust and the Q of Sapphire," *Social Studies of Science* 31, no. 1 (2001): 71–85. For examples of tacit knowledge in biological research, see Michael Lynch, "Protocols, Practices, and the Reproduction of Technique in Molecular Biology," *British Journal of Sociology* 53, no. 2 (2002): 203–20; Alberto Cambrosio and Peter Keating, "Going Monoclonal: Art, Science and Magic in Day-to-Day Use of Hybridoma Technology," *Social Problems* 35, no. 3 (1988): 244–60; Kathleen Jordan and Michael Lynch, "The Sociology of a Genetic Engineering Technique: Ritual and Rationality in the Performance of the Plasmid Prep," in *The Right Tools for the Job: At Work in Twentieth-Century Life Sciences,* ed. Adele E. Clarke and Joan H. Fujimura (Princeton, NJ: Princeton University Press, 1992): 77–114.

35 U.S. National Academies of Science, *An International Perspective on Advancing Technologies and Strategies for Managing Dual-Use Risks: Report of a Workshop* (Washington, DC: U.S. National Academies of Science Press, 2005): 35–36.

36 ETC group, *Extreme Genetic Engineering: An Introduction to Synthetic Biology* (January 2007), http://www.etcgroup.org/en/issues/synthetic_ biology.html (accessed August 3, 2007).

37 U.S. National Academies of Science, Biotechnology Research in an Age of Terrorism (Washington, DC: U.S. National Academies Press, 2004): 18.

38 Roger Roffey, "Biological Weapons and Potential Indicators of Offensive Biological Weapon Activities," in *SIPRI Yearbook 2004: Armaments, Disarmament and International Security* (Oxford: Oxford University Press, 2004): 557.

39 All three of the following case studies draw on my previous and current research. For the purposes of this discussion I will focus only on a few core elements of these cases that are especially germane to the transparency discussion.

40 For more details see, Kathleen M. Vogel, "Bioweapons Proliferation: Where Science Studies and Public Policy Collide," *Social Studies of Science* 36, no. 5 (October 2006): 659–90.

41 Jeronimo Cello, Aniko V. Paul, and Eckard Wimmer, "Chemical Synthesis of Poliovirus cDNA: Generation of Infectious Virus in the Absence of Natural Template," *Science* 297 (August 9, 2002): 1016–18.

42 HeLa cell-free cytoplasmic extract is derived from HeLa cells, which are a type of human cancer cell. The extracts contain the cytoplasm, cellular proteins, organelles (e.g., ribosomes), and chemicals; however, the nuclei,

mitochondria, and some other cellular organelles have been removed.

43 Hamilton O. Smith et al., "Generating a Synthetic Genome by Whole Genome Assembly: phiX174 Bacteriophage from Synthetic Oligonucleotides," *PNAS* 100, no. 26 (December 23, 2003): 15440–45.

44 For a description of this PCR method, see W. P. C. Stemmer et al., "Single-step Assembly of a Gene and Entire Plasmid from Large Numbers of Oligodeoxyribonucleotides," *Gene* 164, no. 1 (1995): 49–53

45 The generation of plaques involves injecting the synthesized phage into plates of *E. coli* and waiting for large plaques to form on the plates; large, robust plaques typically signify accurate, infectious phage.

46 It is important to note that Hutchinson is considered to be one of the world's foremost experts on DNA and has spent over forty years studying and working with the phiX bacteriophage.

47 Sarah J. Kodumal et al., "Total Synthesis of Long DNA Sequences: Synthesis of a Contiguous 32-kb Polyketide Synthase Gene Cluster," *PNAS* 101, no. 44 (2004): 15573–78; Peter A. Carr et al., "Protein-mediated Error Correction for de novo DNA Synthesis," *Nucleic Acids Research* 32, no. 20 (2004): 1–9; Brock F. Binkowski et al., "Correcting Errors in Synthetic DNA through Consensus Shuffling," *Nucleic Acids Research* 33, no. 6 (2005): 1–8; Ai-Sheng Xiong et al., "A Simple, Rapid, High-fidelity and Cost-effective PCR-based Two-step DNA Synthesis Method for Long Gene Sequences," *Nucleic Acids Research* 32, no. 12 (2004): 1–10; Lei Young and Qihan Dong, "Two-step Total Gene Synthesis Method," *Nucleic Acids Research* 32, no. 7 (2004): 1–6.

48 Although these studies do not specifically look at bioweapons, they do cover a range of biotechnologies and biological techniques and processes, such as genetic engineering, monoclonal antibodies, drug discovery, drug development, genomics, and postgenomics research. See Roberta Joppi, Vittorio Bertele, and Silvio Garattini, "Disappointing Biotech," *British Medical Journal* 331 (2005): 895–97; Michael M. Hopkins et al., "The Myth of the Biotech Revolution: An Assessment of Technological, Clinical, and Organizational Change," *Research Policy* 36 (2007): 566–89; Gary Pisano, *Science Business: The Promise, The Reality, and the Future of Biotech* (Boston: Harvard Business School Press, 2006); Paul Nightingale and Paul Martin, "The Myth of the Biotech Revolution," *TRENDS in Biotechnology* 22, no. 11 (2004): 564–69; Adam Hedgcoe and Paul Martin, "The Drugs Don't Work: Expectations and the Shaping of Pharmacogenetics," *Social Studies of Science* 33, no. 3 (2003): 327–64; David F. Horrobin, "Modern Biomedical Research: An Internally Self-Consistent Universe with Little Contact with Medical Reality?" *Nature Reviews* 2 (2003): 151–54; David F. Horrobin, "Realism in Drug Discovery—Could Cassandra Be Right?" *Nature Biotechnology* 19 (2001): 1099–1100.

49 For example, David Edgerton's book emphasizes that one should think of technological development more in terms of a "technology-in-use" narrative that takes into account contingency and sociotechnical understandings; see *Shock of the Old: Technology & Global History Since 1900* (Oxford: Oxford University Press, 2006).

50 Ember, "Testing the Limits," 29.

51 Michael Aaron Dennis, "Secrecy and Science Revisited: From Politics to Historical Practice and Back," in *Secrecy and Knowledge Production, Peace Studies Program Occasional Paper #23*, ed. Judith V. Reppy (Ithaca, NY: Cornell University

Peace Studies Program, October 1999): 1–16.

52 Also, this kind of approach would likely hinder accurate assessment of state-level offensive programs.

53 Each individual U.S. government agency is responsible for conducting its own internal biodefense review for BTWC compliance.

54 David L. Huxsoll, Testimony to the U.S. Senate Committee on Governmental Affairs, *Hearings on Global Spread of Chemical and Biological Weapons*, 101st Cong., 1st sess. (May 1989).

55 Ibid.

56 Leitenberg, *Biological Weapons Arms Control*, 74–78.

57 Although "end-to-end" biodefense assessments have been undertaken (e.g., in 2005 by the Homeland Security Council), they tend to focus, again, on specific activities and programs, instead of taking a more holistic look at how knowledge production and transfer is occurring within the U.S. biodefense enterprise.

58 For example, in the 1990s the Clinton Administration set up a special commission to evaluate declassification policies on radiation and nuclear issues. See https://www.osti.gov/opennet/ (accessed March 25, 2008).

59 Also see Richard Kerr, Thomas Wolfe, Rebecca Donegan, and Aris Pappas, "Issues for the U.S. Intelligence Community: Collection and Analysis on Iraq," *Studies in Intelligence* 49, no. 3 (2005), https://www.cia.gov/library/center-for-the-study-of-intelligence/csi-publications/csi-studies/studies/vol49no3/html_files/Collection_Analysis_Iraq_5.htm (accessed March 25, 2008).

60 I take this idea of "transactional" knowledge from Benjamin Sims, Los Alamos National Laboratory, from his talk, "The Uninvention of the Nuclear Weapons Complex? A Transactional View of Tacit Knowledge," at the 2007 Society for Social Studies of Science annual Conference in Montreal, Canada, 13 October 2007, http://www.4sonline.org/documents/AbstractsAll090907.pdf (accessed March 26, 2008). Sims defines "transactional knowledge" as that which is necessary to coordinate practice across multiple technical communities, such that the knowledge of each community can effectively contribute to a larger technological goal.

61 David Huxsoll, Testimony, U.S. Senate, Committee on Governmental Affairs, *Hearings on Global Spread of Chemical and Biological Weapons*, 101st Cong., 1st sess. (May 1989).

62 Interview with a former commander of USAMRIID, Frederick, MD, August, 2, 2007.

63 Leitenberg, *Assessing the Biological Weapons*, 54–55.

64 Judith Reppy, email communication, July 31, 2007.

65 Pearson, "Federal Funding."

66 My current research on the pre- and postwar assessments of Iraq's BW program suggest how a more contextualized approach could be carried out to reform intelligence assessments. Also see Kerr et al., "Issues for the U.S. Intelligence Community."

67 Richard Kerr, Thomas Wolfe, Rebecca Donegan, Aris Pappas, "Intelligence Analysis: A Holistic Vision for the Analytic Unit," *Studies in Intelligence* 50, no. 2 (2006), https://www.cia.gov/library/center-for-the-study-of-intelligence/csi-publications/csi-studies/studies/vol50no2/html_files/Holistic_Vision_5.htm (accessed March 25, 2008).

68 The White House, *Biodefense*, 1.

CHAPTER TEN

Anticipations of Biosecurity

Carlo Caduff

In memory of Allan Pred
(1936–2007)

In the United States, a series of recent events, including the terrorist attacks of September 11, 2001, and the ensuing, and still unresolved, discovery of the mailing of four letters containing anthrax, have come to serve as stable points of reference vindicating the apparent necessity of ever more biosecurity initiatives.[1] These events are commonly said to have wrought "a new sense of vulnerability" upon the post–Cold War era, prompting the U.S. government to initiate the Patriot Act and the Public Health Security and Bioterrorism Preparedness and Response Act of 2002.[2] As is well known, the concerted legislative effort gave birth to an unparalleled number of biodefense projects launched in the name of anticipating, preventing, and mitigating potentially catastrophic incidents. In addition, a series of elaborate biosecurity rules and guidelines were put into practice and new review and advisory boards were established, among them, and most prominently, the National Science Advisory Board for Biosecurity.[3] Scholars in the social sciences and the humanities have approached these developments in the past few years from a variety of perspectives and have responded with a growing body of critical work that reveals the contradictions and contestations generously elided by the built-in self-descriptions of biosecurity.[4]

This chapter looks at the future. It looks at the future, I should say, as it is currently envisioned by biosecurity experts whose aim is to intervene in the present. My focus is specifically on how infectious disease research has been problematized in the United States as a "potential threat to national security."[5] As biosecurity experts Ronald M. Atlas and Judith Reppy succinctly put it in a 2005 article, "in the current paradigm, all infectious disease research is potentially relevant to bioterror-ism and may be implicated in controversies over the motivation and possible uses of the research."[6] Of course, infectious disease research has always been a politically charged territory, as both past and present experience clearly demonstrate, but it now is even more so and in a very particular way.[7] While the scientific study of suf-ficiently understood agents like anthrax and smallpox is being actively promoted by the federal government, experimental investigations of polio and influenza now face new obstacles. All I will have to say here, it is important to underline, refers primarily to this partial and yet salient and unnerving aspect of the problematic of biosecurity, its concern with infectious disease research, and its potentially unlim-ited scope of regulatory intervention.

As an anthropologist I am predisposed to engage specific situations where concrete issues have come to matter to people. In this chapter, I draw in particular on my fieldwork among public health professionals and biomedical scientists in the United States. In this ongoing ethnographic research, I explore the current attempt to anticipate the next influenza pandemic from an anthropological per-spective that pays attention to the material infrastructure of biomedical research. Two recent events at the juncture of public health and scientific research provide the empirical substance of this chapter. The first event concerns the distribution of scores of samples containing a "pandemic flu virus" to a number of clinical laboratories in late 2004. The dissemination of these samples was immediately considered a serious violation of fundamental principles of biosafety. The second event pertains to the publication of a landmark research article in 2005 announc-ing the successful reconstruction of the flu virus that caused the devastating pan-demic of 1918–19. I have selected these two cases as a contrasting pair contrived to illustrate the fundamental difference between biosafety and biosecurity. In the first case, it was the distribution of biological *matter* that caused considerable concern; in the second case, by contrast, it was primarily the dissemination of biological *information* that generated anxiety among government officials and biosecurity experts. Biosafety, as we shall see, is first and foremost concerned with the possibil-ity of *accidental infection* of laboratory personnel, while biosecurity predominantly envisions the potential of *deliberate abuse* of information.[8] As we might imagine, in the context of biotechnology's capacity to convert almost any kind of living matter into molecular information, it is indeed not surprising that concerns with biosecurity have taken center stage over and against the traditional framework of biosafety. The reason for this development, however, is not biotechnology's miraculous transformative capacity itself but rather the ability attributed to information to circulate and reproduce faster and more easily than matter. Information is bodiless, or is at least said to be so, and thus appears to escape the universal law of gravity.

Conflict between biosafety and biosecurity most often arises in relation to questions of signage. A biohazard notice on an entrance to a lab, for instance, is designed to prevent hazardous accidents. From a different perspective, however, the notice may acquire a different meaning and appear as a sign that facilitates the successful execution of a nefarious plot. Whatever the intended audience of a sign, insofar as it is a sign it can always come under the influence of unforeseen readers. There is forever the possibility of other hermeneutic commitments according to which other meanings may prevail. Biosecurity can thus be described as an effort to actively search semiotic materials for a certain type of unintended meanings. What comes into being as a result of this peculiar effort that builds on the fundamental ambiguity of signs is a map of deliberate misreading. The question is not how a scientist might respond to a claim made by her colleague in a paper (she might critique it, doubt it, check it, reject it, trust it, forget it, think or laugh about it) but how a bioterrorist might reengineer the published information for malicious purposes. In the ominous hermeneutic regime of biosecurity, all descriptions are systematically approached as potential prescriptions for a certain type of action.[9] It is critical that engagements of biosecurity attend to not only the political but also the semiotic work that it is doing. Not surprisingly, the penchant of biosecurity is to subtract layers of information so as to make things more secure (the sign on the door has to disappear, a materials and methods section has to be removed from a paper, the genetic sequence of a virus must be withdrawn from a database). Biosafety, by contrast, seeks to add layer upon layer so as to make things safer (a virus is enclosed in a cell culture, the cell culture is enclosed in a test tube, the test tube is enclosed in a safety cabinet, the safety cabinet is enclosed in a safety lab). The critical question is either how much to add, or, as in the case of biosecurity, how much to remove.

The stakes involved in establishing ever more biosecurity guidelines, review boards, and advisory committees for the control of infectious disease research are considerable and many scientists are worried about the dramatic consequences that may ensue when provisional rules, vague obligations, and impossible demands are systematically imposed on biomedical research in the name of national security, while concomitantly biodefense labs with a significantly higher risk profile continue to mushroom all over the United States. Yet as critical social scientists, our task is to push our effort beyond the bare intuition that the problem of biosecurity merely constitutes a welcome opportunity for a powerful coalition of political and economic interests. However accurate that immediate intuition may be, it is nonetheless analytically insufficient.

In the past decade, anthropologists and historians have explored in a number of fascinating studies the constitutive role of secrecy in the nuclear project.[10] Biosecurity, however, does not simply index an extension of existing state practices of classification from nuclear physics to molecular biology. Biosecurity's central concern with the political implications of scientific investigation rather suggests an elective affinity with the emerging culture of research regulation that calls upon scientists to take into account the "ethical, legal, and social issues" of their work. As a matter of fact, the U.S. government already has the sovereign right to classify any kind of information in the name of national security. The reason for the recent proliferation of biosecurity rules, guidelines, review boards, and advisory committees is thus not immediately obvious. In terms of analysis, at any rate, the bureaucratic effort to internalize the implications of a certain kind of scientific investigation is more adequately framed as the articulation of an ethical form of research governance rather than as the extension of a legal system of security classification.[11] For biomedical scientists who are involved in infectious disease research the challenge is primarily to navigate a politically charged territory that threatens to disable their work. But before I explore a specific research project that successfully steered through the contingent concerns and unpredictable demands of biosecurity by animating a few things in the laboratory, let me first turn to biosafety.

Matter Comes to Matter

The modern state with its territorial boundaries has always been aware of the promise and peril that the seamless flow of persons and things represents.[12] Over and over, modern states have been deeply involved in both promoting and channeling, and thus controlling, such flows by a variety of means. Infectious diseases such as influenza constitute an interesting site for anthropological inquiry, for they index a fascinating field of potent flows, both tamed and untamed. Among those numerous things that travel the globe on dry ice are patient specimens.[13] Clinical laboratories, large and small, are at the receiving end of this generative circuit. The critical task of clinical laboratories is to process high volumes of samples efficiently and perform diagnostic procedures accurately so as to turn biological matter into meaningful medical information. Equipped with an elaborate instrumental architecture of safety cabinets, centrifuges, refrigerators, microscopes, and the reagents necessary to identify a certain number of pathogens, clinical labs are not supposed (nor do they have the means) to detect and determine any kind of agent. In late February of 2005, the specimen of a patient suffering from a respiratory disease made its way to a lab in Vancouver. Standard diagnostic tests soon revealed the presence of an unknown strain of the flu virus. Following standard procedure, the specimen was sent on for further investigation to the National Microbiology Laboratory in Winnipeg, Manitoba, where it was identified as a flu virus of the H2N2 subtype. This particular subtype of the flu virus had not been seen in people for decades and its appearance in the bodily fluids of a patient was troubling indeed. Confronted with the terrifying prospect of a pandemic in the making, the Canadian public health authorities immediately informed the communicable disease section of the World Health Organization (WHO) in Geneva as well as the influenza branch of the U.S. Centers for Disease Control and Prevention (CDC) in Atlanta.

The H2N2 subtype of the flu virus enjoys pride of place in medical history and is known among biomedical scientists and public health experts as the pathogenic agent that caused the mild pandemic of 1957. The virus originally emerged in Asia in February. It arrived in the United States in the summer, and continued to cause annual epidemics in humans for roughly a decade.[14] Then, in 1968, it vanished abruptly and was replaced by a new subtype of the flu virus, H3N2, and was isolated henceforth in birds only, the "natural reservoir" of the flu virus, as it were. Alerted by the unexpected emergence and spread of SARS in 2003, the Canadian experts anxiously wondered in those days of March 2005 if they had just received the ominous signal announcing the return of a notorious virus and the onset of a deadly pandemic.[15]

In the end, the dreaded event didn't occur, as we all now know. Nervously tracking down the origin of the unusual specimen, the Canadian authorities soon concluded that the ailing body from which the specimen had been extracted failed to present the characteristic symptoms generally associated with an influenza infection. But if it was not present in the patient's blood, where had the virus come from? What was its source? As an extensive epidemiological investigation revealed, the patient's specimen had inadvertently been contaminated in the course of the initial analysis performed in the clinical lab in Vancouver. It was, as it turned out, a panel of proficiency testing samples provided by the College of American Pathologists that in fact contained the H2N2 virus.

Certified clinical labs are required to regularly demonstrate that they are able to identify a certain number of pathogenic agents accurately and efficiently. Proficiency testing programs are mandatory and customary in the United States and must be administered by private nonprofit organizations as mandated under the Clinical Laboratory Improvement Amendments of 1988. The oldest and largest provider of proficiency testing programs in the United States is the College of American Pathologists, a medical society with nearly sixteen thousand members. In late September of 2004, the nonprofit organization (in addition to a few other organizations) routinely delivered forty-four hundred panels containing samples of various influenza viruses to participating laboratories mainly in the United States and Canada.[16] These samples were designed to mimic as best as possible actual patient specimens that labs regularly receive and process. Manufactured by a contractor, Meridian Bioscience of Cincinnati, Ohio, the samples were supposed to contain strains of the two subtypes of the flu virus known as H1N1 and H3N2. Strains of these two subtypes are currently infecting humans every year and are therefore considered low risk for laboratory personnel and the public. For reasons that have remained unclear, Meridian decided in 2004 to include strains of the H2N2 virus in their proficiency testing samples.

Due to the contamination, the initial diagnosis of the patient specimen was clearly compromised. However, the detection of the clinical error generated its own effect: the "imminent crisis" that seemed to have been unfolding changed its form and became a "potential crisis" that might have occurred. Confronted with the new circumstances of a potential crisis, public health authorities resolved to deal with it in advance. A flurry of action and a frantic effort to destroy all of the panels that had been sent out to laboratories followed. However, except for the accidental contamination and the compromised diagnosis, it is unlikely that the potential crisis would ever have been anticipated at all. In fact, not a single lab to which the thousands of testing kits had been delivered actually remarked, or found it remarkable, that the samples turned out to contain a strain of the H2N2 flu virus. It was, as we have seen, the analysis of the contaminated patient specimen that generated the alert, not the analysis of the proficiency testing samples. Indeed, the H2N2 strain caused considerable concern precisely because it was discovered in a patient specimen. The accidental contamination and the compromised diagnosis played a constitutive role obliging public health officials to recognize the potential crisis. Ironically, the consequential error occurred in the context of a program designed to evaluate the ability of clinical laboratories to identify microbiological matter accurately.

CONTAINMENT INSIDE-OUT

The frantic attempts mandated by public health authorities to immediately destroy all proficiency testing samples were accompanied by an avalanche of equally frantic media commentaries invoking the specter of a "killer flu virus" sent out to "thousands of labs all over the world."[17] The distribution of the pathogenic agent across the world was deemed a violation of standard biosafety principles. But what, in fact, is biosafety and how is it different from more recent concerns with biosecurity?

In the United States, responsibility for biosafety is dispersed among a number of diverse federal agencies, ranging from the Centers for Disease Control to the National Institutes of Health (NIH), the Department of Homeland Security, the Department of Agriculture, the Environmental Protection Agency, and the Food and Drug Administration. A large number of biosafety protocols issued by various international organizations, governmental agencies, and institutional committees is currently available, but the key guidelines regularly consulted by public and private labs alike, as well as institutional biosafety committees, are formulated in a prominent manual entitled *Biosafety in Microbiological and Biomedical Laboratories* (*BMBL*), published by the CDC and the NIH.[18]

The *BMBL* manual describes a number of microbiological practices, safety equipment, and facility safeguards recommended for work with specific pathogenic agents. These recommendations, it is important to underscore, are advisory and voluntary. *BMBL* fashions itself as a professional code of practice "that all members of a laboratory community will together embrace to safeguard themselves and their colleagues, and to protect the public health and environment."[19] According to the manual, the key principle of biosafety is "containment." Its purpose is "to reduce or eliminate exposure of laboratory workers, other persons, and the outside environment to potentially hazardous agents." The problem to which containment primarily responds is unintentional infection of laboratory personnel during experimental research. The manual renders the risk of infection tangible with a long list of reported accidents involving a broad range of infectious agents including typhoid, tetanus, tuberculosis, brucellosis, cholera, and hepatitis. Indeed, the history of microbiology is also a history of unintentionally infected scientists and lab technicians. Containment thus responds to the very tangible risk posed by the handling of infectious biological matter in the laboratory in the course of experimental work. As a professional code of practice, the kind of biosafety formulated in *BMBL* pertains not to the governmental domain of sovereign law but to the ethical domain of professional self-regulation. Biosafety refers to a particular purpose, a particular principle, a particular place, and is concerned with a particular kind of subject. To wit: its purpose is protection, its principle is containment, its place is the laboratory, and its subject is the laboratory worker engaged in research practices.

In order to reduce the risk of exposing lab workers unnecessarily to the H2N2 flu virus, public health authorities ordered clinical labs to destroy the samples immediately. Meanwhile, scientists were accused of failing to consider biosafety issues seriously and to prevent such incidents systematically. The disease control centers responded to the crisis by upgrading the H2N2 virus from a biosafety level 2 to a biosafety level 3 pathogen. Handling a biosafety level 3 pathogen requires a combination of laboratory practices, safety equipment, and facility design that provides a higher level of protection to scientists, lab technicians, and the public. Research with such a pathogen becomes, accordingly, more cumbersome. In order to minimize moments of exposure and reduce potential occasions of accidental infection, barriers are established that draw a line and keep things separate and contained. The four different levels of biosafety outlined by the *BMBL* manual refer to four distinctive combinations of practices, devices, and facilities contrived to ensure that things are enclosed and remain enclosed within other things. With its automatic doors and sealed windows, its air treatment and waste management systems, the lab facility functions as the most encompassing container. On its inside, the lab facility contains a series of additional containers, among them safety cabinets which contain safety centrifuge cups which contain test tubes which contain cell cultures which contain pathogens. Gloves keep human skin separate from infected matter and face masks protect people from inhaling dangerous aerosols. Biosafety thus entails a complex assemblage of architectural structure, artifact design, and deeply ingrained practices aimed at enclosing things materially within other things.

The purpose of containment is to *prevent* infection, as we have seen. But there is also another form of containment that is central in influenza research. This form of containment *presumes* infection. Viruses, as is well known, are not autonomous living beings; they are, rather, parasites that depend on the genetic machinery of host cells in order to reproduce and propagate their own kind. Viruses therefore primarily exist as things contained in other things. In the natural environment, it is mainly cells in human and animal bodies, or bodily fluids that contain flu viruses. In the artificial environment of the lab, it is monkey kidney cells and fertilized chicken eggs that keep them forever replicating. Ever since my first visit to a lab, I have been and continue to be fascinated by the fact that influenza researchers still work with eggs as their primary medium to isolate and grow their biological research material. The influenza branch at CDC, as Dr. Amanda Balish explained to me one afternoon, consumes approximately three hundred dozen eggs per week. These eggs, of course, are not the kind one buys in a neighborhood grocery store. The eggs on which influenza researchers draw are ten-day-old fertilized chicken eggs with a living embryo inside. The egg is swabbed with alcohol and then a small hole is punched in its top. A needle is introduced into the egg and the virus is inoculated into both the amniotic and the allantoic fluid. The hole in the egg is then sealed with wax and it is put into an incubator for two to three days. In the meantime, influenza viruses bind to sialic acids on the surface of the fertilized chicken egg cells to initiate replication.[20] This form of containment is thus predicated on infection. The entities that are contained are not separate from their containers; they become part of it. In their journey from fertilized chicken egg to fertilized chicken egg, influenza viruses begin to adapt to their new host and reproduce and propagate more efficiently. As a consequence of this process, reference strains adapted to eggs are unlikely to induce clinical influenza when given to humans.

If labs can be said to contain viruses, viruses can also be said to contain labs. Once made to exist in the artificial environment of the lab, flu viruses comprise the conditions of their existence. The H2N2 strain isolated in Japan in 1957 and disseminated as proficiency testing samples in 2004 was not a patient specimen but a reference strain. It had spent half a century in labs passing numerous times through fertilized chicken eggs. Adapted to its artificial environment, the strain was growing well and had become easy to work with. Interacting with its new animal host under laboratory conditions, the virus gradually adjusted to its container and partially changed its features. As scientists pointed out, when the 1957 flu strain was sent out to clinical labs nothing was known about its infectivity and virulence for humans. Paradoxically, then, the virus that was said to be in urgent need of containment already was contained. Nonetheless, things abruptly changed in 2005 and the H2N2 influenza virus was set apart from other influenza viruses by actors eager to demonstrate to the public that they were taking responsible action.

OF THINGS NONCONTEMPORARY

The first successful isolation of a human influenza virus was achieved in 1933 by Wilson Smith, Christopher Andrewes, and Patrick Laidlaw at the National Institute for Medical Research in Mill Hill. In a much celebrated set of experiments, the British scientists were able to accomplish what had been attempted many times before but to no avail, namely to infect animals in the laboratory with the pathogenic agent suspected to be responsible for recurring flu epidemics. The procedure followed by the scientists was comparatively simple: in the midst of an ongoing epidemic, Smith, Andrewes, and Laidlaw obtained throat washings from a number of recent patients which they dropped into the noses of a couple of ferrets.[21] The scientists succeeded primarily because they were able to work with a stock of naïve ferrets bred and kept in complete isolation. Originally, the ferrets were raised at the institute for a research project on dog distemper made possible by a large financial contribution solicited by *The Field* magazine, a sporting weekly. Due to the affective investment of the British aristocracy, not in people suffering from influenza but in hounds plagued by dog distemper, scientists at the National Institute for Medical Research were able to conduct extensive research and to design, construct, and maintain a costly technical infrastructure that contributed in no small part to the success of the first experimental transmission of the influenza virus from human to animal bodies. Not surprisingly, the ability to work with naïve animal bodies bred and kept in complete isolation was of the essence for a research endeavor designed to identify the unknown cause of a widely circulating, highly infectious disease.

Since 1933, biomedical scientists and public health experts have invested considerable resources in generating and channeling a seamless flow of viral strains not only across species, bodies, and tissues but also across countries, institutions, and disciplines. It was this controlled flow of biological matter that allowed influenza research to become independent of the seasonal occurrence of epidemic disease. Laboratories were eager to assemble and maintain their own stockpile of strains available for experimental research around the clock. Methods of cultivation and circuits of exchange were established and a vigorous flow of viral things was set in motion. As a consequence, influenza research became partially autonomous by imposing its own temporal norms and forms on things natural. Techniques of isolating, cultivating, and passing flu viruses in naïve animals (usually ferrets and mice), fertilized chicken eggs, and kidney cells (as well as other tissue cultures) generated matter that began to live differently in time.[22] Strains as famous as A/PR/8 and A/WSN/34, originally isolated in 1933 and 1934, respectively, are still used today in experimental research due to their complete assimilation to laboratory conditions. Released from the selective pressure of natural evolution, the viruses adapted to their new hosts and began to change slowly but steadily in a process that scientists call "laboratory drift." A new category of biological matter emerged: "noncontemporary human influenza strains." Scientific techniques developed in the late 1980s even allow the reconstruction of flu viruses that are not in circulation anymore and that have never been isolated by scientists. It is to the recent re-creation of the flu virus that caused the pandemic of 1918–19 that I now turn. As biosecurity experts argue, the reconstruction of this virus poses problems that cannot be solved within the traditional framework of standard biosafety safeguards.

Information Comes to Matter

In early 1995, Dr. Jeffery Taubenberger and Dr. Ann Reid of the Armed Forces Institute of Pathology in Rockville, Maryland, embarked on an uncertain research project that took nearly ten years to complete. Snips of lung soaked in formalin enclosed in paraffin and stored at the Armed Forces Institute of Pathology, in addition to a few tissue samples recovered by Johann Hultin from a frozen corpse of an Inuit woman in Brevig Mission, Alaska, made it feasible to sequence, piece by piece, the entire genome of the virus that caused the devastating pandemic of 1918–19.[23] A widely used reverse genetics technique initially developed in the esteemed lab of Dr. Peter Palese at Mount Sinai School of Medicine in New York made it possible to re-create the virus in cell culture using the genetic information provided by Taubenberger and Reid.[24] Chunks of matter, thus, were first turned into chunks of information, following which the information was assembled like a puzzle, and then turned into matter again with the help of plasmids. The landmark paper announcing the successful reconstruction of the 1918 virus in a biosafety level 3+ lab at the CDC in Atlanta was published in *Science* on October 7, 2005.[25] The publication was the result of a close collaboration between three groups of researchers: Dr. Taubenberger and his colleagues at the Armed Forces Institute in Rockville worked on the sequences, Dr. Palese and his group at Mount Sinai School of Medicine in New York provided the genetic technology and the necessary plasmids, and Dr. Terrence Tumpey and his collaborators at the CDC in Atlanta recreated the virus in the lab under stringent biosafety rules.

Given the contentious debate that the synthesis of the polio virus encountered in 2002, Palese, Taubenberger, and Tumpey clearly understood that their research project was unlikely to go unnoticed. And indeed, upon publication their paper immediately created a stir, causing great anxiety among government officials, biomedical scientists, and biosecurity experts alike. The concern was that someone might abuse the published information for nefarious purposes and "cause another pandemic."[26] In advance of publication, the authors had taken precautionary action by consulting with the director of the disease control centers, Julie Gerberding, informing the director of the National Institute of Allergy and Infectious Disease, Anthony Fauci, and notifying Amy Patterson, director of the Office of Biotechnology Activities at the National Institutes of Health.[27] As *Science* editor-in-chief Donald Kennedy reported in a comment, "all three felt that the public health benefits of the study far outweighed any biosecurity risks."[28] On September 17, however, the editorial board received an unexpected call from the Office of the Secretary of the U.S. Department of Health and Human Services (HHS) signaling serious biosecurity concerns regarding the peer-reviewed paper. A flurry of anxious conference calls followed in which Assistant Secretary Stewart Simonson declared that HHS Secretary Michael Leavitt insisted on additional review of the paper by the recently established National Science Advisory Board for Biosecurity (NSABB). As the issue of *Science* was being printed, Simonson announced that he had ordered the advisory board to be polled. It voted in favor of publication, asking the journal to add a note explaining the general purpose of the research in question.

The paper was published as planned, the stir kept on, and articles began to appear. In its News section, *Nature* reported that the 1918 virus would be sent to other labs by regular mail.[29] The CDC immediately denied the sensationalist allegation.[30] In a critical piece published in the *Washington Post,* journalist Wendy Orent warned that once all the genetic information was in the public domain "the entire 1918 flu could be built from scratch by anyone, anywhere, who has sufficient resources and skill."[31] She added the speculation that "it is quite conceivable that resurrected 1918 flu could someday be used as a bioterrorist [sic] agent." A group of supposedly irresponsible and naïve scientists dared to open the "gates of hell," as *Washington Post* op-ed columnist Charles Krauthammer dramatically put it.[32] In the meantime, Richard Ebright of Rutgers University granted a number of interviews and positioned himself among the most vocal opponents of the attempt to reconstruct the 1918 virus. The research should not have been performed in the first place, he authoritatively declared: "If this virus was to be accidentally or intentionally released, it is...quite possible that the threat of a pandemic that is in the news daily would become a reality."[33] Except, of course, that the 1918 virus is not able to cause a pandemic because viruses of the same subtype continue to circulate today.

More recently, Jan van Aken, a biosecurity expert, took issue with Tumpey and his colleagues questioning the basic purpose of the research. He maintained that "the tangible societal benefits of sequencing and reconstructing the 1918 virus remain poorly defined." And he concluded: "Considering the high risk of abuse, the availability of alternative research avenues and the limited added value to public health, this particular research project seems to be one of the few cases in which the risks outweigh the benefits and that therefore should not have proceeded."[34] Van Aken summoned scientists to "increase awareness of any potential security implications of their work" and he suggested that "the discussion of potential biosecurity implications of proposed experiments" be made "a mandatory prerequisite for grant proposals."[35] Scientific research has not only ethical, legal, and social but also, and increasingly, biosecurity implications.

POLITICALLY MODIFIED ORGANISMS

Although the reconstruction of the 1918 virus encountered considerable contention, the biosecurity concerns and anxieties soon subsided and the influenza researchers were able to continue with their work and explore fundamental questions of virulence, pathogenicity, and transmissibility. Tumpey and his colleagues successfully navigated a politically charged territory and prevented biosecurity concerns from undermining a significant research project designed to establish a new experimental system. This success was largely due to a series of earlier experiments conducted before the 1918 virus was fully reconstructed in one of the safest labs at CDC in 2005. Anticipating potential biosecurity concerns, the researchers conducted a form of risk assessment by constructing a set of recombinant viruses that contained only part of the genes of the 1918 virus (the sequencing of all genes took several years and was accomplished in 2005). Starting in 2002, Tumpey and his colleagues crafted recombinant viruses with one to five genes from the 1918 virus, while the remaining genes were taken from another H1N1 influenza virus. Experiments were then designed in order to test if current vaccines for regular seasonal influenza would provide protection against these newly created recombinant viruses that contained genes from the 1918 virus.[36] Since all current vaccines for seasonal influenza include antibodies against the most recent strain of the H1N1 virus and since the 1918 virus belongs to this particular subtype of the influenza virus, it was obvious from the outset that current vaccines would provide a partial protection. Experiments conducted with mice fully confirmed this assumption and provided the necessary data for a publication. In addition, the efficacy of four FDA–approved antiviral agents were tested.[37] A comparison of the chemical structures on the computer screen already indicated that these drugs would indeed be effective. Nonetheless a series of experiments was conducted with actual viruses both in tissue culture as well as in mice in order to confirm what was already known.

This series of experiments conducted in advance of the full reconstruction of the 1918 virus accomplished in 2005 was not supposed to generate unexpected results or new insights. Indeed, nothing was surprising about their actual outcome. The point, of course, is not their scientific value but their political significance. As a matter of fact, the experiments were designed as a sort of public risk assessment and with a political question firmly in mind; they were carried out in anticipation of potential biosecurity concerns. The experimental results provided authoritative arguments, literally tried and tested in tissue culture and mice. The study was successful not only because it generated relevant and conclusive data but also because it effectively preempted a political contestation that might have disabled any future research on and with the fully reconstructed 1918 virus. A set of recombinant viruses, some tissue culture, and a couple of inbred mice, in other words, were animated to perform a political demonstration. The experiments conducted by Tumpey and his colleagues, however, were not political in the sense of being biased in some way. Rather, they were political because they were designed as a public risk assessment conducted *in vitro* and *in vivo*. Scientifically valid inscriptions were generated to make a point. By enrolling a few recombinant viruses, some tissue culture, and a couple of inbred mice a truth was performed to open up rather than close down the future of a research project.

Recent concerns with biosecurity, articulated primarily by government officials and biosecurity experts, have politicized influenza research (and infectious disease research more generally) in particular ways. New rules have been established, new obligations and demands have been formulated, and new review boards and advisory committees have been institutionalized. The mandates of these review boards and advisory committees have been shifting, as have the rules, obligations, and demands. The paradigmatic change from a concern with research that involves "select agents," a clearly defined group of dangerous pathogens, to the invocation of the ever-elusive category of "dual-use research" practically means that any kind of study may come under review for potential abuse. Since no definite criteria have been formulated up until now that would indicate what kind of research activities the new category of "dual-use research" includes, the potential scope of regulatory intervention is in fact infinitely expandable. The terrain of biosecurity is chronically uncertain. Scientists with an interest in molecular factors that impact the virulence, pathogenicity, and transmissibility of viruses are constantly creating new strains with new properties in their labs and they now face new political liabilities that make a specific kind of work necessary.

Scientific knowledge production, as many anthropologists, sociologists, and historians have pointed out, is a situated practice. The political liabilities that are now being inscribed into infectious disease research have led researchers to design experiments that carry out a certain kind of work that is neither purely chemical nor biological but also, and sometimes primarily, political.[38] This chapter has briefly explored the reconstruction of the virus that caused the pandemic of 1918–19. While biosecurity experts raised concerns focusing on intrinsic viral virulence, influenza researchers were aware that virulence constitutes only one side of the equation. On the other side lies the human host and the partial immunity that this host has today, in contrast to 1918, to viruses of the H1N1 subtype.

As one of my interlocutors, an epidemiologist once told me in a somewhat different but nonetheless related context, many experts implicitly draw on the model of smallpox when considering the case of influenza. Smallpox indeed occupies a special place in the public health and biosecurity community.[39] It was the first and only serious infectious disease that was eradicated due to a successful worldwide vaccination campaign. Confronted with a pandemic flu virus that killed twenty to fifty million people in 1918–19, the implicit analogy with smallpox impels experts to extrapolate and forecast a similar or even higher mortality rate for the case of a deliberate release of the 1918 virus today. This translation, however, is a rather fragile one. The point is simply that an eradicated disease such as smallpox with an immunologically naïve population as its potential host is not necessarily a good model for an annually recurring pathogenic agent that infects a large part of the human population each year. For better or worse, flu viruses travel through a complex, historically saturated, and ever-changing biosocial landscape composed of hosts that come with all kinds of naturally produced and artificially induced immunities.

My aim here has been to weave an anthropological narrative of sorts that highlights the embedded nature of things, not unlike the practice of biosafety itself and its distinctive logic of layering. Specifically, I have put what appeared to be a free-floating, disembodied, and out-of-control H2N2 virus back into the allantoic and amniotic fluids of fertilized chicken eggs in which influenza viruses are grown. The consideration of the material infrastructure required to promote and control the traffic of influenza viruses has led us to a different kind of assessment. Turning to biosecurity and its prime concern with the free flow of information and the intrinsic ambiguity of signs, I have explored how a group of researchers, in addition to rigorous adherence to stringent biosafety standards, successfully preempted potential biosecurity contestations by embedding political lines of argument into the virus itself. Once government officials and biosecurity experts arrived on stage, belated, hurried, and troubled, they realized that the reconstructed 1918 virus had been politically modified in a way that made it immune to the prospect of a certain kind of influence. The strategic animation of a few recombinant viruses, some tissue culture, and a couple of inbred mice had already done the necessary work.

NOTES

Acknowledgment: I am indebted to Andrew Lakoff and Stephen Collier for kindly inviting me to a workshop on biosecurity held at the Social Science Research Council in New York City. I would like to thank all participants as well as the organizers for two days of thoughtful, delightful, and engaged discussion. Thanks for encouragement and suggestions are also due to Melinda Cooper, Nicolas Langlitz, Onur Ozgode, Paul Rabinow, Tobias Rees, Arpita Roy, Meg Stalcup, and Anthony Stavrianakis. All claims made in this paper are solely my responsibility.

1 The anthrax mail attacks occurred just two months after the Bush administration rejected the draft verification protocol of the Biological and Toxin Weapons Convention.

2 National Research Council, *Biotechnology Research in an Age of Terrorism* (Washington, DC: National Academies Press, 2004), 79.

3 The Patriot Act passed Congress in late October 2001. The Bioterrorism Act was signed into law in June 2002. Project BioShield was launched two years later. For an overview of recent U.S. federal biodefense funding, see Filippa Lentzos, "Rationality, Risk and Response: A Research Agenda for Biosecurity," *BioSocieties* 1 (2006): 453–64. Biosecurity concerns had already emerged in the early 1990s; see Susan Wright, "Terrorists and Biological Weapons: Forging the Linkage in the Clinton Administration," *Politics and the Life Sciences* 25, no. 1–2 (2007): 57–115.

4 Stephen J. Collier, Andrew Lakoff, and Paul Rabinow, "Biosecurity: Towards an Anthropology of the Contemporary," *Anthropology Today* 20, no. 5 (2004): 3–7; Melinda Cooper, "Preempting Emergence: The Biological Turn in the War on Terror," *Theory, Culture & Society*

23, no. 4 (2006): 113–35; Lentzos, "Rationality, Risk and Response"; Jeanne Guillemin, *Anthrax: The Investigation of a Deadly Outbreak* (Berkeley: University of California Press, 2001) and *Biological Weapons: From the Invention of State-Sponsored Programs to Contemporary Bioterrorism* (New York: Columbia University Press, 2006); Philipp Sarasin, *Anthrax: Bioterror as Fact and Fantasy,* trans. Giselle Weiss (Cambridge, MA: Harvard University Press, 2006); Kathleen Vogel, "Bioweapons Proliferation: Where Science Studies and Public Policy Collide," *Social Studies of Science* 36, no. 5 (2006): 659–90. Also see the contributions to this volume.

5 On the so-called dual-use dilemma, see Kathleen Vogel's essay in this volume.

6 Ronald M. Atlas and Judith Reppy, "Globalizing Biosecurity," *Biosecurity and Bioterrorism: Biodefense Strategy, Practice, and Science* 3, no. 1 (2005): 51–60.

7 On the politics of infectious disease control, see, among many others, Peter Baldwin, *Contagion and the State in Europe, 1830–1930* (Cambridge: Cambridge University Press, 1999); João Biehl, "The Activist State: Global Pharmaceuticals, AIDS, and Citizenship in Brazil," *Social Text* 22, no. 3 (2004): 105–32; François Delaporte, *Disease and Civilization: The Cholera in Paris (1832)* (Cambridge, MA: The MIT Press, 1986); Steven Epstein, *Impure Science: AIDS, Activism, and the Politics of Knowledge* (Berkeley, Los Angeles, London: University of California Press, 1996); Paul Farmer, *AIDS and Accusation: Haiti and the Geography of Blame* (Berkeley, Los Angeles, London: University of California Press, 1992); Arthur Kleinman and James L. Watson, eds., *SARS in China: Prelude to Pandemic?* (Stanford, CA: Stanford University

Press, 2006); Bruno Latour, *The Pasteurization of France*, trans. Alan Sheridan and John Law (Cambridge, MA; London: Harvard University Press, 1988); Nicholas B. King, "Security, Disease, Commerce: Ideologies of Postcolonial Global Health," *Social Studies of Science* 32, no. 5-6 (2002): 763–89; Emily Martin, *Flexible Bodies: Tracking Immunity in American Culture from the Days of Polio to the Age of AIDS* (Boston: Beacon Press, 1994); and Paul Rabinow, *French Modern: Norms and Forms of the Social Environment*, 2nd ed. (Chicago, London: University of Chicago Press, 1995).

8 The concepts of safety, security, and preparedness have recently been explored in the context of synthetic biology. See Paul Rabinow, Gaymon Bennett, and Anthony Stavrianakis, "Response to 'Synthetic Genomics: Options for Governance,'" http://openwetware.org/images/3/3f/Response_to_Draft_Governance_Report.pdf (accessed February 15, 2008).

9 I borrow this notion of prescriptions from Strathern. See Marilyn Strathern, *Commons and Borderlands: Working Papers on Interdisciplinarity, Accountability and the Flow of Knowledge* (Wantage: Sean Kingston Pub., 2004).

10 Hugh Gusterson, *Nuclear Rites: A Weapons Laboratory at the End of the Cold War* (Berkeley, Los Angeles, London: University of California Press, 1996); Joseph Masco, "Lie Detectors: On Secrets and Hypersecurity in Los Alamos," *Public Culture* 14, no. 3 (2002): 441–67, and *The Nuclear Borderlands: The Manhattan Project in Post–Cold War New Mexico* (Princeton, NJ: Princeton University Press, 2006); Peter Galison, "Removing Knowledge," *Critical Inquiry* 31 (2004): 229–43.

11 Ethical forms of governance have been explored in recent years by Paul Rabinow, *French DNA: Trouble in Purgatory* (Chicago, London: University of Chicago Press, 1999);

Marilyn Strathern, ed., *Audit Cultures: Anthropological Studies in Accountability, Ethics and the Academy* (London, New York: Routledge, 2000); Cori Hayden, *When Nature Goes Public: The Making and Unmaking of Bioprospecting in Mexico* (Princeton, NJ: Princeton University Press, 2003); Lawrence Cohen, "Where It Hurts: Indian Material for an Ethics of Organ Transplantation," *Daedalus* 128, no. 4 (1999): 135–65; Aihwa Ong and Stephen J. Collier, eds., *Global Assemblages: Technology, Politics, and Ethics as Anthropological Problems* (Oxford: Blackwell, 2005). See as well a series of essays and comments on institutional review boards published in a recent issue of the *American Ethnologist* (33, no. 4 [2006]).

12 Michel Foucault, *Security, Territory, Population: Lectures at the Collège de France, 1977-78*, trans. Graham Burchell (London: Palgrave, 2006); Hayden, *When Nature Goes Public*.

13 For a salient anthropological analysis of the trafficking in sputum samples in Georgia, see Erin Koch, "Beyond Suspicion: Evidence (Un)Certainty, and Tuberculosis in Georgian Prisons," *American Ethnologist* 33, no. 1 (2006). Rayna Rapp has paid attention to the preparation of amniocentesis samples in a well-known study; see Rayna Rapp, *Testing Women, Testing the Fetus: The Impact of Aminocentesis in America* (London: Routledge, 2000). Informed by recent work in science studies and the anthropology of science, Cori Hayden has forged a remarkable ethnographic account out of the traffic in plant specimens; see *When Nature Goes Public*. The material infrastructure, finally, that allows biological matter to travel near and far, is the object of Hannah Landecker's formidable exploration of tissue culture. See Hannah Landecker, *Culturing Life: How Cells Became Technologies* (Cambridge, MA: Harvard University Press, 2007).

14 Edwin D. Kilbourne, "Influenza Pandemics of the 20th Century," *Emerging Infectious Diseases* 12, no. 1 (2006): 9–14.

15 In 2005, of course, the focus of public health officials and the media was predominantly and almost exclusively on the avian influenza H5N1, or "bird flu" virus. The appearance of an H2N2 virus came as a surprise to many.

16 The proficiency testing samples produced by Meridian Bioscience were distributed by the College of American Pathologists, the American College of Physicians, the American Academy of Family Physicians, and the American Association of Bioanalysts. Although a number of countries were involved, 98% of the labs were located in the United States and Canada.

17 See, among many others, Marc Santora, "50s Killer Flu Is Still Here. Why?" *New York Times*, April 17, 2005; Sarah Boseley, Suzanne Goldenberg, and Luke Harding, "Scientists Hunt Thousands of Vials of Deadly Flu Virus Sent across World," *Guardian*, April 14, 2005.

18 Prior to the publication of the first edition of *BMBL* in 1984, the CDC edited a report, *Classification of Etiologic Agents on the Basis of Hazards,;* in 1974. In the same year, the NIH published the more limited *National Cancer Institute Safety Standards for Research Involving Oncogenic Viruses,* followed two years later by the important *NIH Guidelines for Research Involving Recombinant DNA Molecules.*

19 *Biosafety in Microbiological and Biomedical Laboratories,* 5th ed. (2007); available at http://www.cdc.gov/OD/ohs/biosfty/bmbl5/bmbl5toc.htm.

20 Peter Palese and Megan L. Shaw, "Orthomyxoviridae: The Viruses and Their Replication," in *Fields Virology,* ed. B.N. Fields and D.M. Knipe (Philadelphia: Lippincott Williams and Wilkins, 2001).

21 Wilson Smith, C.H. Andrewes, and P.P. Laidlaw, "A Virus Obtained from Influenza Patients," *Lancet* 2 (1933): 66–74.

22 Hannah Landecker, "Living Differently in Time: Plasticity, Temporality and Cellular Biotechnologies," *Culture Machine* 7 (2005), http://www.culturemachine.net. On the development of tissue cultures, see Landecker's brilliant study *Culturing Life.*

23 Not surprisingly, two journalistic accounts of Johann Hultin's attempts to recover tissue samples in Alaska have been published. The story fits nicely into the stereotypic narrative of science as the great adventure of a heroic individual. The collective effort and technical skill it actually took to sequence the genes and develop a reverse genetics technique that would allow the reconstitution of the virus has not made it into the accounts. Gina Kolata, *Flu: The Story of the Great Influenza Pandemic of 1918 and the Search for the Virus That Caused It* (New York: Simon & Schuster, 2005); Pete Davies, *The Devil's Flu* (New York: Henry Holt & Company, 2000).

24 Willem Luytjes et al., "Amplification, Expression, and Packaging of a Foreign Gene by Influenza Virus," *Cell* 59 (1989): 1107–13; Ervin Fodor et al., "Rescue of Influenza A Virus from Recombinant DNA," *Journal of Virology* 73, no. 11 (1999): 9679–82.

25 Terrence M. Tumpey et al., "Characterization of the Reconstructed 1918 Spanish Influenza Pandemic Virus," *Science* 310 (2005): 77–80.

26 Andreas von Bubnoff, "Spanish Flu Papers Put Spotlight on 'Dual Use' Decisions," *Nature* 11, no. 11 (2005): 1130.

27 Joceyln Kaiser, "Resurrected Influenza Virus Yields Secrets of Deadly 1918 Pandemic," *Science* 310 (2005): 28–29.

28 Donald Kennedy, "Better Never Than Late," *Science* 310 (2005): 195.

29 Andreas von Bubnoff, "Deadly Flu Virus Can

Be Sent through the Mail," *Nature* 438 (2005): 134–35.

30 Julie Louise Gerberding, "Flu Virus Will Not Be Sent in the Regular U.S. Mail," *Nature* 438 (2005): 738.

31 Wendy Orent, "Playing with Viruses: Replicating This Flu Strain Could Get Us Burned," *Washington Post*, April 17, 2005.

32 Charles Krauthammer, "A Flu Hope, or Horror?," *Washington Post*, October 14, 2005.

33 Jamie Shreeve, "Why Revive a Deadly Flu Virus?," *New York Times*, January 29, 2006.

34 Jan van Aken, "When Risk Outweighs Benefit: Dual-Use Research Needs a Scientifically Sound

Risk-Benefit Analysis and Legally Binding Biosecurity Measures," *EMBO Reports* 7 (2006): S10–S13.

35 Ibid., S13.

36 Terrence M. Tumpey et al., "Pathogenicity and Immunogenicity of Influenza Viruses with Genes from the 1918 Pandemic Virus," *PNAS* 101, no. 9 (2004): 3166–71.

37 Terrence M. Tumpey et al., "Existing Antivirals Are Effective against Influenza Virus with Genes from the 1918 Pandemic Virus," *PNAS* 99, no. 21 (2002): 13849–54.

38 See Hayden, *When Nature Goes Public*.

39 See Dale Rose's chapter in this volume.

Episodes or Incidents

SEEKING SIGNIFICANCE

Paul Rabinow

*Episode: "A significant incident: an event that is part of but distinct from
a greater whole and that often has specific significance."*
Incident: "Something that happens...an event that may result in a crisis."

The essays collected here display an extravagant range, depth, and scale of insights, reflections, and explorations covering an extensive array of topics. At first blush, these topics appear to form a quite heterogeneous set, if they form a set at all. That being said, these chapters and their topics cluster around the question of what to make of a burgeoning constellation of experts and the frequently incongruous (or inconclusive) claims to expertise that these experts produce. That clustering of claims and interpretations grouping episodes and incidents so as to make sense of them operates at a second-order level. These papers are acute observations of other observers observing. Such second-order observation provides something that the majority of other experts, in their claims to immediate relevance and significance, seem unable to do: intelligently and tentatively provide the contours of those milieus into which they intervene, with attention to the fact that their interventions might contribute to shaping those milieus. Of equal import, the chapters convincingly provide a preliminary identification of the venues for the analysis and evaluation of the flow of data these experts are authorized to contend with, make sense of, and propose responses for—in first-order terms.

Such clustering, such set-making, such second-order ordering, of course, is no accident. The chapters in this volume have been assembled precisely with an awareness of the existing heterogeneity of topics as well as the need to be attentive to the rationality or rationalities that may well be linking them now or in the near future. The editors have brought together authors who proceed from a broadly common working hypothesis, or orientation, to wit that these heterogeneous topics provide salient sounding points for an early cartography of an emergent problem-space. The chapters provide evidence and arguments that this problem-space, if it is such, contains numerous indications of its significance—scientifically, politically and ethically. These soundings advance through detailed attention to and accounts of incidents and episodes; they rightly eschew claims to epochs or wholly formed fields of significance. Their rigorous abstention from pushing the material farther than it actually deserves is, to my mind, the strength of these reports. These chapters are starting points for inquiry; they are serious initial formulations, not conclusions.

Thus, we learn about a vast range of incidents and episodes: the framing of debates over the safety of food in France; the mutually contested understandings of global bird migration patterns; the tacit knowledge required to build a polio virus from its DNA sequence; how nurses and doctors ready themselves for potential epidemics; the multiple aspects of containment procedures and preparedness tactics; the different undertakings of diverse NGOs; the state of play of organization and reorganization in federal and international bureaucracies; the role of shadow organizations in the world and the place of such knowledge in the imagination of self-styled hard-headed and sincere experts; the production of an imaginary of virtual terrorists, and the practices of official counterterrorists; the growth of vast budgets for security planning and implementation. Throughout, we learn of the ever accelerating expansion of expertise and more expertise, and the war-like rumblings of diverse organizational contests over territory and authority.

In sum, reading these chapters in and of themselves provides an education. They are instructive about how knowledge-dependent are major sectors of the contemporary world; how these knowledge-dependent sectors interface with and ramify from the micropractices of everyday life as well as strategic global initiatives. In these pages we encounter an ever growing and seemingly neverending tsunami of data, facts, interpretations, contestations, disputations, demonstrations, inter-correlations, inferences, deductions, obfuscations, and a pervasive sense of confusion, cloaked for the public—and most tellingly, for many of the experts themselves—in declarations of assurance and reassurance.

This cacophony of experts and expertise is permeated with and molded by affect waves of urgency and vigilance. The imperative to be attentive to that which might be or is emerging (or in some cases, we suspect, is probably already present) is heartfelt (as the old metaphor would have it) and deeply cathected (as an older knowledge system would put it). The range of affects associated with this urgent need to know covers and inflects an equally impressively wide spectrum of other affects, sentiments, passions and moods ranging from fear, care, shame, guilt, pride, arrogance, humility, and the like, to the occasional touch of despair. Now and then, infrequently it seems, there are touches of humor and splashes of ironic distancing from the utter self-importance of it all.

What is one to make of this porridge of affect and truth claims? One must never lose sight of the fact that these experts operate within a partially self-constructed set of milieus and venues characterized by a vertiginous whipping motion of too much information countered but not complemented by too little information. There are too many incidents and too few events; too many episodes and too few plausible narratives. This information imbalance as well as its associated significance vacuum is hardly restricted to security domains but it does attain a specific salience there. That assemblages are taking shape and being recomposed, projected, and critiqued is certain. The significance of all this activity remains far from clear even though there is a constant and insistent demand to make it so. Thus, we learn about a range of diverse yet seemingly consonant preparedness practices in domains concerning what we eat, what we drink, how we travel—the ecology of our innards as well as of spatial configurations large and small. At the same time we learn about the industry of insurance and its steady probability series, painstakingly built over the decades of construction of social modernity (both capitalist and socialist) when avalanches of numbers may have stripped individual acts and the cosmos of their semantic underpinnings but at least demonstrated regular and repeated patterns. What good is probability thinking if events do not occur and recur? Today, while such probability-based insurance rationality is certainly still present in certain well swept corners like life insurance, more recently—as the chapters in this volume demonstrate—attention and technical firepower has been turned instead toward incidents and episodes that do not belong to such verifiable series and whose consequences are not only not strictly calculable but imagined on the basis of the aforementioned work's being catastrophic or disastrous or traumatic or vital or crucial or critical. Of course, which of these qualifiers is the right one is not yet stabilized either in an institutional sense or in the cultural imaginary. No one can say with certainty what to think about security; but that does not prevent an ever increasing body of experts from being paid, trained, cultivated, and incited to recite what they know or claim to know. The best of them may deploy subjunctives but nevertheless continue to speak and write and prognosticate and imagine and plot and critique in a crescendo of production of serious speech acts. For the most part, such truth claims are cast analytically and affectively in outdated modes. What, after all, is the mathematics appropriate to incidents and episodes?

As old Luhmann seemed to have taken great pleasure in saying: the future is uncertain and contingent, so act now! Or prepare to act as soon as possible or whenever it is the right time to do so. That time might be soon, or gone, or never to come, or just around the corner, or about to happen, or eventually certain to appear, it seems. On the second anniversary of Hurricane Katrina, there had not been any major hurricanes passing through New Orleans. There will be, of that we are certain. But are we prepared? Are we secure? Are we safe? To pose the question is to answer it but not yet to respond appropriately. Was Katrina an event? An episode? Or an incident? Which models and which strategy will provide the best answer to those questions? Act now! The future depends on it.

Today, the situation seems to be the opposite of Purgatory. In the Christian purgatory, souls waited for an indefinite amount of time—divine temporality—before passing on to the heavenly spheres that eventually awaited them. In a purgatorial regime, intercession might or might not help; but it certainly could not hurt. Hence there seemed to be something to do. And regardless of who was acting, and whose influence might or might not count, one thing was apparently certain: if you made it to purgatory you could only remain there or ascend. Purgatory was the Christian answer to tragedy.

Today we seem to be in another kind of antechamber, awaiting the descent into catastrophe through the single episode whose virtualities were and are incalculable and which may or may not be part of a series or regular pattern. We are not even certain when we might descend or where we might descend to. Today we seem to have moved from the narrative simplicities of Christian purgatory into some contemporary Buddhist space of seemingly endless hells with their demons, antechambers, imagined trials, and travails, all the while not knowing whether this is all the torment of the soul or the tumultuous end of some airport, city, water supply, nesting pattern, viral mutation, or vaccine run amok. We do not know whether we have encountered bureaucracies unleashed or in utter stasis, and lessons learned or mutilated from an earlier Armageddon that did not take place, perhaps because it was prevented and contained or deterred. In the contemporary world, *The Tibetan Book of the Dead* seems more relevant than Seneca's notebooks.

So, let's plan, interpret, decipher, decode, analyze, synthesize, diagnose, contest, approve, improve, convince, decry, denounce, and raise holy hell. And above all, act now! Not acting has consequences even if they are not knowable. Given that, let's imagine, script, narrate, role play: the theater of the virtual has never been more apropos. And if nothing happens? Perhaps something ominous has been forestalled. Who knows for sure?

As billions of dollars circulate in venues of expert uncertainty, one might wonder whether the ocean's temperature continues to rise, as reports emerge of glaciers cascading sheets of ice into the waters of what used to be the Gulf Stream. One might wonder whether obscure terrorists in Islamic lands are transmitting and teaching that tacit knowledge of viral manipulation they learned at MIT or Stanford; or whether the potential unleashers of viral threats are the brilliant graduate students who have trained their whole lives to succeed and can no longer stand the delay of living, choosing to accelerate things by hacking their way into ignominy and fame. Is that new unclassified bacteria an escapee from a lab; or is it simply the evolutionary product of the vast gorging markets of the prosperous Chinese, where untold bounty of vital things yield both error and selectivity before flying parasitically along trans-Siberian and trans-Polar routes, eventually dropping their feces over the industrialized chicken farms of Egypt—or was it in Egypt that they picked up the mutations in the first place?

And has your grant been approved by the Committee on Human Subjects? And is your patent application being submitted to the DoD or to the U.S. Patent Office? And what if intellectual property is being infringed in the mountains of

Waziristan? Or Chicago? Shall we sue them? Blocking patents are the prudent path to follow: who knows, they might actually be upheld.

Beware the Ides of March. Incidentally, this or that episode might be an event! Or it might presage an event!

Perhaps today the take-home message is: Only the second-order observers know for sure that they don't know. Yet.

Acknowledgments

We are grateful to the Social Science Research Council for its generous support of this project, especially to Craig Calhoun, Paul Price, and Melissa Aronczyk. We also acknowledge the National Science Foundation (Award #0450975) for support of the project on "The Global Biopolitics of Security."

Contributors

Nick Bingham is a lecturer in human geography at the Open University in the UK. He has published widely on the challenging geographies that emerge when the nonhuman elements of our collectives—from technologies to plants—are taken seriously. Most recently this has involved a series of pieces on the controversies around genetically modified crops, including publications in the journals *Environment and Planning A* and *Geoforum*. His current work addresses the making of biosecurities and the cosmopolitics of coexistence.

Carlo Caduff is a PhD candidate in anthropology at the University of California, Berkeley. His current research focuses on pandemic influenza in the United States and draws on ethnographic fieldwork among American public health professionals and biomedical scientists. He works as a regular contributor to the newspaper *Neue Zürcher Zeitung*.

Stephen J. Collier is an assistant professor at the program in international affairs at The New School. He received his PhD in anthropology from the University of California, Berkeley in 2001, and held research and teaching positions at Columbia University. He is the co-editor (with Aihwa Ong) of *Global Assemblages: Technology, Politics and Ethics as Anthropological Problems* (Blackwell, 2004). His articles have appeared in *Theory, Culture, and Society*, *Economy and Society*, *Environment and Planning D*, *Anthropology Today*, *Anthropological Theory*, and *Post-Soviet Affairs*. He is currently finishing a book manuscript on urbanism and neoliberal reform in post-Soviet Russia.

Lyle Fearnley is a PhD candidate in the department of medical anthropology, University of California, Berkeley. He is a contributing member of the Anthropology of the Contemporary Research Collaboratory. A forthcoming article, entitled "Signals Come and Go: Syndromic Surveillance and Styles of Biosecurity," will appear in the journal *Environment and Planning A*.

Steve Hinchliffe is a reader in environmental geography at the Open University in the UK. He has written and edited a number of books and journal special editions, including, most recently, "Geographies of Nature: Societies, Environments, Ecologies" (2007) and a special issue of *Environment and Planning A* entitled "Biosecurity: Spaces, Practices and Boundaries" (2008). He is currently working on biosecurity practices in the UK, and on a European Union-funded "Science in Society" project which develops research collaborations with civil society organizations on environmental problems in Europe.

Frédéric Keck is a researcher at the Centre National de Recherche Scientifique in Paris. He belongs to the Groupe de sociologie politique et morale, a laboratory of the Ecole des hautes études en sciences sociales. He has published *Lévi-Strauss et la pensée sauvage* (2004), *Claude Lévi-Strauss, une introduction* (2005) and *Lucien Lévy-Bruhl, entre philosophie et anthropologie* (2008). He currently works on the security apparatuses against bird flu in Hong Kong.

Erin Koch is an assistant professor of anthropology at the University of Kentucky. Her most recent publication is "Recrafting Georgian Medicine: The Politics of Standardization and Tuberculosis Control in Postsocialist Georgia," in *Caucasus Paradigms: Anthropologies, Histories and the Making of a World Area,* edited by Bruce Grant and Lale Yalçin-Heckman (2007). She is currently working on a book entitled *Free Market Tuberculosis: Georgia and the Management of Disease after the Soviet Union.*

Andrew Lakoff is an associate professor of sociology and science studies at the University of California, San Diego. He received a PhD in anthropology from the University of California, Berkeley, and was a postdoctoral fellow in the department of social medicine at Harvard University. His publications include *Pharmaceutical Reason: Knowledge and Value in Global Psychiatry* (2005) and *Global Pharmaceuticals: Ethics, Markets, Practices,* co-edited with Adriana Petryna and Arthur Kleinman (2006). His current research concerns the historical emergence and global extension of techniques of biological preparedness.

Paul Rabinow is a professor of anthropology at the University of California, Berkeley. He has written many articles and books on biotechnology, including *Making PCR: A Story of Biotechnology* (1996), *French DNA: Trouble in Purgatory* (1999), and, with Talia Dan-Cohen, *A Machine to Make a Future: Biotech Chronicles* (2004). Rabinow has also written extensively on conceptual and theoretical questions relating to anthropology and science and technology studies, including *Essays on the Anthropology of Reason* (1996), *Anthropos Today: Reflections on Modern Equipment* (2001), and, most recently, *Marking Time: On the Anthropology of the Contemporary* (2007).

Peter Redfield is an associate professor of anthropology at the University of North Carolina, Chapel Hill. The author of *Space in the Tropics: From Convicts to Rockets in French Guiana* (2000), he is currently finishing a book about the organization Doctors Without Borders/ Médecins Sans Frontières (MSF). A related article, "Doctors, Borders and Life in Crisis" (*Cultural Anthropology,* 2005), won the 2006 Cultural Horizons Prize from the Society for Cultural Anthropology.

Dale A. Rose completed his PhD in sociology at the University of California, San Francisco. His dissertation focused on emergent sites of public health preparedness at national and local levels. He has been a researcher and practitioner in areas related to emergency services and public health preparedness since 2001, when he became an emergency medical technician. Dale works with Fritz Institute in San Francisco as a Preparedness Analyst, where he manages or contributes to three programs to improve community preparedness, focusing on the Bay Area's non-profit service providers to at-risk populations.

Kathleen M. Vogel is an assistant professor at Cornell University, with a joint appointment in the department of science and technology studies and the peace studies program. Before coming to Cornell, Vogel worked with the U.S. Department of State as a William C. Foster Fellow in the Bureau of Nonproliferation in the Office of Proliferation Threat Reduction. She holds a PhD in biological chemistry from Princeton University. Her current research explores the technical and social factors influencing the proliferation of biological weapons technology to terrorist groups and countries of proliferation concern.

Index

dual use research, 232, 234, 252n27, 272

dual use strategy, 61, 70

Due Process Vetting System, 232

Dufour, Barbara, 207

Dye, Christopher, 135

E. coli, 11, 67–68

   food safety and, 22

early warning systems, 73

eating, 197

Ebola virus, 46, 165–166

Ebright, Richard, 269

Ecole Vétérinaire, 207

ecologies of practice, 186

Egypt

   avian flu in, 174, 176–187, 189, 190–191

Egypt Today (newspaper), 180

Electronic Surveillance System for the Early

   Notification of Community-Based Epidemics

   (ESSENCE), 71, 74–76

El-Halaj, Zuheir, 180

Eliaszewicz, Muriel, 196, 207, 208

emergency management techniques, 17–19

Emerging Infections: Microbial Threats to Health

   in the United States (U.S. Institute of Medicine

   report), 176

emerging infectious disease, 9–10, 17, 29n9,

   46, 67

   as a national security threat, 48

Emerging Viruses (Horowitz), 46

England. See Britain

environmental movement, 23

Environmental Protection Agency (EPA), 263

epidemic detection, 77

epidemiologic response, 72

epidemiology, 36, 40, 69

   lack of funding for, 82

epizootia point of view, 195, 205, 212

Epstein, Gerald, 242

equation, 101

ESSENCE. See Electronic Surveillance System for

the Early Notification of Community-Based

   Epidemics (ESSENCE)

ESSENCE II, 75–76

Estacio, Peter, 83

Ethiopia, 153

Europe, 11, 133, 137, 155

   biosecurity in, 173

European Union, 22

Ewald, François, 211

experts, 199, 221, 223–224n17

   conflicts of interest of, 208–209

   controversies between, 195, 197

   of food safety, 202

   reaction time of, 219

   See also physicians; veterinarians

extensively drug-resistant tuberculosis (XDR-TB),

   124, 143n17

factory farms, 178, 179, 180, 189

   subsidies for, 184

Falkenrath, Richard, 35–36, 53–54

false alerts, 79–80

family planning, 18

famine, 153–154

farm-based practices, 197

farmers, 20, 198

farming, 173, 177–178

   avian influenza and, 181, 183–187

   See also poultry

Fauci, Anthony, 269

Fearnley, Lyle, 13, 15, 61

Federal Emergency Management Agency (FEMA),

   52

first aid kits, 157

first-line antibiotics, 126, 142n1, 144–145n36

first-order actors, 12, 26–27

first responders, 93, 105

   vaccination of, 14, 51–52, 102

1918 flu virus, 25, 69

Foege, William, 47

Food and Agriculture Organization of the United

global, 47–48
management of, 80
tuberculosis and, 125, 131, 133
See also syndromic surveillance
surveillance technologies, 174
SVP. *See* Smallpox Vaccination Program (SVP)
swine flu, 39–42, 55–56
syndromic surveillance, 15–16, 27, 61–63, 65,
73–76, 84
BioSense and, 76–78
bioterrorism and, 69, 72–73, 81
calibration problems of, 65
development of, 67, 68–69, 70–71
ESSENCE and, 71
infrastructure of, 82
public health and, 84
structural dilemma facing, 82–83
synthetic biology, 10

Tamiflu (avian influenza vaccine), 179
Taubenberger, Jeffery, 268
territorial versions of security, 179, 181
terrorist organizations, 10, 283
Thacker, S., 66
Thailand, 152, 158
third worldism, 152–153
thirdworldization, 47
Tibetan Book of the Dead, The, 283
TOPOFF (Top officials) exercise, 53, 72–73, 81, 84
Toyota Land Cruisers, 160
transparency, 227, 228
See also secrecy/transparency debate
tropical disease experts, 47
tuberculosis, 7, 9, 46, 121, 124–125, 136–137,
144n26
antibiotics used to treat, 126
extensively drug-resistant (XDR-TB), 124,
143n17
in Georgia, 122, 138–139, 140, 144n31
global response to, 122–123, 128
HIV and, 143n15

management of, 140–141
medical care responses to, 128, 130
multidrug resistant (MDR-TB), 121–122, 137–
138, 142n1
social stigma and, 126, 135, 138
Soviet methods of control, 129–130, 131–134,
140, 144n34
See also Global Tuberculosis Emergency
tuberculosis control programs, 18–20, 132
See also DOTS (Directly-Observed Treatment,
Short-Course); National Tuberculosis
Program (NTP)
Tucker, Jonathan, 232
Tumpey, Terrence, 268, 270–271
Turck, Dominique, 208
Tuskegee Syphilis Experiment, 23

Uganda, 20, 153–154, 162–163, 165–166, 169n20
United Nations, 151
United States, 22
biodefense program of, 227–228, 229–231, 235,
242–245, 248–249, 252n20
biosecurity initiatives of, 257
disease outbreaks in, 33
food safety crises in, 11, 21
history of public health in, 65–67, 107
national security concerns of, 36, 260
preparedness efforts in, 52
public health in, 13–14, 80
public health infrastructure of, 74, 100
responsibility for biosafety in, 263–264
treaty commitments of, 227, 242, 250n2
tuberculosis in, 144n31
vaccination policy in, 95
vulnerability to terrorism of, 89, 246, 257
United States Agency for International Development (USAID), 128
in Georgia, 131, 140
United States Department of Agriculture, 21, 263
United States Department of Defense (DoD), 54,
69–71, 73–74, 227